Essential Psychiatry for the Aesthetic Practitioner

Essential Psychiatry for the Aesthetic Practitioner

Edited by

Evan A. Rieder, MD
The Ronald O. Perelman Department
of Dermatology
New York University Grossman School
of Medicine
New York, NY
USA

Richard G. Fried, MD, PhD
Yardley Dermatology Associates
Yardley, PA
USA

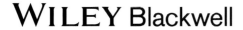

Registered Office(s)
John Wiley & Sons, Inc., 111 River Street, Hoboken, NJ 07030, USA
John Wiley & Sons Ltd, The Atrium, Southern Gate, Chichester, West Sussex, PO19 8SQ, UK

Editorial Office
9600 Garsington Road, Oxford, OX4 2DQ, UK

For details of our global editorial offices, customer services, and more information about Wiley products visit us at www.wiley.com.

Wiley also publishes its books in a variety of electronic formats and by print-on-demand. Some content that appears in standard print versions of this book may not be available in other formats.

Library of Congress Cataloging-in-Publication Data

Names: Rieder, Evan A., editor. | Fried, Richard G., editor.
Title: Essential psychiatry for the aesthetic practitioner / edited by Evan
  A. Rieder, Richard G. Fried.
Description: Hoboken, NJ : Wiley Blackwell 2021. | Includes bibliographical
  references and index.
Identifiers: LCCN 2020045467 (print) | LCCN 2020045468 (ebook) | ISBN
  9781119680123 (hardback) | ISBN 9781119680130 (adobe pdf) | ISBN
  9781119680062 (epub)
Subjects: MESH: Cosmetic Techniques–psychology | Skin |
  Patients–psychology | Body Image–psychology | Stress,
  Psychological–complications | Physician-Patient Relations
Classification: LCC RD119 (print) | LCC RD119 (ebook) | NLM WR 650 | DDC
  617.9/520651–dc23
LC record available at https://lccn.loc.gov/2020045467
LC ebook record available at https://lccn.loc.gov/2020045468

Cover Design: Wiley
Cover Image: © Di Yan

Set in 9.5/12.5pt STIXTwoText by SPi Global, Pondicherry, India
Printed and bound by CPI Group (UK) Ltd, Croydon, CR0 4YY

C9781119680123_250321

Contents

List of Contributors

Michael Abrouk, MD
Dr Phillip Frost Department of Dermatology
& Cutaneous Surgery
University of Miami Miller School of
Medicine
Miami, FL
USA

Mathew M. Avram, MD, JD
Dermatology Laser and Cosmetic Center
Massachusetts General Hospital
Harvard Medical School
Boston, MA,
USA

and

Wellman Center for Photomedicine
Massachusetts General Hospital
Harvard Medical School
Boston, MA
USA

Nicholas Brownstone, MD
Department of Dermatology
University of California San Francisco
San Francisco, CA
USA

Vanessa J. Cutler, MD, MPH
Department of Psychiatry
New York University Grossman School of
Medicine
New York, NY
USA

Doris Day, MD, MA
Day Dermatology & Aesthetics
New York, NY
USA

and

The Ronald O. Perelman Department of
Dermatology
New York University Grossman School of
Medicine
New York, NY
USA

Zoe Diana Draelos, MD
Dermatology Consulting Services
PLLC
High Point, NC
USA

Richard G. Fried, MD, PhD
Yardley Dermatology Associates
Yardley, PA
USA

Brian Ginsberg, MD
Chelsea Skin & Laser
New York, NY
USA

and

Department of Dermatology
Icahn School of Medicine at Mount Sinai
New York, NY
USA

Leslie Harris, MA
Cosmetics and Fragrance Marketing and
Management
Fashion Institute of Technology
New York, NY
USA

Brian P. Hibler, MD
Dermatology Laser and Cosmetic
Center
Massachusetts General Hospital
Harvard Medical School
Boston, MA
USA
and
Wellman Center for Photomedicine
Massachusetts General Hospital
Harvard Medical School
Boston, MA
USA

Josie Howard, MD
Private practice
San Francisco, CA
USA
and
Department of Dermatology
University of California San Francisco
San Francisco, CA
USA

Michael S. Kaminer, MD
SkinCare Physicians, Inc.
Chestnut Hill, MA
USA
and
Department of Dermatology
Brown University School of Medicine
Providence, RI
USA
and
Department of Dermatology
Yale University School of Medicine
New Haven, CT
USA

Prasanthi Kandula, MD
Department of Dermatology
Brown University School of
Medicine
Providence, RI
USA
and
SkinCare Physicians, Inc.
Chestnut Hill, MA
USA

John Koo, MD
Department of Dermatology
University of California San Francisco
San Francisco, CA
USA

Nathaniel Lampley III, BS
University of Cincinnati College of
Medicine
Cincinnati, OH
USA

Michelle Magid, MD
Department of Psychiatry
University of Texas Dell Medical School
Austin, TX
USA
and
Texas A&M Health Science Center
Round Rock, TX
USA

Emily C. Milam, MD
The Ronald O. Perelman Department of
Dermatology
New York University Grossman School of
Medicine
New York, NY
USA

Bridget Myers, BS
Department of Dermatology
University of California San Francisco
San Francisco, CA
USA

Mio Nakamura, MD
Department of Dermatology
University of Michigan
Ann Arbor, MI
USA

Karen M. Ong, MD, PhD
Department of Internal Medicine
University of Texas Medical Health
Galveston, TX
USA

Catherine Pisano, MD
Department of Dermatology
University of Texas Dell Medical School
Austin, TX,
USA

Susruthi Rajanala, MD
Department of Dermatology
Boston University School of Medicine
Boston, MA,
USA

Jason Reichenberg, MD, MBA
Department of Dermatology
University of Texas Dell Medical School
Austin, TX
USA

Evan A. Rieder, MD
The Ronald O. Perelman Department of
Dermatology
New York University Grossman School of
Medicine
New York, NY
USA

Anthony Rossi, MD
Department of Dermatology
Weill Cornell Medicine
New York, NY
USA
and
Dermatology Service
Department of Medicine
Memorial Sloan Kettering Cancer Center
New York, NY
USA

Jacob Sacks, MD
Private practice
San Francisco, CA
USA
and
Department of Psychiatry
University of California San Francisco
San Francisco, CA
USA

Kalee Shah, MD
Department of Dermatology
Weill Cornell Medicine
New York, NY
USA

Payal Shah, BS
The Ronald O. Perelman Department
of Dermatology
New York University Grossman School of
Medicine
New York, NY, USA

Philip D. Shenefelt, MD
Department of Dermatology
University of South Florida
Tampa, FL
USA

Noëlle S. Sherber, MD
Sherber and Rad
Washington, DC, USA
and
Department of Dermatology
George Washington University
School of Medicine & Health Sciences
Washington, DC,
USA

Mary D. Sun, BSE, BA
Icahn School of Medicine at Mount Sinai
New York, NY
USA

Neelam A. Vashi, MD
Department of Dermatology
Boston University School of Medicine
Boston, MA
USA

Jill S. Waibel, MD
Miami Dermatology & Laser
Institute
Miami, FL
USA

Jacqueline Watchmaker, MD
Department of Dermatology
Boston University School of Medicine
Boston, MA
USA

Danielle Weitzer, DO
Department of Psychiatry
Rowan University School of Osteopathic
Medicine
Stratford, NJ
USA

Eagan Zettlemoyer, MS
Drexel University College of Medicine
Philadelphia, PA
USA

Preface

When we endeavored to write this book, we knew that there was a clear voice lacking in the field of aesthetics. While the field of cosmetic medicine has enjoyed rapid expansion, all of the available texts focus on products, devices, techniques, cosmetic concerns, and/or assessment. While technical prowess, procedural expertise, and an understanding of anatomy are fundamental, so much of the aesthetic experience is based on interpersonal relations between the aesthetic practitioner and patient and an understanding of human behavior. However, this is not a textbook designed to understand human behavior to maximize aesthetic practice viability or profits. Instead, through common clinical scenarios, this book aims to improve practitioner–patient relations and answer common questions such as:

Is this patient a good candidate for a cosmetic procedure?

Why am I feeling ill-at-ease during this consultation – and what can I do about it?

How can I make this person feel better about themself?

How can I protect myself and my patient in this tricky situation?

How can I enhance the patient experience in this visit and beyond?

We knew that we had to write a book that could best help our colleagues navigate the complexities of the aesthetic world. And we knew we had to do it in a way that was easy-to-read, practical, and digestible for people of all training and experience levels.

This book would not be possible without the contributions of our co-authors, all of whom have attained expertise in the mental health professions or aesthetics, some of them in both fields. They discuss the science and psychology of beauty, giving historical context to human and societal behaviors concerning appearance. They emphasize the importance of recognizing and screening for common psychological comorbidities, as aesthetic practitioners are commonly forced to triage and provide initial management for several psychiatric conditions. They discuss how aesthetic interventions can help our patients to feel better about themselves and also be perceived better by others across multiple social and occupational domains. They discuss how to optimize the provider–patient relationship and how to protect our patients and ourselves. They detail common and easy-to-perform psychological modalities that can be of great utility during the cosmetic visit and readily adopted by patients outside of the office setting. And finally, they close the arc in moving from a discussion of the history of beauty to more contemporary concepts: how a social-media-obsessed world may be causing a crisis in beauty and appearance; how fluidity in gender and variations in ethnicity are changing the ways we approach the aesthetic patient; and how we must evolve and propose novel guidelines to best treat a rapidly evolving patient population.

We thank you for taking the time to read this text and hope that you find it to be helpful as you guide your patients through their aesthetic journeys.

New York, NY   *Evan A. Rieder*
Yardley, PA   *Richard G. Fried*

Part I

The Basics

1

Stress, Skin, and Beauty

The Basic Science Base

Mary D. Sun[1] and Evan A. Rieder[2]

[1] Icahn School of Medicine at Mount Sinai, New York, NY, USA
[2] The Ronald O. Perelman Department of Dermatology, New York University Grossman School of Medicine, New York, NY, USA

The relationship between stress and skin health has been documented since ancient times. Today, patients of aesthetic medical providers continue to cite psychological stress as a common precipitating factor of exacerbations in skin diseases such as acne, eczema, and psoriasis. This connection is invoked in scientific literature and frequently discussed in the lay media, with implications for general wellness practices as well as the provision of appropriate medical care. Despite this long history, the precise mechanisms through which stress impacts the skin are not yet well understood. However, recent advancements have illuminated multifactorial and bidirectional interactions between the brain, nervous system, microbiome, and skin, with key implications for the inflammatory and microbiological milieu. This area of investigation has the potential to significantly inform aesthetic care and should be regarded with great interest.

Basic Science Principles

Introduction

In this section, we provide an overview of the biological pathways believed to play a role in the relationship between psychosocial stress and the physical appearance of skin. Stress is defined as any set of aversive stimuli that provoke an associated response, which can be thought of as a coping mechanism in an individual [1, 2]. Clinically significant effects caused by stress are primarily due to impacts on the internal processes that maintain and restore skin homeostasis. We consider only psychosocial stress and do not include somatic forms of stress such as chronological aging, photoaging, and/or physical shear stress, unless the effects of somatic stressors are facilitated or potentiated by psychological stress. We further emphasize the role of chronic stress.

Our discussion occurs in the context of known neuroendocrine effects of stress. Stress increases levels of cortisol [3], known as the "fight-or-flight" hormone, which activates the hypothalamic-pituitary-adrenal (HPA) axis [4, 5]. For this reason, the HPA axis is also referred to as the central stress axis. Overactivation of the stress axis can have consequences across multiple levels of molecular function, affecting the sympathetic nervous system [4, 6], immune response [7, 8], cholinergic response [9], and microbiome [10–12]. There is also strong epidemiological evidence that the presence and exacerbation of many skin conditions such as acne [13], chronic itch [14], and psoriasis [15] have an emotional component. Progression of such skin diseases is often comorbid with negative outcomes in mental health and quality of life, suggesting a bidirectional relationship [16, 17]. Indeed, nearly one-third of skin disorders are estimated to occur with or be worsened by psychiatric disorders and/or psychological distress [17]. The recent discovery of a fully functional, peripheral HPA axis in the skin [18] further clarifies this relationship and suggests impacts across the inflammatory and atopic responses, skin barrier dysfunction, vulnerability to cutaneous infection, and impairment of wound healing and melanogenesis. Additionally, emerging evidence from studies of the cutaneous microbiome suggests that stress can act through the "gut-brain-skin" axis to induce dysbiosis [19]. This gives us further insight into how lifestyle factors such as diet, personal care (hygiene), and sleep can mediate the effects of stress on skin health and appearance. This chapter summarizes these clinically important relationships and emphasizes areas of significant academic, clinical, and commercial impact.

The Central (Systemic) HPA Stress Axis

In times of psychological stress, the body mounts a neuroendocrine-mediated immune response controlled by the sympathoadrenal and central nervous systems. Increased cytokine levels [20] activate the locus coeruleus–norepinephrine sympathetic adrenomedullary (LC-NE/SAM) system, which secretes epinephrine and norepinephrine that further upregulate the immune response, as well as the HPA axis [21]. Notably, the results of these changes differ by stress duration. During acute stress, cytokine proliferation increases and lymphocytes are mobilized from the blood to the surface of the skin [22]. This creates conditions of sympathetic hypersensitivity and generates inflammation through the actions of various proinflammatory factors [7, 21].

Conversely, chronic stress actually suppresses the inflammatory response. The HPA axis negatively feeds back to the LC-NE/SAM system, where secretion of corticotropin-releasing hormone (CRH) and arginine vasopressin (AVP) [23] stimulates the release of anti-inflammatory peptides from the anterior pituitary [21]. Adrenocorticotropic hormone (ACTH) is also released, causing the adrenal medulla to secrete cortisol and prolactin [21, 24]. Cortisol downregulates inflammatory cytokines and upregulates anti-inflammatory factors [25], suppressing Th-1 mediated cellular immunity in favor of Th-2 mediated humoral immunity. At the same time, ACTH upregulates glucocorticoid response elements (GREs) and increases expression levels of anti-inflammatory genes [26]. Under conditions of high glucocorticoids, prolactin attenuates the reactivity of the HPA axis by reducing input to the hypothalamus [27]. Therefore, the chronic stress response mobilizes resources within the body while mitigating potentially dangerous levels of inflammation [28].

The Cutaneous (Peripheral) HPA Stress Axis

We have recently discovered that the skin has its own HPA stress axis made up of intracutaneous, crosstalking peripheral networks. The cutaneous axis is a fully functional analog of the central axis [29, 30], able to locally upregulate inflammatory cytokines [31, 32], release cortisol and catecholamines [5, 6, 33–36], and express a complete CRH/ACTH signaling system [34, 37]. Furthermore, melanocytes and keratinocytes differentially express regulators of the CRH/ACTH system as well as other molecules important to neuroendocrine signaling [18, 38–41]. The skin also locally expresses CRH [31] and ACTH [40, 42], where receptors for CRH are found in epidermis, dermis, and subcutis cells [43]. These receptors have been implicated in the development of several chronic skin diseases [25, 44].

The cutaneous stress axis is organized through regulatory feedback loops that mirror those in the central axis [5, 30, 36, 45]. Increases in cutaneous CRH caused by acute stress [43] are associated with increased ACTH and glucocorticoid levels in human skin cell populations [37]. ACTH increases, while CRH decreases the expression of proinflammatory factors [39, 46]. Therefore, the cutaneous stress axis similarly increases cortisol levels through CRH/POMC/ACTH pathways and negatively feeds back on itself through interepithelial CRH and POMC.

Though research is ongoing, evidence points to bidirectional interaction between the central and peripheral HPA axes. Namely, stress-induced glucocorticoid elevation alters skin barrier function [47, 48] and is known to contribute to inflammatory skin diseases like atopic dermatitis, chronic urticaria [49, 50], and psoriasis [51]. While there are numerous preclinical examples of the connectivity between these axes, further research into the mechanisms of this crosstalk will improve our understanding of how stressed skin attempts to restore homeostasis.

Clinical Correlates

The molecular factors that comprise the central (systemic) and cutaneous (peripheral) stress axes provide important background for the clinical effects of stress on skin health. The role of stress in inflammatory skin conditions is particularly noteworthy, given the link that has been established between psychosocial stress and the development and exacerbation of these conditions. In the following, we summarize significant clinical findings that have been linked to psychosocial stress and are of interest to the aesthetic practitioner. While there are numerous clinical correlates in the processes of psoriasis, atopic dermatitis, and vitiligo, we will limit our discussion to cosmetic concerns, including the skin barrier, skin aging, wound healing, infection, and lifestyle factors. While research is still ongoing, many of these impacts are likely affected if not caused by the downstream

effects of interactions between the central and peripheral stress axes.

Stress Impairs the Skin Barrier and Increases Skin Thinning, Skin Aging, and Sebum Production

Psychosocial stress is consistently associated with impairment of the skin barrier in both healthy individuals and those with preexisting skin conditions [52, 53]. The skin barrier is a permeable layer in the outermost layer of the skin, called the stratum corneum (SC), that prevents transepidermal water loss (TEWL) and protects the skin from outside elements. Lipid bilayers fill the internal barrier space and sit between lamellae composed of ceramides, cholesterol, and fatty acids [54]. Barrier health is characterized by factors such as skin pH, hydration, and sebum excretion, which are often targeted by various clinical treatments and impact skin health. Psychosocial stress, as experienced through challenging social and romantic relationships [55, 56], is associated with decreases in skin barrier function including TEWL and epidermal hyperplasia. Additionally, hormones produced by the HPA stress axes can damage the structural lipids and proteins necessary for maintaining skin hydration [57]. Increased endogenous glucocorticoids negatively affect epidermal growth and lipid synthesis needed to restore the SC [58, 59]; indeed, glucocorticoid blockade reverses stress-induced SC damage [60, 61]. Topical and emulsion-formulated treatments that replenish lipids and ceramides [62–64], as well as psychological relaxation techniques [65–67] that may inhibit the HPA response have proven effective for skin conditions like atopic dermatitis, where there is a known barrier defect.

The stress-activated reductase 11β-hydroxysteroid dehydrogenase (11β-HSD) has been implicated in the relationship between glucocorticoid levels and skin barrier function. 11β-HSD1 is directly activated by psychological stress [68] and induces the active form of cortisol in keratinocytes [68, 69]. Under conditions of stress, its activity is associated with itch [70], delayed wound healing [71], impaired skin cell proliferation [72], and TEWL [73, 74]. 11β-HSD1 also modulates the effects of steroidal products on sebocytes and has been linked to excess sebum production and acne development [74]. Blockades of 11β-HSD1 restore glucocorticoid levels [75, 76], epidermal integrity [77], and wound healing [78], and are also found to increase collagen content in the skin [79]. In patients with anxiety, stress-relieving medications (selective serotonin reuptake inhibitors, SSRIs) similarly reverse the effects of 11β-HSD1 through attenuation of the HPA axis [68].

Stress Suppresses Mechanisms that Protect the Skin from Infection

Psychosocial stressors are a well-documented risk factor for the development and recurrence of viral cutaneous infections like herpes simplex [80] as well as skin diseases such as acne, atopic dermatitis, and psoriasis [81–85]. The disease processes of these conditions share an important feature: microbial colonization. Emerging research suggests that chronic stress downregulates the expression of antimicrobial peptides (AMPs) on the epidermis, compromising cutaneous defenses that leave the skin more susceptible to infection [86, 87]. Under normal circumstances, AMPs help destroy foreign microbes and are a critical part of infection prevention. AMPs are delivered to the SC by lamellar bodies, which cannot be produced as effectively in the high adrenergic and glucocorticoid conditions caused by stress [88–91]. Excess glucocorticoids also impair the production of lipids, which are needed for encapsulation of AMPs [92]. While stress appears to increase the expression of AMPs and beta-defensins, the actual delivery of these peptides is impaired and causes reduced clearance of skin bacterial pathogens like *Staphylococcus aureus* and *Staphylococcus pyogenes* [93–95].

Therapies that reduce the physiological effects of stress appear to restore normal levels of AMPs and reduce the risk of cutaneous infection. These findings are demonstrated in studies of glucocorticoid inhibitors, CRH inhibitors, and topical lipid-containing treatments [86]. Psychological stress-reduction techniques, including cognitive behavioral stress management, relaxation training, biofeedback, and visualization similarly reduce the severity of several chronic cosmetically challenging skin conditions [96–99].

Chronic Stress Impairs Wound Healing in Skin

The immunosuppressive effects of chronic psychological stress delay wound healing [100]. While regulating inflammation can be protective, this response also disrupts the inflammatory environment needed to initiate the healing process. Specifically, high glucocorticoid levels downregulate components of the immune response that play a critical role in early healing [101]. These include inflammatory cytokines and chemoattractants that act quickly at wound sites. Accordingly, psychological stressors such as hostile marital interactions, extended housing insecurity, and examination stress reduce these inflammatory components and delay cutaneous healing [7, 102–105]. Conversely, the inhibition of glucocorticoids improves healing rates in situations of stress [106], as do anti-anxiety medications [107], social supports, and psychological interventions [108, 109].

The Gut-Brain-Skin Axis: Probiotics and the Promise of Treating the Skin Microbiome

New advances in our understanding of the cutaneous microbiome have established a link between dysbiosis and the development of skin disease. For instance, the bacterium *Cutibacterium acnes* makes up the vast majority of microbiota colonizing sebum-rich areas of the skin, can be pathologic in acne patients, and is affected by treatment with retinoids and antibiotics [110–112]. There is also interplay with other bacterial species; for example, the acne-inducing effects of *C. acnes* seem to be inhibited by *S. epidermidis* [113]. The cutaneous microbiomes of patients with conditions including acne and seborrheic dermatitis show higher proportions of *Malassezia* species [114–116], while *Firmicutes* is overrepresented in vitiligo lesions [117]. Disproportionate colonization by *S. aureus* correlates with immune dysfunction in psoriasis [118], dysbiosis in eczema [119], and inflammatory flares in atopic dermatitis [120–122].

Disturbances to the skin microbiome are clearly useful signals of skin disease. However, certain shifts in the structure and diversity of microbiota can actually be therapeutic in a variety of conditions [123]. Specifically, increased colonization with commensal bacteria appears to protect against inflammatory allergic reactions and the development of atopic dermatitis [124–126]. These species play an important role in maintaining the skin barrier and help immunize the skin from external pathogens [127]. Similarly protective effects are observed in adults and their children [125, 128], implicating the maternal microbiome in the health of offspring [129].

Studies of probiotics show promise for therapeutic use in acne [130, 131] and have been shown to have other positive effects such as reducing inflammatory skin conditions and increasing hair growth [19, 132, 133]. Treatments that affect microbiota also have implications for disease development and wound healing [134–136].

The gut-brain-skin axis theory describes a relationship between emotional states and changes in gastrointestinal function, microbial colonization, and systemic inflammation that has been validated in translational research [130, 137]. Differences in microbiota appear to drive differential activity of the HPA stress axis in response to psychological stress [138–141] and in cases of psychiatric illness [142]. This response

has been explained by two stress-related pathways: (i) steroid/glucocorticoid-associated regulation and (ii) the increased permeability of epithelial barriers. In animal models, the absence of commensal bacteria results in higher corticosterone levels and thus hyperreactivity of the HPA axes upon exposure to stress [9, 143, 144]. Stress also facilitates the crossing of external bacterial material through barriers that usually prevent entry into the skin and gut. These components can trigger or upregulate inflammation, as has been observed in the brain, intestinal tract, and hair and skin disease [145–149].

Stress Impacts Lifestyle Factors Including Diet, Personal Care, and Sleep that Have Consequences for Skin and Hair Health

Diet

In addition to directly affecting neuro-immuno-endocrine systems, psychosocial stress impacts lifestyle factors that have implications for skin and hair health [150–153]. Diet is particularly important, given its influence on the aging processes of skin cells, skin inflammation, and the cutaneous microbiome. For instance, studies of the transcriptome find that high-fat diets lead to the accumulation of pro-adipogenic traits in dermal cells [154]. These traits indicate accelerated aging of the upper layers of skin [154], a process that can be partially prevented through caloric restriction [155]. High-fat diets, coupled with increased alcohol intake also disrupt collagen fibers, impair wound repair [156], and reduce adhesion proteins needed to maintain the connective integrity of skin [157, 158]. In mice models, western diets rich in cholesterol and fat are linked to decreased ceramide levels, increased skin inflammation, hair loss, and hair discoloration [159]. Other studies have found similar associations with increases in sebum, altered skin pH, and decreased skin hydration [160]. These factors influence the physical environments required for skin microbiota to survive and such changes can leave the microbiome vulnerable to dysbiosis [161].

Consuming foods that cause high glycemic loads, such as dairy, red meat, refined carbohydrates, and sugary foods, is correlated with increased acne severity [156, 162]. High glycemic indexes are known to increase concentrations of insulin and insulin-like growth factor, known contributors to acne [163]. These foods also frequently contain advanced glycation end products (AGEs), byproducts of modern food processing procedures. Higher AGE levels are linked to inflammatory skin responses that are implicated in psoriasis development and severity [164]. In the general population, decreased AGE levels tend to occur with avoidance of sugary foods, adequate sleep duration, and low psychological stress [165]. Conversely, diets with low glycemic loads and high protein improve biochemical measures of acne [166, 167].

Nordic and Mediterranean diets that instead feature plant-based foods, whole grains, and seafood appear to improve skin health. Short- and long-term diet interventions improve cutaneous blood flow, oxygen tension, and lipid profiles, and are associated with less sebum [168–170]. These eating patterns are also linked to a lower risk of malignant skin tumors and cancer [171, 172]. In particular, fruit-derived metabolites improve skin function and attenuate skin disease [173, 174], while polyphenols found in coffee and green tea improve skin smoothness and blood flow [175, 176]. These compounds also protect against sun-related pigmentation [172] and improve rates of skin barrier recovery [177]. In animals, polyphenols from whole fruits and vegetables reduce oxidative stress, which aids in microvascular function, and upregulate cellular antiproliferation, potentially reducing cancer risk [178]. Furthermore, extracts from grapes, apples, and tomatoes are chemoprotective due to their facilitation of appropriate cell death and DNA repair [179–181].

Personal Care

Personal hygiene and self-care practices are often negatively affected by psychological stress. Such behavioral changes can have varying impacts, as the contemporary use of various skincare and cosmetic products can be beneficial or detrimental to the skin. Some of these consequences are mediated by the cutaneous microbiome, which can be disturbed [182, 183] by a wide range of products including antibiotics, hand sanitizers [184], toothpaste [112, 185, 186], hygiene items like antiperspirants, deodorants, and foot powders [187, 188], skincare items [189, 190], cosmetics [191], specific laundering methods and clothing types [192–194], and even fitness routines [195, 196]. The use of these products involves physical interaction with the upper layers of the epidermis, where most microbial species are found [197]. In particular, cosmetics that alter the diversity of microflora are associated with reduced differences between well- and poorly hydrated facial skin [198]. Liquid carriers and detergents in facial cleansers induce changes in cellular components, disturbing the acidic environment necessary for sustaining native microbes [183, 199]. Surfactants in bar soaps, some deodorants, face and body washes, and micelle waters strip the skin of moisturizing factors and can lead to dry, scaly, and/or red skin [189, 200]. On the other hand, "anti-aging" products like skin creams and skin massagers can increase the expression of dermal proteins important to maintaining skin elasticity [201]. Moisturizers can be beneficial for skin barrier function and are useful in the prevention and management of skin disease [202, 203].

Sleep

Psychosocial stress is a risk factor for impaired sleep [204], which mediates direct effects on the HPA axes and therefore immune and microbial dysfunction. Experiencing insufficient or lower-quality sleep blunts the cortisol response in settings of acute stress, potentiating hyperreactivity of the stress axis and increasing sensitivity to future stress [205–207]. Chronically poor sleep is associated with higher TEWL, lower levels of immune cells, and slower skin barrier recovery [208, 209], while sufficient sleep is associated with faster wound healing [210]. Poor sleep due to shift work and sleep disorders is also linked to increased inflammation [211] and a higher incidence of inflammatory skin conditions and skin cancer [212, 213]. A number of microbial compounds, including polyphenols and vitamins, help regulate circadian rhythms and mood [214, 215]. By disrupting these rhythms, poor sleep can directly alter the microbial environment and predispose individuals to metabolic and mood disorders [216, 217]. Disruptions to circadian rhythms also accelerate the aging processes and can predispose age-related pathologies [218].

Conclusions

Psychosocial stress affects skin health through complex interactions with neuroendocrine, immune, and microbial networks. Our understanding of the classic HPA stress axis has expanded to include its cutaneous analog, considering a likely bidirectional relationship between the systemic and local stress response. Molecular mediators of this relationship are being investigated as potential targets for pharmacologic therapies in skin conditions involving a dysfunctional stress response. Inflammatory reactions and skin conditions are disproportionately observed in chronically stressed patients. Stress also impairs the skin's innate defenses against foreign microbes and infection and can disturb its structural integrity. Higher levels of glucocorticoids and catecholamines produced by the stress response negatively affect wound healing. Emerging studies of the skin microbiome highlight the importance of commensal bacteria and demonstrate microbial activation of the stress axis. Given this context, aesthetic providers should also be aware of lifestyle factors impacted by stress, including diet, personal care practices, and sleep, and their therapeutic value. These behaviors impact skin and hair health and can inform lifestyle-based treatment recommendations.

References

1 Hodo, D.W. (2006). Kaplan and Sadock's comprehensive textbook of psychiatry, eighth edition. *American Journal of Psychiatry* 163 (8): 1458.

2 Lazarus, R.S. and Folkman, S. (1987). Transactional theory and research on emotions and coping. *European Journal of Personality* 1 (3): 141–169.

3 Munck, A., Guyre, P.M., and Holbrook, N.J. (1984). Physiological functions of glucocorticoids in stress and their relation to pharmacological actions. *Endocrine Reviews* 5 (1): 25–44.

4 Allen, A.P., Kennedy, P.J., Cryan, J.F. et al. (2014). Biological and psychological markers of stress in humans: focus on the trier social stress test. *Neuroscience and Biobehavioral Reviews* 38: 94–124.

5 Slominski, A.T., Zmijewski, M.A., Skobowiat, C. et al. (2012). *Corticotropin Signaling System in the Skin. Sensing the Environment: Regulation of Local and Global Homeostasis by the Skin's Neuroendocrine System*, 41–50. Berlin: Springer.

6 Romana-Souza, B., Santos Lima-Cezar, G., and Monte-Alto-Costa, A. (2015). Psychological stress-induced catecholamines accelerates cutaneous aging in mice. *Mechanisms of Ageing and Development* 152: 63–73.

7 Kiecolt-Glaser, J.K., Loving, T.J., Stowell, J.R. et al. (2005). Hostile marital interactions, proinflammatory cytokine production, and wound healing. *Archives of General Psychiatry* 62 (12): 1377.

8 Curtis, B.J. and Radek, K.A. (2012). Cholinergic regulation of keratinocyte innate immunity and permeability barrier integrity: new perspectives in epidermal immunity and disease. *Journal of Investigative Dermatology* 132 (1): 28–42.

9 Tetel, M.J., de Vries, G.J., Melcangi, R.C. et al. (2018). Steroids, stress and the gut

microbiome-brain axis. *Journal of Neuroendocrinology* 30 (2): e12548.

10 Rea, K., Dinan, T.G., and Cryan, J.F. (2016). The microbiome: a key regulator of stress and neuroinflammation. *Neurobiology of Stress* 4: 23–33.

11 Kelly, J.R., Kennedy, P.J., Cryan, J.F. et al. (2015). Breaking down the barriers: the gut microbiome, intestinal permeability and stress-related psychiatric disorders. *Frontiers in Cellular Neuroscience* 9: 392.

12 Zouboulis, C.C. and Bohm, M. (2004). Neuroendocrine regulation of sebocytes – a pathogenetic link between stress and acne. *Experimental Dermatology* 13 (s4): 31–35.

13 Jović, A., Marinović, B., Kostović, K. et al. (2017). The impact of pyschological stress on acne. *Acta Dermatovenerologica Croatica* 25 (2): 1133–1141.

14 Reszke, R. and Szepietowski, J.C. (2020). Itch and psyche: bilateral associations. *Acta Dermato-Venereologica* 100 (2): adv00026.

15 Tampa, M., Sarbu, M.-I., Mitran, M.-I. et al. (2018). The pathophysiological mechanisms and the quest for biomarkers in psoriasis, a stress-related skin disease. *Disease Markers* 2018: 1–14.

16 Huynh, M., Gupta, R., and Koo, J. (2013). Emotional stress as a trigger for inflammatory skin disorders. *Seminars in Cutaneous Medicine and Surgery* 32 (2): 68–72.

17 Shenefelt, P.D. (2011). Psychodermatological disorders: recognition and treatment. *International Journal of Dermatology* 50 (11): 1309–1322.

18 Slominski, A., Wortsman, J., Tuckey, R.C., and Paus, R. (2007). Differential expression of HPA axis homolog in the skin. *Molecular and Cellular Endocrinology* 265–266: 143–149.

19 Arck, P., Handjiski, B., Hagen, E. et al. (2010). Is there a 'gut-brain-skin axis'? *Experimental Dermatology* 19 (5): 401–405.

20 Hayashi, T. (2015). Conversion of psychological stress into cellular stress response: roles of the sigma-1 receptor in the process. *Psychiatry and Clinical Neurosciences* 69 (4): 179–191.

21 Elenkov, I.J. and Chrousos, G.P. (2006). Stress system – organization, physiology and immunoregulation. *Neuroimmunomodulation* 13 (5–6): 257–267.

22 Dhabhar, F.S. (2006). Acute stress enhances while chronic stress suppresses skin immunity: the role of stress hormones and leukocyte trafficking. *Annals of the New York Academy of Sciences* 917 (1): 876–893.

23 Kane, M.O., Murphy, E.P., and Kirby, B. (2006). The role of corticotropin-releasing hormone in immune-mediated cutaneous inflammatory disease. *Experimental Dermatology* 15 (3): 143–153.

24 Torner, L. (2016). Actions of prolactin in the brain: from physiological adaptations to stress and neurogenesis to psychopathology. *Frontiers in Endocrinology* 7: 25.

25 Arck, P.C., Slominski, A., Theoharides, T.C. et al. (2006). Neuroimmunology of stress: skin takes center stage. *Journal of Investigative Dermatology* 126 (8): 1697–1704.

26 Zen, M., Canova, M., Campana, C. et al. (2011). The kaleidoscope of glucorticoid effects on immune system. *Autoimmunity Reviews* 10 (6): 305–310.

27 Donner, N., Bredewold, R., Maloumby, R., and Neumann, I.D. (2007). Chronic intracerebral prolactin attenuates neuronal stress circuitries in virgin rats. *European Journal of Neuroscience* 25 (6): 1804–1814.

28 Xanthos, D.N. and Sandkühler, J. (2014). Neurogenic neuroinflammation: inflammatory CNS reactions in response to neuronal activity. *Nature Reviews. Neuroscience* 15 (1): 43–53.

29 Slominski, A. (2000). Neuroendocrinology of the skin. *Endocrine Reviews* 21 (5): 457–487.

30 Ito, N., Ito, T., Kromminga, A. et al. (2005). Human hair follicles display a functional equivalent of the hypothalamic-pituitary-adrenal (HPA) axis and synthesize cortisol. *The FASEB Journal* 19 (10): 1332–1334.

31 Theoharides, T.C., Donelan, J.M., Papadopoulou, N. et al. (2004). Mast cells as

targets of corticotropin-releasing factor and related peptides. *Trends in Pharmacological Sciences* 25 (11): 563–568.

32 Park, H.J., Kim, H.J., Lee, J.Y. et al. (2007). Adrenocorticotropin hormone stimulates interleukin-18 expression in human HaCaT keratinocytes. *Journal of Investigative Dermatology* 127 (5): 1210–1216.

33 Slominski, A., Zbytek, B., Nikolakis, G. et al. (2013). Steroidogenesis in the skin: implications for local immune functions. *Journal of Steroid Biochemistry and Molecular Biology* 137: 107–123.

34 Slominski, A., Pisarchik, A., Wortsman, J. et al. (2002). Expression of hypothalamic–pituitary–thyroid axis related genes in the human skin. *Journal of Investigative Dermatology* 119 (6): 1449–1455.

35 Vukelic, S., Stojadinovic, O., Pastar, I. et al. (2011). Cortisol synthesis in epidermis is induced by IL-1 and tissue injury. *Journal of Biological Chemistry* 286 (12): 10265–10275.

36 Slominski, A., Zbytek, B., Szczesniewski, A., and Wortsman, J. (2006). Cultured human dermal fibroblasts do produce cortisol. *Journal of Investigative Dermatology* 126 (5): 1177–1178.

37 Slominski, A., Zbytek, B., Szczesniewski, A. et al. (2005). CRH stimulation of corticosteroids production in melanocytes is mediated by ACTH. *American Journal of Physiology. Endocrinology and Metabolism* 288 (4): E701–E706.

38 Rousseau, K., Kauser, S., Pritchard, L.E. et al. (2007). Proopiomelanocortin (POMC), the ACTH/melanocortin precursor, is secreted by human epidermal keratinocytes and melanocytes and stimulates melanogenesis. *The FASEB Journal* 21 (8): 1844–1856.

39 Roloff, B., Fechner, K., Slominski, A. et al. (1998). Hair cycle-dependent expression of corticotropin-releasing factor (CRF) and CRF receptors in murine skin. *The FASEB Journal* 12 (3): 287–297.

40 Slominski, A., Wortsman, J., and Tobin, D.J. (2005). The cutaneous serotoninergic/melatoninergic system: securing a place

under the sun. *The FASEB Journal* 19 (2): 176–194.

41 Kim, J., Cho, B., Cho, D., and Park, H. (2013). Expression of hypothalamic–pituitary–adrenal axis in common skin diseases: evidence of its association with stress-related disease activity. *Acta Dermato-Venereologica* 93 (4): 387–393.

42 Schauer, E., Trautinger, F., Köck, A. et al. (1994). Proopiomelanocortin-derived peptides are synthesized and released by human keratinocytes. *Journal of Clinical Investigation* 93 (5): 2258–2262.

43 Kaneko, K., Kawana, S., Arai, K., and Shibasaki, T. (2003). Corticotropin-releasing factor receptor type 1 is involved in the stress-induced exacerbation of chronic contact dermatitis in rats. *Experimental Dermatology* 12 (1): 47–52.

44 Katsarou-Katsari, A., Singh, L.K., and Theoharides, T.C. (2001). Alopecia areata and affected skin CRH receptor upregulation induced by acute emotional stress. *Dermatology* 203 (2): 157–161.

45 Slominski, A., Zbytek, B., Semak, I. et al. (2005). CRH stimulates POMC activity and corticosterone production in dermal fibroblasts. *Journal of Neuroimmunology* 162 (1–2): 97–102.

46 Mazurkiewicz, J.E., Corliss, D., and Slominski, A. (2000). Spatiotemporal expression, distribution, and processing of POMC and POMC-derived peptides in murine skin. *Journal of Histochemistry and Cytochemistry* 48 (7): 905–914.

47 Lin, T.-K., Man, M.-Q., Santiago, J.-L. et al. (2014). Paradoxical benefits of psychological stress in inflammatory dermatoses models are glucocorticoid mediated. *Journal of Investigative Dermatology* 134 (12): 2890–2897.

48 Tausk, F.A. and Nousari, H. (2001). Stress and the skin. *Archives of Dermatology* 137 (1): 78–82.

49 Lin, T.-K., Zhong, L., and Santiago, J. (2017). Association between stress and the HPA axis in the atopic dermatitis. *International Journal of Molecular Sciences* 18 (10): 2131.

50 Kong, L., Wu, J., Lin, Y. et al. (2015). BuShenYiQi granule inhibits atopic dermatitis via improving central and skin hypothalamic-pituitary-adrenal axis function. *PLoS One* 10 (2): e0116427.

51 Chen, K., Wang, G., Jin, H. et al. (2017). Clinic characteristics of psoriasis in China: a nationwide survey in over 12000 patients. *Oncotarget* 8 (28): 46381–46389.

52 Maarouf, M., Maarouf, C.L., Yosipovitch, G., and Shi, V.Y. (2019). The impact of stress on epidermal barrier function: an evidence-based review. *British Journal of Dermatology* 181 (6): 1129–1137.

53 van Smeden, J. and Bouwstra, J.A. (2016). Stratum corneum lipids: their role for the skin barrier function in healthy subjects and atopic dermatitis patients. *Current Problems in Dermatology* 49: 8–26.

54 Boer, M., Duchnik, E., Maleszka, R., and Marchlewicz, M. (2016). Structural and biophysical characteristics of human skin in maintaining proper epidermal barrier function. *Postepy Dermatologii i Alergologii* 33 (1): 1–5.

55 Robles, T.F., Brooks, K.P., Kane, H.S., and Schetter, C.D. (2013). Attachment, skin deep? Relationships between adult attachment and skin barrier recovery. *International Journal of Psychophysiology* 88 (3): 241–252.

56 Robinson, H., Ravikulan, A., Nater, U.M. et al. (2017). The role of social closeness during tape stripping to facilitate skin barrier recovery: preliminary findings. *Health Psychology* 36 (7): 619–629.

57 Choi, E.-H., Brown, B.E., Crumrine, D. et al. (2005). Mechanisms by which psychologic stress alters cutaneous permeability barrier homeostasis and stratum corneum integrity. *Journal of Investigative Dermatology* 124 (3): 587–595.

58 Sheu, H.M., Lee, J.Y.Y., Chai, C.Y., and Kuo, K.W. (1997). Depletion of stratum corneum intercellular lipid lamellae and barrier function abnormalities after long-term topical corticosteroids. *British Journal of Dermatology* 136 (6): 884–890.

59 Kao, J.S., Fluhr, J.W., Man, M.-Q. et al. (2003). Short-term glucocorticoid treatment compromises both permeability barrier homeostasis and stratum corneum integrity: inhibition of epidermal lipid synthesis accounts for functional abnormalities. *Journal of Investigative Dermatology* 120 (3): 456–464.

60 Choi, E.-H., Demerjian, M., Crumrine, D. et al. (2006). Glucocorticoid blockade reverses psychological stress-induced abnormalities in epidermal structure and function. *American Journal of Physiology. Regulatory, Integrative and Comparative Physiology* 291 (6): R1657–R1662.

61 Demerjian, M., Choi, E.-H., Man, M.-Q. et al. (2009). Activators of PPARs and LXR decrease the adverse effects of exogenous glucocorticoids on the epidermis. *Experimental Dermatology* 18 (7): 643–649.

62 Xu, Z., Liu, X., Niu, Y. et al. (2020). Skin benefits of moisturising body wash formulas for children with atopic dermatitis: a randomised controlled clinical study in China. *Australasian Journal of Dermatology* 61 (1): e54–e59.

63 Kircik, L., Hougeir, F., and Bikowski, J. (2013). Atopic dermatitis, and the role for a ceramide-dominant, physiologic lipid-based barrier repair emulsion. *Journal of Drugs in Dermatology* 12 (9): 1024–1027.

64 Sugarman, J.L. and Parish, L.C. (2009). Efficacy of a lipid-based barrier repair formulation in moderate-to-severe pediatric atopic dermatitis. *Journal of Drugs in Dermatology* 8 (12): 1106–1111.

65 Robinson, H., Jarrett, P., and Broadbent, E. (2015). The effects of relaxation before or after skin damage on skin barrier recovery. *Psychosomatic Medicine* 77 (8): 844–852.

66 Robles, T.F., Brooks, K.P., and Pressman, S.D. (2009). Trait positive affect buffers the effects of acute stress on skin barrier recovery. *Health Psychology* 28 (3): 373–378.

67 Fukada, M., Kano, E., Miyoshi, M. et al. (2012). Effect of "rose essential oil" inhalation on stress-induced skin-barrier disruption in rats and humans. *Chemical Senses* 37 (4): 347–356.

68 Choe, S.J., Kim, D., Kim, E.J. et al. (2018). Psychological stress deteriorates skin barrier function by activating 11β-hydroxysteroid dehydrogenase 1 and the HPA axis. *Scientific Reports* 8 (1): 6334.

69 Terao, M., Itoi, S., Matsumura, S. et al. (2016). Local glucocorticoid activation by 11β-hydroxysteroid dehydrogenase 1 in keratinocytes. *American Journal of Pathology* 186 (6): 1499–1510.

70 Matsumoto, A., Murota, H., Terao, M., and Katayama, I. (2018). Attenuated activation of homeostatic glucocorticoid in keratinocytes induces alloknesis via aberrant artemin production. *Journal of Investigative Dermatology* 138 (7): 1491–1500.

71 Tiganescu, A., Hupe, M., Uchida, Y. et al. (2014). Increased glucocorticoid activation during mouse skin wound healing. *Journal of Endocrinology* 221 (1): 51–61.

72 Hammami, M.M. and Siiteri, P.K. (1991). Regulation of 11β-hydroxysteroid dehydrogenase activity in human skin fibroblasts: enzymatic modulation of glucocorticoid action. *Journal of Clinical Endocrinology & Metabolism* 73 (2): 326–334.

73 Itoi-Ochi, S., Terao, M., Murota, H., and Katayama, I. (2016). Local corticosterone activation by 11β-hydroxysteroid dehydrogenase 1 in keratinocytes: the role in narrow-band UVB-induced dermatitis. *Dermato-Endocrinology* 8 (1): e1119958.

74 Lee, S.E., Kim, J.M., Jeong, M.K. et al. (2012). 11β-Hydroxysteroid dehydrogenase type 1 is expressed in human sebaceous glands and regulates glucocorticoid-induced lipid synthesis and toll-like receptor 2 expression in SZ95 sebocytes. *British Journal of Dermatology* 168 (1): 47–55.

75 Tiganescu, A., Hupe, M., Uchida, Y. et al. (2017). Topical 11β-hydroxysteroid dehydrogenase type 1 inhibition corrects cutaneous features of systemic glucocorticoid excess in female mice. *Endocrinology* 159 (1): 547–556.

76 Choi, J., Lee, S., Lee, E. et al. (2017). 258 11β-Hydroxysteroid dehydrogenase type 1 inhibition attenuates the adverse effects of glucocorticoids on dermal papilla cells. *Journal of Investigative Dermatology* 137 (10): S237.

77 Tiganescu, A., Tahrani, A.A., Morgan, S.A. et al. (2013). 11β-Hydroxysteroid dehydrogenase blockade prevents age-induced skin structure and function defects. *Journal of Clinical Investigation* 123 (7): 3051–3060.

78 Zou, X., Ramachandran, P., Kendall, T.J. et al. (2018). 11Beta-hydroxysteroid dehydrogenase-1 deficiency or inhibition enhances hepatic myofibroblast activation in murine liver fibrosis. *Hepatology* 67 (6): 2167–2181.

79 Terao, M., Tani, M., Itoi, S. et al. (2014). 11β-Hydroxysteroid dehydrogenase 1 specific inhibitor increased dermal collagen content and promotes fibroblast proliferation. *PLoS One* 9 (3): e93051.

80 Chida, Y. and Mao, X. (2009). Does psychosocial stress predict symptomatic herpes simplex virus recurrence? A meta-analytic investigation on prospective studies. *Brain, Behavior, and Immunity* 23 (7): 917–925.

81 Stewart, T.J., Tong, W., and Whitfeld, M.J. (2018). The associations between psychological stress and psoriasis: a systematic review. *International Journal of Dermatology* 57 (11): 1275–1282.

82 Dashko, M.O., Syzon, O.O., Chaplyk-Chyzho, I.O., and Turkevych, S.A. (2019). Pathogenetic peculiarities of neuroendocrine and metabolic disorders in patients with acne associated with chronic stress. *Wiad Lek* 72 (5 cs 2): 997–1001.

83 Pancar Yuksel, E., Durmus, D., and Sarisoy, G. (2019). Perceived stress, life events, fatigue and temperament in patients with psoriasis. *Journal of International Medical Research* 47 (9): 4284–4291.

84 Nakano-Tahara, M., Murota, H., and Katayama, I. (2017). *Psychological Stress in*

Atopic Dermatitis. *Evolution of Atopic Dermatitis in the 21st Century*, 157–163. Singapore: Springer.

85 Fortune, D.G., Richards, H.L., Kirby, B. et al. (2003). Psychological distress impairs clearance of psoriasis in patients treated with photochemotherapy. *Archives of Dermatology* 139 (6): 752–756.

86 Aberg, K.M., Radek, K.A., Choi, E.-H. et al. (2007). Psychological stress downregulates epidermal antimicrobial peptide expression and increases severity of cutaneous infections in mice. *Journal of Clinical Investigation* 117 (11): 3339–3349.

87 Niyonsaba, F., Kiatsurayanon, C., Chieosilapatham, P., and Ogawa, H. (2017). Friends or foes? Host defense (antimicrobial) peptides and proteins in human skin diseases. *Experimental Dermatology* 26 (11): 989–998.

88 Oren, A., Ganz, T., Liu, L., and Meerloo, T. (2003). In human epidermis, β-defensin 2 is packaged in lamellar bodies. *Experimental and Molecular Pathology* 74 (2): 180–182.

89 Braff, M.H., Nardo, A.D., and Gallo, R.L. (2005). Keratinocytes store the antimicrobial peptide cathelicidin in lamellar bodies. *Journal of Investigative Dermatology* 124 (2): 394–400.

90 Menon, G.K., Lee, S.E., and Lee, S.-H. (2018). An overview of epidermal lamellar bodies: novel roles in biological adaptations and secondary barriers. *Journal of Dermatological Science* 92 (1): 10–17.

91 Martin-Ezquerra, G., Man, M.-Q., Hupe, M. et al. (2011). Psychological stress regulates antimicrobial peptide expression by both glucocorticoid and β-adrenergic mechanisms. *European Journal of Dermatology* 21 (S1): 48–51.

92 Teixeira, V., Feio, M.J., and Bastos, M. (2012). Role of lipids in the interaction of antimicrobial peptides with membranes. *Progress in Lipid Research* 51 (2): 149–177.

93 Schittek, B., Paulmann, M., Senyurek, I., and Steffen, H. (2008). The role of antimicrobial peptides in human skin and in skin infectious diseases. *Infectious Disorders: Drug Targets* 8 (3): 135–143.

94 Rojas, I.-G., Padgett, D.A., Sheridan, J.F., and Marucha, P.T. (2002). Stress-induced susceptibility to bacterial infection during cutaneous wound healing. *Brain, Behavior, and Immunity* 16 (1): 74–84.

95 Heilborn, J.D., Nilsson, M.F., Sørensen, O. et al. (2003). The cathelicidin anti-microbial peptide LL-37 is involved in re-epithelialization of human skin wounds and is lacking in chronic ulcer epithelium. *Journal of Investigative Dermatology* 120 (3): 379–389.

96 Vieira, B.L., Lim, N.R., Lohman, M.E., and Lio, P.A. (2016). Complementary and alternative medicine for atopic dermatitis: an evidence-based review. *American Journal of Clinical Dermatology* 17 (6): 557–581.

97 Raychaudhuri, S.K., Bagchi, D., and Raychaudhuri, S.P. (2017). *Concept of Total Care. Psoriasis and Psoriatic Arthritis*, 271–280. Boca Raton: CRC Press.

98 Shenefelt, P.D. (2003). Biofeedback, cognitive-behavioral methods, and hypnosis in dermatology: is it all in your mind? *Dermatologic Therapy* 16 (2): 114–122.

99 Cruess, S., Antoni, M., Cruess, D. et al. (2000). Reductions in herpes simplex virus type 2 antibody titers after cognitive behavioral stress management and relationships with neuroendocrine function, relaxation skills, and social support in HIV-positive men. *Psychosomatic Medicine* 62 (6): 828–837.

100 Walburn, J., Vedhara, K., Hankins, M. et al. (2009). Psychological stress and wound healing in humans: a systematic review and meta-analysis. *Journal of Psychosomatic Research* 67 (3): 253–271.

101 Willenborg, S. and Eming, S.A. (2018). Cellular networks in wound healing. *Science* 362 (6417): 891–892.

102 Connor, T.J., Brewer, C., Kelly, J.P., and Harkin, A. (2005). Acute stress suppresses

pro-inflammatory cytokines TNF-α and IL-1β independent of a catecholamine-driven increase in IL-10 production. *Journal of Neuroimmunology* 159 (1–2): 119–128.

103 Koschwanez, H., Vurnek, M., Weinman, J. et al. (2015). Stress-related changes to immune cells in the skin prior to wounding may impair subsequent healing. *Brain, Behavior, and Immunity* 50: 47–51.

104 Marucha, P.T., Kiecolt-Glaser, J.K., and Favagehi, M. (1998). Mucosal wound healing is impaired by examination stress. *Psychosomatic Medicine* 60 (3): 362–365.

105 Vegas, O., Vanbuskirk, J., Richardson, S. et al. (2008). Stress and wound healing: effects of housing conditions and coping with a psychological stress. *Brain, Behavior, and Immunity* 22 (4): 12.

106 Youm, J.-K., Park, K., Uchida, Y. et al. (2013). Local blockade of glucocorticoid activation reverses stress- and glucocorticoid-induced delays in cutaneous wound healing. *Wound Repair and Regeneration* 21 (5): 715–722.

107 Curtin, N.M., Boyle, N.T., Mills, K.H.G., and Connor, T.J. (2009). Psychological stress suppresses innate IFN-γ production via glucocorticoid receptor activation: reversal by the anxiolytic chlordiazepoxide. *Brain, Behavior, and Immunity* 23 (4): 535–547.

108 Robinson, H., Norton, S., Jarrett, P., and Broadbent, E. (2017). The effects of psychological interventions on wound healing: a systematic review of randomized trials. *British Journal of Health Psychology* 22 (4): 805–835.

109 Detillion, C.E., Craft, T.K.S., Glasper, E.R. et al. (2004). Social facilitation of wound healing. *Psychoneuroendocrinology* 29 (8): 1004–1011.

110 Barnard, E., Shi, B., Kang, D. et al. (2016). The balance of metagenomic elements shapes the skin microbiome in acne and health. *Scientific Reports* 6 (1): 39491.

111 Kelhälä, H.-L., Aho, V.T.E., Fyhrquist, N. et al. (2017). Isotretinoin and lymecycline treatments modify the skin microbiota in acne. *Experimental Dermatology* 27 (1): 30–36.

112 Xu, H. and Li, H. (2019). Acne, the skin microbiome, and antibiotic treatment. *American Journal of Clinical Dermatology* 20 (3): 335–344.

113 Christensen, G.J.M., Scholz, C.F.P., Enghild, J. et al. (2016). Antagonism between *Staphylococcus epidermidis* and *Propionibacterium acnes* and its genomic basis. *BMC Genomics* 17 (1): 152.

114 Soares, R.C., Zani, M.B., Arruda, A.C.B.B. et al. (2015). *Malassezia* intra-specific diversity and potentially new species in the skin microbiota from Brazilian healthy subjects and seborrheic dermatitis patients. *PLoS One* 10 (2): e0117921.

115 Soares, R.C., Camargo-Penna, P.H., de Moraes, V.C.S. et al. (2016). Dysbiotic bacterial and fungal communities not restricted to clinically affected skin sites in dandruff. *Frontiers in Cellular and Infection Microbiology* 6: 157.

116 O'Neill, A.M. and Gallo, R.L. (2018). Host–microbiome interactions and recent progress into understanding the biology of acne vulgaris. *Microbiome* 6 (1).

117 Ganju, P., Nagpal, S., Mohammed, M.H. et al. (2016). Microbial community profiling shows dysbiosis in the lesional skin of vitiligo subjects. *Scientific Reports* 6 (1): 18761.

118 Chang, H.-W., Yan, D., Singh, R. et al. (2018). Alteration of the cutaneous microbiome in psoriasis and potential role in Th17 polarization. *Microbiome* 6 (1): 154.

119 Thomas, C.L. and Fernández-Peñas, P. (2016). The microbiome and atopic eczema: more than skin deep. *Australasian Journal of Dermatology* 58 (1): 18–24.

120 Kobayashi, T., Glatz, M., Horiuchi, K. et al. (2015). Dysbiosis and *Staphylococcus aureus* colonization drives inflammation in atopic dermatitis. *Immunity* 42 (4): 756–766.

121 Kong, H.H., Oh, J., Deming, C. et al. (2012). Temporal shifts in the skin microbiome

associated with disease flares and treatment in children with atopic dermatitis. *Genome Research* 22 (5): 850–859.

122 Ellis, S.R., Nguyen, M., Vaughn, A.R. et al. (2019). The skin and gut microbiome and its role in common dermatologic conditions. *Microorganisms* 7 (11): 550.

123 Dréno, B., Araviiskaia, E., Berardesca, E. et al. (2016). Microbiome in healthy skin, update for dermatologists. *Journal of the European Academy of Dermatology and Venereology* 30 (12): 2038–2047.

124 Hong, S.-W., Kim, K.S., and Surh, C.D. (2017). Beyond hygiene: commensal microbiota and allergic diseases. *Immune Network* 17 (1): 48.

125 Kennedy, E.Λ., Connolly, J., Hourihane, J.O.B. et al. (2017). Skin microbiome before development of atopic dermatitis: early colonization with commensal staphylococci at 2 months is associated with a lower risk of atopic dermatitis at 1 year. *Journal of Allergy and Clinical Immunology* 139 (1): 166–172.

126 Paller, A.S., Kong, H.H., Seed, P. et al. (2019). The microbiome in patients with atopic dermatitis. *Journal of Allergy and Clinical Immunology* 143 (1): 26–35.

127 Nakamizo, S., Egawa, G., Honda, T. et al. (2014). Commensal bacteria and cutaneous immunity. *Seminars in Immunopathology* 37 (1): 73–80.

128 Schoch, J.J., Monir, R.L., Satcher, K.G. et al. (2019). The infantile cutaneous microbiome: a review. *Pediatric Dermatology* 36 (5): 574–580.

129 Croitoru, D.O. and Piguet, V. (2019). A mother's touch: emerging roles in development of the cutaneous microbiome. *Journal of Investigative Dermatology* 139 (12): 2414–2416.

130 Bowe, W., Patel, N.B., and Logan, A.C. (2014). Acne vulgaris, probiotics and the gut-brain-skin axis: from anecdote to translational medicine. *Beneficial Microbes* 5 (2): 185–199.

131 Mottin, V.H.M. and Suyenaga, E.S. (2018). An approach on the potential use of probiotics in the treatment of skin conditions: acne and atopic dermatitis. *International Journal of Dermatology* 57 (12): 1425–1432.

132 Prakoeswa, C.R.S., Herwanto, N., Prameswari, R. et al. (2017). *Lactobacillus plantarum* IS-10506 supplementation reduced SCORAD in children with atopic dermatitis. *Beneficial Microbes* 8 (5): 833–840.

133 Schmidt, R.M., Pilmann Laursen, R., Bruun, S. et al. (2019). Probiotics in late infancy reduce the incidence of eczema: a randomized controlled trial. *Pediatric Allergy and Immunology* 30 (3): 335–340.

134 Holmes, C.J., Plichta, J.K., Gamelli, R.L., and Radek, K.A. (2015). Dynamic role of host stress responses in modulating the cutaneous microbiome: implications for wound healing and infection. *Advances in Wound Care* 4 (1): 24–37.

135 Johnson, T., Gómez, B., McIntyre, M. et al. (2018). The cutaneous microbiome and wounds: new molecular targets to promote wound healing. *International Journal of Molecular Sciences* 19 (9): 2699.

136 Williams, H., Crompton, R.A., Thomason, H.A. et al. (2017). Cutaneous Nod2 expression regulates the skin microbiome and wound healing in a murine model. *Journal of Investigative Dermatology* 137 (11): 2427–2436.

137 O'Neill, C.A., Monteleone, G., McLaughlin, J.T., and Paus, R. (2016). The gut-skin axis in health and disease: a paradigm with therapeutic implications. *BioEssays* 38 (11): 1167–1176.

138 Huo, R., Zeng, B., Zeng, L. et al. (2017). Microbiota modulate anxiety-like behavior and endocrine abnormalities in hypothalamic-pituitary-adrenal axis. *Frontiers in Cellular and Infection Microbiology* 7: 489.

139 Vodička, M., Ergang, P., Hrnčíř, T. et al. (2018). Microbiota affects the expression of genes involved in HPA axis regulation and local metabolism of glucocorticoids in

chronic psychosocial stress. *Brain, Behavior, and Immunity* 73: 615–624.

140 Wang, S.-X. (2005). Effects of psychological stress on small intestinal motility and bacteria and mucosa in mice. *World Journal of Gastroenterology* 11 (13): 2016.

141 Gur, T.L. and Bailey, M.T. (2016). *Effects of Stress on Commensal Microbes and Immune System Activity. Microbial Endocrinology: Interkingdom Signaling in Infectious Disease and Health*, 289–300. Basel: Springer.

142 Petra, A.I., Panagiotidou, S., Hatziagelaki, E. et al. (2015). Gut-microbiota-brain axis and its effect on neuropsychiatric disorders with suspected immune dysregulation. *Clinical Therapeutics* 37 (5): 984–995.

143 Mackos, A.R., Galley, J.D., Eubank, T.D. et al. (2015). Social stress-enhanced severity of *Citrobacter rodentium*-induced colitis is CCL2-dependent and attenuated by probiotic Lactobacillus reuteri. *Mucosal Immunology* 9 (2): 515–526.

144 Sudo, N., Chida, Y., Aiba, Y. et al. (2004). Postnatal microbial colonization programs the hypothalamic-pituitary-adrenal system for stress response in mice. *Journal of Physiology* 558 (1): 263–275.

145 de Punder, K. and Pruimboom, L. (2015). Stress induces endotoxemia and low-grade inflammation by increasing barrier permeability. *Frontiers in Immunology* 6: 223.

146 Iwamoto, K., Moriwaki, M., Miyake, R., and Hide, M. (2019). *Staphylococcus aureus* in atopic dermatitis: strain-specific cell wall proteins and skin immunity. *Allergology International* 68 (3): 309–315.

147 Bailey, M.T. (2014). Influence of stressor-induced nervous system activation on the intestinal microbiota and the importance for immunomodulation. *Advances in Experimental Medicine and Biology* 814: 255–276.

148 Mohajeri, M.H., La Fata, G., Steinert, R.E., and Weber, P. (2018). Relationship between the gut microbiome and brain function. *Nutrition Reviews* 76 (7): 481–496.

149 Polak-Witka, K., Rudnicka, L., Blume-Peytavi, U., and Vogt, A. (2019). The role of the microbiome in scalp hair follicle biology and disease. *Experimental Dermatology* 29 (3): 286–294.

150 Dalton, E.D., Hammen, C.L., Brennan, P.A., and Najman, J.M. (2016). Pathways maintaining physical health problems from childhood to young adulthood: the role of stress and mood. *Psychology and Health* 31 (11): 1255–1271.

151 Millar, S.E. (2018). Revitalizing aging skin through diet. *Cell* 175 (6): 1461–1463.

152 Schultchen, D., Reichenberger, J., Mittl, T. et al. (2019). Bidirectional relationship of stress and affect with physical activity and healthy eating. *British Journal of Health Psychology* 24 (2): 315–333.

153 Wong, M.L., Lau, E.Y.Y., Wan, J.H.Y. et al. (2013). The interplay between sleep and mood in predicting academic functioning, physical health and psychological health: a longitudinal study. *Journal of Psychosomatic Research* 74 (4): 271–277.

154 Salzer, M.C., Lafzi, A., Berenguer-Llergo, A. et al. (2018). Identity noise and adipogenic traits characterize dermal fibroblast aging. *Cell* 175 (6): 1575–1590.

155 Forni, M.F., Peloggia, J., Braga, T.T. et al. (2017). Caloric restriction promotes structural and metabolic changes in the skin. *Cell Reports* 20 (11): 2678–2692.

156 Rosa, D.F., Sarandy, M.M., Novaes, R.D. et al. (2017). Effect of a high-fat diet and alcohol on cutaneous repair: a systematic review of murine experimental models. *PLoS One* 12 (5): e0176240.

157 Rosa, D.F., Sarandy, M.M., Novaes, R.D. et al. (2018). High-fat diet and alcohol intake promotes inflammation and impairs skin wound healing in Wistar rats. *Mediators of Inflammation* 2018: 1–12.

158 Leguina-Ruzzi, A., Ortiz, R., and Velarde, V. (2018). The streptozotocin-high fat diet induced diabetic mouse model exhibits severe skin damage and alterations in local

lipid mediators. *Biomedical Journal* 41 (5): 328–332.

159 Bedja, D., Yan, W., Lad, V. et al. (2018). Inhibition of glycosphingolipid synthesis reverses skin inflammation and hair loss in ApoE−/− mice fed western diet. *Scientific Reports* 8 (1): 11463.

160 Karadağ, A.S., Balta, İ., Saricaoğlu, H. et al. (2019). The effect of personal, familial, and environmental characteristics on acne vulgaris: a prospective, multicenter, case controlled study. *Giornale Italiano di Dermatologia e Venereologia* 154 (2): 177–185.

161 Mukherjee, S., Mitra, R., Maitra, A. et al. (2016). Sebum and hydration levels in specific regions of human face significantly predict the nature and diversity of facial skin microbiome. *Scientific Reports* 6 (1): 36062.

162 Dai, R., Hua, W., Chen, W. et al. (2018). The effect of milk consumption on acne: a meta-analysis of observational studies. *Journal of the European Academy of Dermatology and Venereology* 32 (12): 2244–2253.

163 Burris, J., Rietkerk, W., Shikany, J.M., and Woolf, K. (2017). Differences in dietary glycemic load and hormones in New York City adults with no and moderate/severe acne. *Journal of the Academy of Nutrition and Dietetics* 117 (9): 1375–1383.

164 Papagrigoraki, A., Maurelli, M., del Giglio, M. et al. (2017). Advanced glycation end products in the pathogenesis of psoriasis. *International Journal of Molecular Sciences* 18 (11): 2471.

165 Isami, F., West, B.J., Nakajima, S., and Yamagishi, S.-I. (2018). Association of advanced glycation end products, evaluated by skin autofluorescence, with lifestyle habits in a general Japanese population. *Journal of International Medical Research* 46 (3): 1043–1051.

166 Burris, J., Shikany, J.M., Rietkerk, W., and Woolf, K. (2018). A low glycemic index and glycemic load diet decreases insulin-like growth factor-1 among adults with moderate and severe acne: a short-duration, 2-week randomized controlled trial. *Journal of the Academy of Nutrition and Dietetics* 118 (10): 1874–1885.

167 Smith, R.N., Mann, N.J., Braue, A. et al. (2007). The effect of a high-protein, low glycemic-load diet versus a conventional, high glycemic-load diet on biochemical parameters associated with acne vulgaris: a randomized, investigator-masked, controlled trial. *Journal of the American Academy of Dermatology* 57 (2): 247–256.

168 Rogerson, D., McNeill, S., Könönen, H., and Klonizakis, M. (2018). Encouraging effects of a short-term, adapted Nordic diet intervention on skin microvascular function and skin oxygen tension in younger and older adults. *Nutrition* 49: 96–101.

169 Klonizakis, M., Grammatikopoulou, M.G., Theodoridis, X. et al. (2019). Effects of long- versus short-term exposure to the Mediterranean diet on skin microvascular function and quality of life of healthy adults in Greece and the UK. *Nutrients* 11 (10): 2487.

170 Lim, S., Shin, J., Cho, Y., and Kim, K.-P. (2019). Dietary patterns associated with sebum content, skin hydration and pH, and their sex-dependent differences in healthy Korean adults. *Nutrients* 11 (3): 619.

171 Yang, K., Fung, T.T., and Nan, H. (2018). An epidemiological review of diet and cutaneous malignant melanoma. *Cancer Epidemiology, Biomarkers and Prevention* 27 (10): 1115–1122.

172 Mintie, C.A., Singh, C.K., and Ahmad, N. (2020). Whole fruit phytochemicals combating skin damage and carcinogenesis. *Translational Oncology* 13 (2): 146–156.

173 Działo, M., Mierziak, J., Korzun, U. et al. (2016). The potential of plant phenolics in prevention and therapy of skin disorders. *International Journal of Molecular Sciences* 17 (2): 160.

174 Woodby, B., Penta, K., Pecorelli, A. et al. (2020). Skin health from the inside out. *Annual Review of Food Science and Technology* 11 (1): 235–254.

175 Ueda, S., Tanahashi, M., Higaki, Y. et al. (2017). Ingestion of coffee polyphenols improves a scaly skin surface and the recovery rate of skin temperature after cold stress: a randomized, controlled trial. *Journal of Nutritional Science and Vitaminology* 63 (5): 291–297.

176 Fukushima, Y., Takahashi, Y., Kishimoto, Y. et al. (2020). Consumption of polyphenols in coffee and green tea alleviates skin photoaging in healthy Japanese women. *Clinical, Cosmetic and Investigational Dermatology* 13: 165–172.

177 Kagawa, D., Fujii, A., Ohtsuka, M., and Murase, T. (2018). Ingestion of coffee polyphenols suppresses deterioration of skin barrier function after barrier disruption, concomitant with the modulation of autonomic nervous system activity in healthy subjects. *Bioscience, Biotechnology, and Biochemistry* 82 (5): 879–884.

178 Cho, B.O., Che, D.N., Shin, J.Y. et al. (2018). Ameliorative effects of fruit stem extract from Muscat Bailey A against chronic UV-induced skin damage in BALB/c mice. *Biomedicine and Pharmacotherapy* 97: 1680–1688.

179 Singh, C.K., Mintie, C.A., Ndiaye, M.A. et al. (2019). Chemoprotective effects of dietary grape powder on UVB radiation-mediated skin carcinogenesis in SKH-1 hairless mice. *Journal of Investigative Dermatology* 139 (3): 552–561.

180 George, V.C. and Rupasinghe, H.P.V. (2017). Apple flavonoids suppress carcinogen-induced DNA damage in normal human bronchial epithelial cells. *Oxidative Medicine and Cellular Longevity* 2017: 1–12.

181 Cooperstone, J.L., Tober, K.L., Riedl, K.M. et al. (2017). Tomatoes protect against development of UV-induced keratinocyte carcinoma via metabolomic alterations. *Scientific Reports* 7 (1): 5106.

182 Maguire, M. and Maguire, G. (2017). The role of microbiota, and probiotics and prebiotics in skin health. *Archives of Dermatological Research* 309 (6): 411–421.

183 McBain, A.J., O'Neill, C.A., Amezquita, A. et al. (2019). Consumer safety considerations of skin and oral microbiome perturbation. *Clinical Microbiology Reviews* 32 (4): e000511–e000551. https://doi.org/10.1128/CMR.00051-19.

184 Babeluk, R., Jutz, S., Mertlitz, S. et al. (2014). Hand hygiene – evaluation of three disinfectant hand sanitizers in a community setting. *PLoS One* 9 (11): e111969.

185 Park, S.-Y., Kim, H.S., Lee, S.H., and Kim, S. (2020). Characterization and analysis of the skin microbiota in acne: impact of systemic antibiotics. *Journal of Clinical Medicine* 9 (1): 168.

186 Kilian, M., Chapple, I.L.C., Hannig, M. et al. (2016). The oral microbiome – an update for oral healthcare professionals. *British Dental Journal* 221 (10): 657–666.

187 Urban, J., Fergus, D.J., Savage, A.M. et al. (2016). The effect of habitual and experimental antiperspirant and deodorant product use on the armpit microbiome. *Peer J* 4: e1605.

188 Callewaert, C., Hutapea, P., Van de Wiele, T., and Boon, N. (2014). Deodorants and antiperspirants affect the axillary bacterial community. *Archives of Dermatological Research* 306 (8): 701–710.

189 Bouslimani, A., da Silva, R., Kosciolek, T. et al. (2019). The impact of skin care products on skin chemistry and microbiome dynamics. *BMC Biology* 17 (1): 47.

190 Blaak, J. and Staib, P. (2018). *The Relation of pH and Skin Cleansing. pH of the Skin: Issues and Challenges*, 132–142. Berlin: S. Karger.

191 Staudinger, T., Pipal, A., and Redl, B. (2011). Molecular analysis of the prevalent microbiota of human male and female forehead skin compared to forearm skin and the influence of make-up. *Journal of Applied Microbiology* 110 (6): 1381–1389.

192 Callewaert, C., Van Nevel, S., Kerckhof, F.-M. et al. (2015). Bacterial exchange in household washing machines. *Frontiers in Microbiology* 6: 1381.

193 Steglińska, J., Szulc, A., Otlewska, A. et al. (2019). Factors influencing microbiological biodiversity of human foot skin. *International Journal of Environmental Research and Public Health* 16 (18): 3503.

194 Lopes, C., Soares, J., Tavaria, F. et al. (2015). Chitosan coated textiles may improve atopic dermatitis severity by modulating skin staphylococcal profile: a randomized controlled trial. *PLoS One* 10 (11): e0142844.

195 Callewaert, C., De Maeseneire, E., Kerckhof, F.-M. et al. (2014). Microbial odor profile of polyester and cotton clothes after a fitness session. *Applied and Environmental Microbiology* 80 (21): 6611–6619.

196 Wood, M., Gibbons, S.M., Lax, S. et al. (2015). Athletic equipment microbiota are shaped by interactions with human skin. *Microbiome* 3 (1): 25.

197 Zlotogorski, A. (1987). Distribution of skin surface pH on the forehead and cheek of adults. *Archives of Dermatological Research* 279 (6): 398–401.

198 Lee, H.J., Jeong, S.E., Lee, S. et al. (2017). Effects of cosmetics on the skin microbiome of facial cheeks with different hydration levels. *Microbiology Open* 7 (2): e00557.

199 Draelos, Z.D. (2017). The science behind skin care: cleansers. *Journal of Cosmetic Dermatology* 17 (1): 8–14.

200 Khosrowpour, Z., Ahmad Nasrollahi, S., Ayatollahi, A. et al. (2018). Effects of four soaps on skin trans-epidermal water loss and erythema index. *Journal of Cosmetic Dermatology* 18 (3): 857–861.

201 Caberlotto, E., Ruiz, L., Miller, Z. et al. (2017). Effects of a skin-massaging device on the ex-vivo expression of human dermis proteins and in-vivo facial wrinkles. *PLoS One* 12 (3): e0172624.

202 Yonezawa, K., Haruna, M., Matsuzaki, M. et al. (2017). Effects of moisturizing skincare on skin barrier function and the prevention of skin problems in 3-month-old infants: a randomized controlled trial. *Journal of Dermatology* 45 (1): 24–30.

203 Elias Peter, M., Wakefield Joan, S., and Man, M.-Q. (2018). Moisturizers versus current and next-generation barrier repair therapy for the management of atopic dermatitis. *Skin Pharmacology and Physiology* 32 (1): 1–7.

204 Kim, E.-J. and Dimsdale, J.E. (2007). The effect of psychosocial stress on sleep: a review of polysomnographic evidence. *Behavioral Sleep Medicine* 5 (4): 256–278.

205 Bassett, S.M., Lupis, S.B., Gianferante, D. et al. (2015). Sleep quality but not sleep quantity effects on cortisol responses to acute psychosocial stress. *Stress* 18 (6): 638–644.

206 Vargas, I. and Lopez-Duran, N. (2017). Investigating the effect of acute sleep deprivation on hypothalamic-pituitary-adrenal-axis response to a psychosocial stressor. *Psychoneuroendocrinology* 79: 1–8.

207 van Dalfsen, J.H. and Markus, C.R. (2018). The influence of sleep on human hypothalamic–pituitary–adrenal (HPA) axis reactivity: a systematic review. *Sleep Medicine Reviews* 39: 187–194.

208 Oyetakin-White, P., Suggs, A., Koo, B. et al. (2014). Does poor sleep quality affect skin ageing? *Clinical and Experimental Dermatology* 40 (1): 17–22.

209 Broadbent, E., Vurnek, M., Weinman, J. et al. (2015). Sleep and skin composition. *Brain, Behavior, and Immunity* 49: 339–340.

210 Koschwanez, H.E., Kerse, N., Darragh, M. et al. (2013). Expressive writing and wound healing in older adults. *Psychosomatic Medicine* 75 (6): 581–590.

211 Opp, M.R. and Krueger, J.M. (2015). Sleep and immunity: a growing field with clinical impact. *Brain, Behavior, and Immunity* 47: 1–3.

212 Krajewska-Włodarczyk, M., Owczarczyk-Saczonek, A., and Placek, W. (2018). Sleep disorders in patients with psoriatic arthritis and psoriasis. *Reumatologia/Rheumatology* 56 (5): 301–306.

213 Heckman, C.J., Kloss, J.D., Feskanich, D. et al. (2016). Associations among rotating night shift work, sleep and skin cancer in Nurses' Health Study II participants. *Occupational and Environmental Medicine* 74 (3): 169–175.

214 Opp, M.R. and Krueger, J.M. (2017). *Sleep and Host Defense. Principles and Practice of Sleep Medicine*, 193–201. Amsterdam: Elsevier.

215 Li, Y., Hao, Y., Fan, F., and Zhang, B. (2018). The role of microbiome in insomnia, circadian disturbance and depression. *Frontiers in Psychiatry* 9: 669.

216 Parkar, S., Kalsbeek, A., and Cheeseman, J. (2019). Potential role for the gut microbiota in modulating host circadian rhythms and metabolic health. *Microorganisms* 7 (2): 41.

217 Ketchesin, K.D., Becker-Krail, D., and McClung, C.A. (2018). Mood-related central and peripheral clocks. *European Journal of Neuroscience* 51 (1): 326–345.

218 De Nobrega, A.K., Luz, K.V., and Lyons, L.C. (2020). Resetting the aging clock: implications for managing age-related diseases. In: *Reviews on New Drug Targets in Age-Related Disorders* (ed. P.C. Guest), 193–265. Cham: Springer International Publishing.

2

The Science and Psychology of Beauty

Vanessa J. Cutler

Department of Psychiatry, New York University Grossman School of Medicine, New York, NY, USA

Beauty may be in the eye of the beholder, as the old adage goes. Yet, it seems that humans across all cultures and ethnicities do have a unified, objective understanding of what exactly it means to be beautiful [1]. Even infants as young as four months, thought to mostly be a blank slate, will tend to dwell longer on more attractive adult faces than on those deemed less attractive [2, 3]. Furthermore, it takes adults only 150 msec to judge a stranger's facial attractiveness [4]. The quest for beauty has spurred multi-trillion-dollar cosmetics, aesthetics, and fitness industries, each one promising a more attractive, youthful, and physically fitter version of self [5]. Beauty also seems to be an important facet of human social interactions and mating behaviors, with more attractive people benefitting from higher long-term socioeconomic status and even being perceived by peers as "better" people. In fact, beautiful people are considered to be friendlier, more intelligent, more interesting, and more socially competent [6]. Beautiful people, too, seem to have better luck attracting romance [7]. Beauty, it seems, confers many advantages. While some have posited that the media is spurring images of what is attractive, it may actually be more likely that the media exploits universal beauty standards. Likewise, social media platforms have influenced beauty standards through instantaneous editing features, filtering, and cropping, allowing people to become the ideal version of themselves.

Evolutionary Explanations for Beauty

From an evolutionary psychology perspective, beauty is likely a beneficial adaptation developed over several hundred thousand years to advertise reproductive fitness to potential mates and ensure the survivability of the human species. However, there are also arguments that beauty, or rather the traits humans find attractive, may just be byproducts of the ways in which human brains process information [8]. On a very primal level, beauty is potentially associated with health and the ability to produce viable offspring [9]. Averageness [10], symmetry [11], and sexual dimorphism [12] are considered to be the qualities that make a face attractive, as well as facial adiposity [13] and carotenoid-based skin color [14], which may be reflective of a diet heavy in vegetables and fruit. Generally, clear skin and shiny, full hair seem to be considered the most attractive features in humans [15]. Hourglass figures, small chins, large eyes, small noses, and high cheekbones are considered to be the most attractive female traits [16].

On the other hand, men with prominent chins, deep-set eyes, and a heavy brow are considered to be most attractive [16].

Though it has been difficult to demonstrate conclusively [17], the immunocompetence handicap hypothesis (ICHH) [18] posits that the most masculine-looking men have hyper-masculinized facial features in order to signal biological hardiness and immunocompetence to potential mates. As males of many species often face considerable mating competition, it is imperative for the male to develop ornamental features for the purposes of attracting a mate, though this ornamentation often comes with a hefty biological price tag [19]. Though crucial for spermatogenesis [20], testosterone (an abundance of which is necessary for male secondary sexual characteristics like chest hair, a strong jaw, and deep baritone voice) can also suppress immune function [21] and increase oxidative stress [22], leading to subsequent risk of damage to multiple organ systems [23]. Due to weaker immune systems, men who are not able to withstand the damaging effects of high levels of testosterone will not appear as masculinized as those with strong immune systems [24] and not be as attractive to potential mates, while the offspring of the most masculine will benefit from greater genetic fitness.

Beauty as a Function of Health

Briefly, it is relevant to note that facial beauty may also be a marker of health and fertility, though there are little data to directly link qualifiers of good health to facial appearance [25]. There is some evidence to suggest that facial symmetry or lack thereof is related to health status [26]; however, the literature is inconsistent when it comes to associations between facial asymmetry and poor health. In women, it seems that the testosterone to estradiol ratio as well as low levels of

testosterone [27] are associated with facial attractiveness. Women with higher levels of estrogen (as measured in the late follicular phase) are judged to have more feminine, attractive, and healthy-appearing faces [28]. A woman's facial attractiveness, however, may fluctuate throughout the menstrual cycle, and women may become more physically attractive during ovulation when estrogen levels and fertility opportunities peak [29]. There is even some evidence to suggest that a woman's facial coloring tracks with estradiol levels throughout the menstrual cycle to indicate higher levels of fertility [30]. Additionally, Lie et al. [31] found that major histocompatibility complex heterozygosity (meaning differences in a set of closely linked genes that code for the immune system in all higher vertebrates, including humans) positively predicted male attractiveness, suggesting a relationship between overall genetic diversity, in some capacity, with attractiveness.

Weight and Attractiveness

Multiple studies [32] have validated 0.7 as being the preferred waist to hip ratio (WHR) in women, potentially because it may signal less risk for cardiovascular disease, diabetes, and cancer [33–35] and possibly greater cognitive ability [36]. Wang et al. [37] found an inverse relationship between perceived female attractiveness and body mass index (BMI) among Caucasian, African, and Asian raters, with the ideal female BMI being somewhere between 22.8 and 24.8, depending on the ethnicity of the rater. In studies taking both the WHR and BMI into account, it seems that lower WHR is more attractive in women while controlling for BMI [38], though BMI seems to be a more important contributor to attractiveness than WHR [39]. Overall, the data suggest that in women, BMIs and WHRs at the lower end of the normal range – BMI around 20 and WHR closer 0.7 – are considered to be the most attractive [40]. For men [41, 42], a WHR around 0.9 seems to be the ideal, and women seem to find a waist to chest ratio of 0.6 to be the most attractive [43].

Facial Proportions

Facial proportions, the distances between features, are important markers of facial attractiveness; the closer to ideal the measurements, the more attractive the face. Likewise, perfect proportion in form is appreciated in art and in nature and has been for centuries. Throughout history, humans have tried to understand what beauty means, as evidenced by the sculpture, painting, and architecture created by prior civilizations – the Egyptians, Greeks, Romans, and Italians – each era struggling to rectify the inherent beauty possessed by the work with the subjective judgment of the passing eye [44]. Today, young artists still perfect their craft by meticulously studying perfect models of symmetry and proportion, spending many an afternoon tucked away in wings of museums around the world, sketching, erasing, and sighing. Fortunately for the aesthetics community, the underpinnings of beautiful proportions are beginning to become understood with the aid of complex mathematical algorithms and sophisticated prediction models [45, 46].

It was the ancient Greek sculptor Polycleitus who established the proportions that eventually gave rise to the neoclassical canons [47], and who modeled his ideals into the statue Doryphorus [48]. The seven original neoclassical canons include measurements of vertical facial proportions (three-section facial profile, naso-aural proportion, naso-aural inclination), as well as horizontal proportions (orbitonasal, orbital, naso-oral, and nasofacial) [49]. Not surprisingly, the canons have less validity for non-North American Caucasian populations [49, 50], including modern Greeks [47] and Brazilians [51].

The golden ratio, also known as the Fibonacci ratio or the "divine proportion," is approximately equal to $1:1.618$ [52]. This ratio appears quite commonly in nature, and, many have argued, may be a key component of facial beauty [52, 53]. Initially recorded in the third century BCE by the Pythagoreans and later by Euclid, it was actually the Egyptians who may have recognized the aesthetically pleasing measurement [48]. Criticisms of standardized approaches to beauty have argued that they do not seem to be applicable across a range of geographic populations [54]. In examining differences in facial proportions between Miss Universe Thailand and Miss Universe winners from all around the world between 2001 and 2015, neither group of women met all measurements as described by the neoclassical canons; however, there were still points of agreement between the two groups and several of the canons, suggesting that they may still hold some relevance [55]. For more on theories of beauty see Chapter 5.

Through machine learning, many have tried to discern key micro measurements and facial landmarks and confirm the importance of these calculations with human raters based on the golden ratio or neoclassical canon or even pure symmetry [56]. Consistently, measures of trichion, menton, nasion, and subnasale [57] seem to be objective measures of importance contributing to facial beauty. Using over 400 computer-generated faces constructed by manipulating facial proportions after averaging the features of Japanese, Chinese, and Korean female celebrities, Shen et al. [58] demonstrated neurophysiologic evidence for human faces with variable attractiveness, even in the absence of skin texture and tone, facial expression, and hairstyle. In both men and women, there seems to be a linear relationship between caudate nucleus and orbitofrontal cortex activity and facial attractiveness. Interestingly, the location where the caudate nucleus shows activity upon recognition of an attractive face is also the region where activity has been observed in studies looking at the association between beauty and romantic love [59], which possibly suggests that specific facial ratios may evoke a "facial attractiveness experience" modulated by the strength of the experience, i.e. the proportions of the face. Accordingly, in both sexes highly attractive faces elicited a response in the lateral orbitofrontal cortex, an area of the brain that is associated with reward; however, only men demonstrated significant neural activity in the amygdala to both highly attractive faces and highly unattractive faces, which may imply that men assign more value to facial proportions than women.

It has been thought previously that facial beauty is directly related to facial symmetry, and yet this may not tell the full truth. There are several examples in the literature [60, 61] that propose facial symmetry to be a key characteristic of the beautiful face, but there are also data to suggest that a small amount of asymmetry may be not only an allowable "flaw" but also preferred [62]. In studies rating the attractiveness of normal full faces to the perfectly symmetrical faces created from them, the perfectly symmetrical face is consistently ranked lower than the asymmetrical face [63]. Likewise, even male and female fashion models, considered to possess at least some attractiveness, have some degree of facial asymmetry.

Absence of symmetry does not necessarily mean absence of beauty, as indicated by asymmetrical scenes in nature and in art [64]. In humans, symmetry is usually conceived of as being directional, or left to right and top to bottom. Functional, directional asymmetries, as opposed to fluctuating asymmetries, have a consistent bias across the population [61], have been found in human smiles and face size [64], and are considered to be the norm and not indicative of any stressors during development. It may be that functional directional asymmetry is a component of human beauty [64], while a perfectly symmetrical face would be considered to be abnormal for lacking in any directional asymmetry [61]. It is unclear, though, how much directional asymmetry is permissible until a face is considered to be unattractive. Conversely, fluctuating asymmetry is a randomly distributed deviation from perfect symmetry in bilaterally paired structures thought to be indicative of developmental instability, like infection or stress [61]. However, it appears that symmetry may actually be a more important quality for male attractiveness [10] than for female attractiveness, and that the quality of male facial symmetry may signify a mate quality that is exclusive to males [10]. Furthermore, bilateral symmetry is considered to be as important as averageness when judging the attractiveness of a face [10].

Averageness confers beauty; however, beautiful faces are not average faces [65]. Facial averageness is a measure of how much a face deviates from the population average, or rather doesn't deviate. Averageness has been noted to be a component of beauty since the nineteenth century when it was found that a composite of faces was actually more attractive than any single face [66], and not much has changed since this initial observation. However, it would be misleading to say that "attractive faces are only average" [67], as the averageness hypothesis asserts. True, average faces are more symmetric and have smoother skin than individual faces, and the quality of averageness persists even when skin texture and symmetry are controlled [68]. Average faces may also be preferred as they are easier for visual systems to process [69]. Perrett et al. [70] were able to demonstrate the contrasting hypothesis – varying face shape along an attractiveness dimension increases attractiveness. They observed that the composites of 60 faces were deemed to be less attractive than composites composed of a subset of 15 of the most attractive faces from the original composite. DeBruine et al. [71] were also able to demonstrate that faces considered to be more attractive were preferred over average faces. However, there does exist a tipping point along the continuum, and increasing attractiveness indefinitely will at some point result in a scenario where the average face is preferred to one that is hyperattractive. While averageness plays a role in discerning attractive from unattractive faces, there seems to be an additional quality independent of averageness that is also an important component of facial attractiveness.

Lastly, facial attractiveness is also a function of sexual dimorphism in human adults. These differences may actually start to appear in infancy as male infants have more globular frontal bones [72]. Key differences between masculinized and feminized faces include differences in jaw shape, eyebrow size, and eye size, with distinct sexual dimorphism appearing in late adolescence [73]. In adolescence, a broadened forehead, chin, jaw, and nose are identified as masculine features and masculinity in a male face is easy to identify and likely associated with free testosterone levels [73]. Large eyes, small noses, and small chins seem to be the hallmarks of feminine beauty [16]. Strikingly, the lower face and jaw seem to be an important component of a feminized face. A hyperfeminized face is distinct due to alveolar prognathism, a horizontal reduction of the chin, and forward movement of the gonion [74], though a hyperfeminized face may not always be rated as more attractive than an average female face with a small chin. What makes for an attractive male face is a little more difficult to pin down and may actually depend on who is being asked to gauge attractiveness. It seems that homosexual men tend to prefer more masculinized male faces, while heterosexual men find feminized versions of male faces to be more attractive [75]. For more on anatomic differences between male and female faces see Chapters 6 and 7.

Age and Youth

Globally, the antiwrinkle products market will be worth nearly $30 billion dollars by 2025, and these products account for only a portion of the anti-aging market [76]. While it may be trite to say that youth is beauty, the appearance of youth is probably implicit to the perception of beauty. Neoteny, or the appearance of babyness [77], as demonstrated by large eyes, small

noses, round cheeks, smooth skin, and lighter coloration, is considered to be attractive [78]. Neoteny is an advantageous quality across the lifespan; infants with greater neoteny receive more attention and are likely to be the recipients of better parental care [79], while infants who are less attractive may be more likely to be subjected to child abuse [80]. Maestripieri et al. [81] found that in both men and women there was a negative association between age and perceived attractiveness; however, the decline in perceived facial attractiveness of 51- to 65-year-old women relative to women aged 35–50 was significantly larger when compared to men of the corresponding age groups. Tatarunaite et al. [82] followed 60 men and women between the ages of 11 and 31 and found that over the course of 20 years, facial attractiveness decreased as the subjects aged.

Enhancing Beauty

Historically, humans have gone to great lengths to cover up facial blemishes. In 1937, Max Factor, the famous makeup artist and namesake of the enduring brand, patented Pan-Cake foundation, the first commercially available foundation created specifically for technicolor film. Released in February 1938 for nonprofessional use, Pan-Cake soon became the most successful product sold by Max Factor and its sales outperformed all of Max Factor's other products combined throughout the 1940s [83]. Today, over a million prescriptions for tretinoin (a form of topical vitamin A) are written annually in the United States [84]. Dermatologists continue to recommend chemical peels [85] and lasers [86] for facial rejuvenation, wrinkles, acne and acne scars, melasma, sun damage, and hyperpigmentation. Healthy looking skin is critical to facial attractiveness and, unsurprisingly, facial texture and degree of pigmentation are key. In a study examining the effect of facial skin quality, attractive men had very healthy appearing skin when judged by a group of women [87]. The same researchers then manipulated the visible skin conditions of the male subjects to make them appear either healthier or unhealthier and found that the unhealthy appearing versions were rated significantly more unattractive than their paired unmanipulated counterparts. Likewise, in women, skin color distribution, independent of face shape or other features, seems to affect perceptions of female facial attractiveness and may signal physiologic health [87].

Knowing the implicit importance of skin texture to physical attractiveness, makeup has been used to enhance attractiveness for over 7000 years, spanning back to 4000 BCE when it is hypothesized that *Homo sapiens* used ground red ochre mineral pigments as body paint [88]. For many, makeup products can be used to augment or improve facial features like facial symmetry [89]. Like many animals, humans, too, utilize adornment as a means of signaling communication to others [90] and use of makeup positively affects ratings of female facial attractiveness. While one would assume that many women use makeup strictly for physical purposes or to fit a primal archetype of beauty, it seems that makeup use may also be related to self-esteem or self-confidence [91] and may be used to improve mood by improving self-confidence [92]. A survey of 70 women among differing age groups revealed that makeup has a dual purpose – either to camouflage the physical or as a means for seduction – and the purpose for use may be dependent on the dominant personality traits of the user [93]. Furthermore, around ovulation, women tend to use more makeup, use makeup more skillfully, and spend more time applying makeup likely because it increases physical attractiveness to potential male suitors [94]. For additional information on the use of cosmetics and makeup and their effects on patient well-being see Chapter 3.

Beauty and the Media

The media, particularly print and television advertisements, have frequently been accused of promoting unattainable beauty standards to impressionable consumers. Historically, these images have targeted females, though, over the past several decades, there has been an uptick in images that are advertising beauty and fitness ideals to men too [95]. As gender roles continue to become more fluid, depictions of the western ideal have also changed, from the soft and subservient housewife of the 1960s to the well-manicured and confident career woman of the 1990s [96]. However, while stereotyped depictions of femininity have softened somewhat, it does not seem as if the beauty messages targeted to women have changed much at all. In fact, while 9.6% of the ads run in the *Australian Women's Weekly* in the 1970s focused on themes of being "more beautiful," so did 9.4% of the ads run in the same magazine in the 1990s [96]. Even across cultures, similar themes resonate. For example, a study [97] comparing skin beauty advertisements in major women's magazines between China and the United States found that "anti-aging," "moisturizing," and "antiwrinkle" were the dominant advertised product functions in both countries. Advertisers also utilize social comparison theory [98] in order to market and sell products, as self-improvement and self-evaluation might motivate an individual to buy a product, especially if it's being modeled by a beautiful individual.

The proliferation of social media applications has allowed people to be in continuous contact. However, social media platforms have also inadvertently created a "selfie-culture" where individuals have come to prefer their own curated mirror image, which may not be a totally accurate reflection of reality [99]. Unfortunately, social media can both affect perceived beauty standards and exacerbate appearance-related dissatisfaction through comparison with heavily altered images [99]. Perceptual adaptation, an experienced-based process that reshapes perceptions of the environment, can happen very quickly on social media where there are thousands of attractive images at a user's fingertips, even if he or she is only "mindlessly scrolling" [99].

While there is ample evidence to suggest strong biological underpinnings for human beauty, repeat exposure to beauty ideals on social media may influence new standards of beauty. However, the desire to enhance one's self either through a filtered selfie or through other methods may also be heavily influenced by one's genes. For additional exploration of the potential negative effects of social media on self-perception and beauty see Chapter 14.

Conclusions

While perspectives on how and why beauty is important differ, the relevance of beauty, particularly facial beauty, endures. From infancy through adulthood, beauty is beneficial to relating to people, moving up the career ladder, and mating. More than what meets the eye, a face is potentially an advertisement for genetic fitness, fertility, and beyond. The right proportions, smooth skin texture, and specific facial features seem to be synonymous with beauty. And yet, with the help of cosmetics, neuromodulators, and aesthetic procedures, beauty may truly only be skin deep. Finally, constant social media presence may be altering personal, if not societal standards of beauty while simultaneously intensifying individual frustrations about appearance.

References

1 Langlois, J.H., Kalakanis, L., Rubenstein, A.J. et al. (2000). Maxims or myths of beauty? A meta-analytic and theoretical review. *Psychological Bulletin* 126: 390–423. https://doi.org/10.1037/0033-2909.126.3.390.

2 Griffey, J.A.F. and Little, A.C. (2014). Infant's visual preferences for facial traits associated with adult attractiveness judgements: data from eye-tracking. *Infant Behavior and Development* 37: 268–275. https://doi.org/10.1016/j.infbeh.2014.03.001.

3 Samuels, C.A., Butterworth, G., Roberts, T. et al. (1994). Facial aesthetics: babies prefer attractiveness to symmetry. *Perception* 23: 823–831. https://doi.org/10.1068/p230823.

4 Goldstein, A.G. and Papageorge, J. (1980). Judgments of facial attractiveness in the absence of eye movements. *Bulletin of the Psychonomic Society* 15: 269–270. https://doi.org/10.3758/BF03334529.

5 Global Wellness Institute. Wellness Industry Statistics & Facts. https://globalwellnessinstitute.org/press-room/statistics-and-facts (accessed 16 August 2020).

6 Hönn, M. and Göz, G. (2007). The ideal of facial beauty: a review. *Journal of Orofacial Orthopedics* 68: 6–16. https://doi.org/10.1007/s00056-007-0604-6.

7 Rhodes, G., Simmons, L.W., and Peters, M. (2005). Attractiveness and sexual behavior: does attractiveness enhance mating success? *Evolution and Human Behavior* 26: 186–201. https://doi.org/10.1016/j.evolhumbehav.2004.08.014.

8 Enquist, M. and Arak, A. (1994). Symmetry, beauty and evolution. *Nature* 372: 169–172. https://doi.org/10.1038/372169a0.

9 Alam, M., Norman, R.A., and Goldberg, L.H. (2002). Dermatologic surgery in geriatric patients: psychosocial considerations and perioperative decision-making. *Dermatologic Surgery* 28: 1043–1050. https://doi.org/10.1046/j.1524-4725.2002.02102.x.

10 Komori, M., Kawamura, S., and Ishihara, S. (2009). Averageness or symmetry: which is more important for facial attractiveness? *Acta Psychologica* 131: 136–142. https://doi.org/10.1016/j.actpsy.2009.03.008.

11 Perrett, D.I., Burt, D.M., Penton-Voak, I.S. et al. (1999). Symmetry and human facial attractiveness. *Evolution and Human Behavior* 20: 295–307. https://doi.org/10.1016/S1090-5138(99)00014-8.

12 Perrett, D.I., Lee, K.J., Penton-Voak, I. et al. (1998). Effects of sexual dimorphism on facial attractiveness. *Nature* 394: 884–887. https://doi.org/10.1038/29772.

13 Coetzee, V., Perrett, D.I., and Stephen, I.D. (2009). Facial adiposity: a cue to health? *Perception* 38: 170011. https://doi.org/10.1068/p6423.

14 Whitehead, R.D., Re, D., Xiao, D. et al. (2012). You are what you eat: within-subject increases in fruit and vegetable consumption confer beneficial skin-color changes. *PLoS One* 7: e32988. https://doi.org/10.1371/journal.pone.0032988.

15 Furnham, A., Lavancy, M., and McClelland, A. (2001). Waist to hip ratio and facial attractiveness: a pilot study. *Personality and Individual Differences* 30: 491–502. https://doi.org/10.1016/S01918869(00)00040-4.

16 Cunningham, M.R., Roberts, A.R., Barbee, A.P. et al. (1995). "Their ideas of beauty are, on the whole, the same as ours": consistency and variability in the cross-cultural perception of female physical attractiveness. *Journal of Personality and Social Psychology* 68: 261–279. https://doi.org/10.1037/0022-3514.68.2.261.

17 Roberts, M.L., Buchanan, K.L., and Evans, M.R. (2004). Testing the immunocompetence handicap hypothesis: a review of the evidence. *Animal Behaviour* 68: 227–239. https://doi.org/10.1016/j.anbehav.2004.05.001.

18 Folstad, I. and Karter, A.J. (1992). Parasites, bright males, and the immunocompetence handicap. *The American Naturalist* 139: 603–622. https://doi.org/10.1086/285346.

19 Andersson, M. and Iwasa, Y. (1996). Sexual selection. *Trends in Ecology & Evolution* 11: 53–58. https://doi.org/10.1016/0169-5347(96)81042-1.

20 Zirkin, B.R. (1998). Spermatogenesis: its regulation by testosterone and FSH. *Seminars in Cell & Developmental Biology* 9: 417–421. https://doi.org/10.1006/scdb.1998.0253.

21 Foo, Y.Z., Nakagawa, S., Rhodes, G., and Simmons, L.W. (2017). The effects of sex hormones on immune function: a meta-analysis: sex hormones and immune function. *Biological Reviews* 92: 551–571. https://doi.org/10.1111/brv.12243.

22 Alonso-Alvarez, C., Bertrand, S., Faivre, B. et al. (2007). Testosterone and oxidative stress: the oxidation handicap hypothesis. *Proceedings of the Royal Society B* 274: 819–825. https://doi.org/10.1098/rspb.2006.3764.

23 Pizzino, G., Irrera, N., Cucinotta, M. et al. (2017). Oxidative stress: harms and benefits for human health. *Oxidative Medicine and Cellular Longevity* 2017: 1–13. https://doi.org/10.1155/2017/8416763.

24 Moore, F.R., Cornwell, R.E., Law Smith, M.J. et al. (2011). Evidence for the stress-linked immunocompetence handicap hypothesis in human male faces. *Proceedings of the Royal Society B* 278: 774–780. https://doi.org/10.1098/rspb.2010.1678.

25 Foo, Y.Z., Simmons, L.W., and Rhodes, G. (2017). Predictors of facial attractiveness and health in humans. *Scientific Reports* 7: 39731. https://doi.org/10.1038/srep39731.

26 Zaidel, D.W., Aarde, S.M., and Baig, K. (2005). Appearance of symmetry, beauty, and health in human faces. *Brain and Cognition* 57: 261–263. https://doi.org/10.1016/j.bandc.2004.08.056.

27 Probst, F., Bobst, C., and Lobmaier, J.S. (2016). Testosterone-to-oestradiol ratio is associated with female facial attractiveness. *Quarterly Journal of Experimental Psychology* 69: 89–99. https://doi.org/10.1080/17470218.2015.1024696.

28 Law Smith, M.J., Perrett, D.I., Jones, B.C. et al. (2006). Facial appearance is a cue to oestrogen levels in women. *Proceedings of the Royal Society B* 273: 135–140. https://doi.org/10.1098/rspb.2005.3296.

29 Puts, D.A., Bailey, D.H., Cárdenas, R.A. et al. (2013). Women's attractiveness changes with estradiol and progesterone across the ovulatory cycle. *Hormones and Behavior* 63: 13–19. https://doi.org/10.1016/j.yhbeh.2012.11.007.

30 Jones, B.C., Hahn, A.C., Fisher, C.I. et al. (2015). Facial coloration tracks changes in women's estradiol. *Psychoneuroendocrinology* 56: 29–34. https://doi.org/10.1016/j.psyneuen.2015.02.021.

31 Lie, H.C., Rhodes, G., and Simmons, L.W. (2008). Genetic diversity revealed in human faces. *Evolution* 62: 2473–2486. https://doi.org/10.1111/j.1558-5646.2008.00478.x.

32 Singh, D. (1994). Waist-to-hip ratio and judgment of attractiveness and healthiness of female figures by male and female physicians. *International Journal of Obesity and Related Metabolic Disorders* 18: 731–737.

33 Sayeed, M.A., Mahtab, H., Latif, Z.A. et al. (2003). Waist-to-height ratio is a better obesity index than body mass index and waist-to-hip ratio for predicting diabetes, hypertension and lipidemia. *Bangladesh Medical Research Council Bulletin* 29: 1–10.

34 Emdin, C.A., Khera, A.V., Natarajan, P. et al. (2017). Genetic association of waist-to-hip ratio with cardiometabolic traits, type 2 diabetes, and coronary heart disease. *JAMA* 317: 626. https://doi.org/10.1001/jama.2016.21042.

35 Connolly, B.S., Barnett, C., Vogt, K.N. et al. (2002). A meta-analysis of published literature on waist-to-hip ratio and risk of breast cancer. *Nutrition and Cancer* 44: 127–138. https://doi.org/10.1207/S15327914NC4402_02.

36 Lassek, W. and Gaulin, S. (2008). Waist-hip ratio and cognitive ability: is gluteofemoral fat a privileged store of neurodevelopmental resources? *Evolution and Human Behavior* 29: 26–34. https://doi.org/10.1016/j.evolhumbehav.2007.07.005.

37 Wang, G., Djafarian, K., Egedigwe, C.A. et al. (2015). The relationship of female physical attractiveness to body fatness. *PeerJ* 3: e1155. https://doi.org/10.7717/peerj.1155.

38 Tovée, M.J. and Cornelissen, P.L. (2001). Female and male perceptions of female physical attractiveness in front-view and profile. *British Journal of Psychology* 92: 391–402. https://doi.org/10.1348/000712601162257.

39 Thornhill, R. and Grammer, K. (1999). The body and face of woman. *Evolution and Human Behavior* 20: 105–120. https://doi.org/10.1016/S1090-5138(98)00044-0.

40 Weeden, J. and Sabini, J. (2005). Physical attractiveness and health in western societies: a review. *Psychological Bulletin* 131: 635–653. https://doi.org/10.1037/0033-2909.131.5.635.

41 Henss, R. (1995). Waist-to-hip ratio and attractiveness. replication and extension. *Personality and Individual Differences* 19: 479–488. https://doi.org/10.1016/0191-8869(95)00093-L.

42 Singh, D. (1995). Female judgment of male attractiveness and desirability for relationships: role of waist-to-hip ratio and financial status. *Journal of Personality and Social Psychology* 69: 1089–1101. https://doi.org/10.1037/0022-3514.69.6.1089.

43 Dixson, A.F., Halliwell, G., East, R. et al. (2003). Masculine somatotype and hirsuteness as determinants of sexual attractiveness to women. *Archives of Sexual Behavior* 32: 29–39. https://doi.org/10.1023/A:1021889228469.

44 Arnheim, R. (1955). A review of proportion. *Journal of Aesthetics and Art Criticism* 14: 44. https://doi.org/10.2307/426640.

45 Schmid, K., Marx, D., and Samal, A. (2008). Computation of a face attractiveness index based on neoclassical canons, symmetry, and golden ratios. *Pattern Recognition* 41: 2710–2717. https://doi.org/10.1016/j.patcog.2007.11.022.

46 Fan, J., Chau, K.P., Wan, X. et al. (2012). Prediction of facial attractiveness from facial proportions. *Pattern Recognition* 45: 2326–2334. https://doi.org/10.1016/j.patcog.2011.11.024.

47 Zacharopoulos, G.V., Manios, A., De Bree, E. et al. (2012). Neoclassical facial canons in young adults: journal of craniofacial. *Surgery* 23: 1693–1698. https://doi.org/10.1097/SCS.0b013e31826b816b.

48 Vegter, F. and Hage, J.J. (2000). Clinical anthropometry and canons of the face in historical perspective. *Plastic and Reconstructive Surgery* 106: 1090–1096. https://doi.org/10.1097/00006534-200010000-00021.

49 Farkas, L.G., Hreczko, T.A., Kolar, J.C., and Munro, I.R. (1985). Vertical and horizontal proportions of the face in young adult North American Caucasians: revision of neoclassical canons. *Plastic and Reconstructive Surgery* 75: 328–337. https://doi.org/10.1097/00006534-198503000-00005.

50 Le, T.T., Farkas, L.G., Ngim, R.C.K. et al. (2002). Proportionality in Asian and North American Caucasian faces using neoclassical facial canons as criteria. *Aesthetic Plastic Surgery* 26: 64–69. https://doi.org/10.1007/s00266-001-0033-7.

51 Gonzales, P.S., Machado, C.E.P., and Michel-Crosato, E. (2020). Analysis of neoclassical facial canons for Brazilian white young adults and comparison with North American Caucasian population. *Journal of Craniofacial Surgery* 31 (5): e432–e435. https://doi.org/10.1097/SCS.0000000000006339.

52 Ricketts, R.M. (1982). The biologic significance of the divine proportion and Fibonacci series. *American Journal of Orthodontics* 81: 351–370. https://doi.org/10.1016/0002-9416(82)90073-2.

53 Pancherz, H., Knapp, V., Erbe, C., and Heiss, A.M. (2010). Divine proportions in attractive and nonattractive faces. *World Journal of Orthodontics* 11: 27–36.

54 Holland, E. (2008). Marquardt's phi mask: pitfalls of relying on fashion models and the golden ratio to describe a beautiful face. *Aesthetic Plastic Surgery* 32: 200–208. https://doi.org/10.1007/s00266-007-9080-z.

55 Burusapat, C. and Lekdaeng, P. (2019). What is the most beautiful facial proportion in the 21st century? Comparative study among Miss Universe, Miss Universe Thailand, neoclassical canons, and facial golden ratios: plastic and reconstructive surgery. *Global Open* 7: e2044. https://doi.org/10.1097/GOX.0000000000002044.

56 Hong, Y.-J., Nam, G., Choi, H. et al. (2017). A novel framework for assessing facial attractiveness based on facial proportions. *Symmetry* 9: 294. https://doi.org/10.3390/sym9120294.

57 Prokopakis, E.P., Vlastos, I.M., and Picavet, V.A. (2013). The golden ratio in facial symmetry. *Rhinology* 51: 18–21. https://doi.org/10.4193/Rhin12.11.

58 Shen, H., Chau, D.K.P., Su, J. et al. (2016). Brain responses to facial attractiveness induced by facial proportions: evidence from an fMRI study. *Scientific Reports* 6: 35905. https://doi.org/10.1038/srep35905.

59 Bartels, A. and Zeki, S. (2000). The neural basis of romantic love. *NeuroReport* 11: 3829–3834. https://doi.org/10.1097/00001756-200011270-00046.

60 Baudouin, J.-Y. and Tiberghien, G. (2004). Symmetry, averageness, and feature size in the facial attractiveness of women. *Acta Psychologica* 117: 313–332. https://doi.org/10.1016/j.actpsy.2004.07.002.

61 Rhodes, G., Proffitt, F., Grady, J.M., and Sumich, A. (1998). Facial symmetry and the perception of beauty. *Psychonomic Bulletin & Review* 5: 659–669. https://doi.org/10.3758/BF03208842.

62 Kowner, R. (1996). Facial asymmetry and attractiveness judgement in developmental perspective. *Journal of Experimental Psychology: Human Perception and Performance* 22: 662–675. https://doi.org/10.1037/0096-1523.22.3.662.

63 Zaidel, D.W. and Deblieck, C. (2007). Attractiveness of natural faces compared to computer constructed perfectly symmetrical faces. *International Journal of Neuroscience* 117: 423–431. https://doi.org/10.1080/00207450600581928.

64 Zaidel, D.W. and Cohen, J.A. (2005). The face, beauty, and symmetry: perceiving asymmetry in beautiful faces. *International Journal of Neuroscience* 115: 1165–1173. https://doi.org/10.1080/00207450590914464.

65 Alley, T.R. and Cunningham, M.R. (1991). Article commentary: averaged faces are attractive, but very attractive faces are not average. *Psychological Science* 2: 123–125. https://doi.org/10.1111/j.1467-9280.1991. tb00113.x.

66 Galton, F. (1879). Composite portraits, made by combining those of many different persons into a single resultant figure. *Journal of the Anthropological Institute of Great Britain and Ireland* 8: 132. https://doi. org/10.2307/2841021.

67 Langlois, J.H. and Roggman, L.A. (1990). Attractive faces are only average. *Psychological Science* 1: 115–121. https://doi. org/10.1111/j.1467-9280.1990.tb00079.x.

68 Valentine, T., Darling, S., and Donnelly, M. (2004). Why are average faces attractive? The effect of view and averageness on the attractiveness of female faces. *Psychonomic Bulletin & Review* 11: 482–487. https://doi. org/10.3758/BF03196599.

69 Webster, M.A., Kaping, D., Mizokami, Y., and Duhamel, P. (2004). Adaptation to natural facial categories. *Nature* 428: 557–561. https://doi.org/10.1038/ nature02420.

70 Perrett, D.I., May, K.A., and Yoshikawa, S. (1994). Facial shape and judgements of female attractiveness. *Nature* 368: 239–242. https://doi.org/10.1038/368239a0.

71 DeBruine, L.M., Jones, B.C., Unger, L. et al. (2007). Dissociating averageness and attractiveness: attractive faces are not always average. *Journal of Experimental Psychology: Human Perception and Performance* 33: 1420–1430. https://doi. org/10.1037/0096-1523.33.6.1420.

72 Bulygina, E., Mitteroecker, P., and Aiello, L. (2006). Ontogeny of facial dimorphism and patterns of individual development within one human population. *American Journal of Physical Anthropology* 131: 432–443. https:// doi.org/10.1002/ajpa.20317.

73 Marečková, K., Weinbrand, Z., Chakravarty, M.M. et al. (2011). Testosterone-mediated sex differences in the face shape during adolescence: subjective impressions and objective features. *Hormones and Behavior* 60: 681–690. https://doi.org/10.1016/j. yhbeh.2011.09.004.

74 Valenzano, D.R., Mennucci, A., Tartarelli, G., and Cellerino, A. (2006). Shape analysis of female facial attractiveness. *Vision Research* 46: 1282–1291. https://doi.org/10.1016/j. visres.2005.10.024.

75 Glassenberg, A.N., Feinberg, D.R., Jones, B.C. et al. (2010). Sex-dimorphic face shape preference in heterosexual and homosexual men and women. *Archives of Sexual Behavior* 39: 1289–1296. https://doi.org/10.1007/ s10508-009-9559-6.

76 Grand View Research. Anti-Wrinkle Products Market Size, Share & Trends Analysis Report by Product (Oils, Serums, Lotions), by Distribution Channel (Hyper & Supermarkets, Online, Specialty Stores, Convenience Stores), and Segment Forecasts, 2019–2025. 2019. https://www. grandviewresearch.com/industry-analysis/ anti-wrinkle-products-market?utm_ source=prnewswire.com&utm_ medium=referral&utm_campaign=prn_ jun05_antiwrinkleproducts_rd2&utm_ content=content (accessed 16 August 2020).

77 Bashour, M. (2006). History and current concepts in the analysis of facial attractiveness. *Plastic and Reconstructive Surgery* 118: 741–756. https://doi. org/10.1097/01.prs.0000233051.61512.65.

78 Barner-Barry, C. (1990). Human ethology[1]. Irenaus Eibl-Eibesfeldt, New York: Aldine de Gruyter, 1989. *Politics and the Life Sciences* 8: 277. https://doi.org/10.1017/ S0730938400010017.

79 Cunningham, M.R., Barbee, A.P., and Philhower, C.L. (2002). Dimensions of Facial Physical Attractiveness: The Intersection of Biology and Culture. Facial Attractiveness: Evolutionary, Cognitive, and Social Perspectives, 193–238. Westport, CT: Ablex Publishing.

80 McCabe, V. (1984). Abstract perceptual information for age level: a risk factor for maltreatment? *Child Development* 55: 267–276. https://doi.org/10.2307/1129851.

81 Maestripieri, D., Klimczuk, A.C.E., Traficonte, D.M., and Wilson, M.C. (2014). A greater decline in female facial attractiveness during middle age reflects women's loss of reproductive value. *Frontiers in Psychology* 5 https://doi.org/10.3389/fpsyg.2014.00179.

82 Tatarunaite, E., Playle, R., Hood, K. et al. (2005). Facial attractiveness: a longitudinal study. *American Journal of Orthodontics and Dentofacial Orthopedics* 127: 676–682. https://doi.org/10.1016/j.ajodo.2004.01.029.

83 Bennett, J. (2020).Cosmetics and skin: Pan-Cake make-up. https://cosmeticsandskin.com/bcb/cake.php (accessed 14 July 2020).

84 ClinCalc DrugStats Database (2020). Tretinoin – Drug Usage Statistics, United States, 2007–2017. https://clincalc.com/drugstats/drugs/tretinoin (accessed 31 May 2020).

85 Landau, M. (2008). Chemical peels. *Clinics in Dermatology* 26: 200–208. https://doi.org/10.1016/j.clindermatol.2007.09.012.

86 Houreld, N.N. (2019). The use of lasers and light sources in skin rejuvenation. *Clinics in Dermatology* 37: 358–364. https://doi.org/10.1016/j.clindermatol.2019.04.008.

87 Jones, B.C., Little, A.C., Burt, D.M., and Perrett, D.I. (2004). When facial attractiveness is only skin deep. *Perception* 33: 569–576. https://doi.org/10.1068/p3463.

88 Watts, I. (2010). The pigments from Pinnacle Point Cave 13B, Western Cape, South Africa. *Journal of Human Evolution* 59: 392–411. https://doi.org/10.1016/j.jhevol.2010.07.006.

89 Etcoff, N.L., Stock, S., Haley, L.E. et al. (2011). Cosmetics as a feature of the extended human phenotype: modulation of the perception of biologically important facial signals. *PLoS One* 6: e25656. https://doi.org/10.1371/journal.pone.0025656.

90 Mulhern, R., Fieldman, G., Hussey, T. et al. (2003). Do cosmetics enhance female Caucasian facial attractiveness? *International Journal of Cosmetic Science* 25: 199–205. https://doi.org/10.1046/j.1467-2494.2003.00188.x.

91 Cash, T.F. and Cash, D.W. (1982). Women's use of cosmetics: psychosocial correlates and consequences. *International Journal of Cosmetic Science* 4: 1–14. https://doi.org/10.1111/j.1467-2494.1982.tb00295.x.

92 Nash, R., Fieldman, G., Hussey, T. et al. (2006). Cosmetics: they influence more than Caucasian female facial attractiveness. *Journal of Applied Social Psychology* 36: 493–504. https://doi.org/10.1111/j.0021-9029.2006.00016.x.

93 Koriche, R., Pelle-de-Queral, D., Gazano, G., and Aubert, A. (2008). Why women use makeup: implication of psychological traits in makeup functions. *International Journal of Cosmetic Science* 59 (2): 127–137.

94 Guéguen, N. (2012). Makeup and menstrual cycle: near ovulation, women use more cosmetics. *Psychological Record* 62: 541–548. https://doi.org/10.1007/BF03395819.

95 Jung, J. (2011). Advertising images of men: body size and muscularity of men depicted in *Men's Health* magazine. *Journal of Global Fashion Marketing* 2: 181–187. https://doi.org/10.1080/20932685.2011.10593096.

96 Brown, A. and Knight, T. (2015). Shifts in media images of women appearance and social status from 1960 to 2010: a content analysis of beauty advertisements in two Australian magazines. *Journal of Aging Studies* 35: 74–83. https://doi.org/10.1016/j.jaging.2015.08.003.

97 Xie, Q. and Zhang, M. (2013). White or tan? A cross-cultural analysis of skin beauty advertisements between China and the United States. *Asian Journal of Communication* 23: 538–554. https://doi.org/10.1080/01292986.2012.756046.

98 Martin, M.C. and Kennedy, P.F. (1994). Social comparison and the beauty of advertising models: the role of motives for comparison. *ACR North American Advances* NA-21: 365–371.

99 Maymone, M.B.C., Laughter, M., Dover, J., and Vashi, N.A. (2019). The malleability of beauty: perceptual adaptation. *Clinics in Dermatology* 37: 592–596. https://doi.org/10.1016/j.clindermatol.2019.05.002.

3

The Use of Cosmetic Products to Improve Self Esteem & Quality of Life

Zoe Diana Draelos

Dermatology Consulting Services, PLLC, High Point, NC, USA

Introduction

The desire to be beautiful in the eyes of peers is a common emotional need that has been consistent throughout history. Both men and women engage in appearance-enhancing activities that are both gender and culture specific. While the concept of outward beauty may change over time, there are four basic genderless concepts that remain consistent: evenly pigmented unblemished skin, large eyes, full lips, and long fingernails. All of these characteristics are consistent with general overall good health and a life of luxury, a surrogate for success.

As importantly, multiple dermatologic conditions can affect the skin in ways that cause pigmentary and contour alterations. In more severe cases, such conditions can result in scars that are both aesthetic and psychological. When in-office treatments and prescriptions are insufficient, it is incumbent upon us to provide our patients with the tools to best normalize and beautify their appearances. The best place to begin our discussion of how cosmetic products can be used to improve our patients' quality of life and self-confidence is to examine historic trends that highlight human appearance-related behavior. We will then discuss cosmetic camouflaging to restore beauty in patients with facial scarring and examine corrective cosmetics and their successful application. Finally, we will close the

chapter with recommendations on how to conduct a cosmetic product consultation.

Human Perceptions of Physical Beauty

Evenly Pigmented Unblemished Skin

The first assessment any human being makes of another is skin health. An interesting study found that the presence of brown spots on the female face increases the perceived apparent age by 10 years. Thus evenly pigmented unblemished skin is a sign of not only health but also youth.

The earliest cosmetic designed to cover facial blemishes and scarring was the beauty patch, which gave way to the current wide range of pigmented facial foundations. The beauty patch was used in the 1600s to cover permanent facial scars from prior smallpox epidemics. The patches were constructed of black silk or velvet shaped like stars, moons, and hearts that were kept in patch boxes. The metal patch box was the forerunner of the facial powder compact with a mirror in the cover. The box was carried everywhere to replace lost patches [1].

The modern concept of a product to create the image of evenly pigmented unblemished skin originated in the theater. The first product was intended to whiten skin, since white skin was considered desirable. Face powder was put

Essential Psychiatry for the Aesthetic Practitioner, First Edition. Edited by Evan A. Rieder and Richard G. Fried.
© 2021 John Wiley & Sons Ltd. Published 2021 by John Wiley & Sons Ltd.

into a liquid and called "wet white" or "French White" [2]. This was considered to be an improvement over simply powdering the skin due to superior adherence. The first major breakthrough in facial foundations for the average woman came when Max Factor developed cake make-up, which he patented in 1936 [3]. This product provided excellent cover for facial blemishes and dyspigmentation while providing velvety skin. Thus it was possible for women to enhance their beauty by creating the illusion of evenly pigmented unblemished skin.

Large Eyes

Another female desire is to capture attention through creating the illusion of large eyes. Since eyes are said to be the mirror to the soul, larger eyes are thought to be more captivating and interesting to the observer. One of the oldest products used to achieve human beauty is mascara: a cosmetic applied to the eyelashes to better frame the eyes. Mascara dates to Biblical times and remains one of the most commonly used methods of adornment today. Its purpose is to darken, thicken, and lengthen the eyelashes, since long eyelashes are considered a prerequisite to female attractiveness.

The original mascara worn by women of many ancient civilizations was kohl, based on antimony trisulfide, which also contained antibacterial qualities and prevented eye infections. The first modern mascara was composed of sodium stearate soaps and lampblack compressed into a cake. The solid was stroked with a wet brushed and applied to the eyelashes. This formulation produced eye irritation, due to the sodium stearate, which resulted in reformulation with triethanolamine stearate and beeswax to make water-resistant mascara [4].

The application of mascara to the eyelashes is said to enlarge and open the eyes by as much as 0.25 inches. The size of the eye can also be enhanced by elongating the eyelashes. Many mascaras contain nylon and rayon fibers that adhere to the eyelashes, making them appear thicker and longer. The wearing of false eyelashes also attests to this need to enlarge the eyes. Thus eye adornment is an activity that is well rooted in history, with a continuing need to exhibit this female behavior in modern times.

Full Lips

After large eyes, full lips are a female facial feature of psychological importance. Full lips are due to the presence of abundant subcutaneous fat in the lip, with larger fat depositions in younger females. To enhance the size and color of the lips, lip adornment has been used since the time of the Sumerians dating to 7000 BCE. This population practice of lip adornment has been seen through many generations from the Egyptians to the Syrians to the Babylonians to the Persians to the Greeks to the Romans to present-day civilizations. A vivid red lip color is a sign of an adequate hematocrit, a sign of physical health, and important when choosing a mate for procreation.

Lip adornment usually comprises red lip color enhancement. In antiquity, plant materials such as hybrid saffron or brazilwood were used to obtain a red stain. The earliest true lipsticks consisted of beeswax, tallow, and pigment [5]. This behavior has persisted into contemporary times. In 1920, an important evolution in the field of lip adornment, the "push-up" lipstick holder, still used today, was invented [6].

Nail Adornment

Long nails are a sign of health and wealth. In order to grow long nails, an adequate supply of protein is necessary, since proteins provide the building blocks for nail keratin. Further, long nails signify someone who does not work in the fields or with their hands doing manual labor, as the nails would be worn away with activity. Nails are a way that humans nonverbally communicate success. This too has led to a cosmetic industry focused on nail adornment, including nail polish.

Nail polish was introduced in the 1920s with the invention of lacquer technology. Nail polish is based on nitrocellulose, created by reacting cellulose fiber, from cotton linters or wood pulp, with nitric acid. When nitrocellulose is boiled, it can be dissolved in organic solvents, forming a hard, glossy film known as a lacquer. Nitrocellulose lacquer was used by the automobile industry as car paint, from which it was adapted to the nail adornment industry [7].

Nails have been adorned through history with stains, many derived from henna, but none possessed the shine and color variety of nail lacquer. Prior to 1920, nails were manicured and then "polished" with abrasive powder to achieve a shine. Color was then added through the use of stains. Modern nail polish was introduced in 1930 by Charles Revson, who later formed Revlon in 1932. These products are still marketed and very popular, judging by the number of females who frequent the nail salons located in almost every strip shopping center. Nail adornment remains a common female behavioral need.

Topical Cosmetic Products for the Patient with Facial Scarring

Introduction and Counseling

The focus of our prior discussion has been on enhancement of important female structures, such as eyes, lips, and nails; however, there is also a need for individuals who do not conform to traditional beauty standards to create the illusion of beauty to present an attractive appearance and to preserve self-esteem. Earlier we discussed the use of facial foundations to create the appearance of unblemished skin; here we will examine the use of a special subset of facial foundations, known as camouflage cosmetics, to create the illusion of skin perfection for patients who need cosmetic counseling. Camouflage cosmetics are designed to minimize facial defects while accentuating attractive features of the face [8]. When applied correctly, such products can make a meaningful impact on patient satisfaction and self-esteem.

Types of Defects

There are two types of facial defects that can be camouflaged: defects of contour/texture and defects of pigmentation. Each of these defects requires a different technique for correction. It is best not to assume the area that the patient is concerned about correcting. It is always best to ask. You may be surprised that the area you think is most obvious is not the problematic area for the patient. Once the area for camouflaging has been identified, it is then necessary to determine the nature of the defect before proceeding to recommend camouflaging techniques.

Contour/Texture Defects

Defects of contour are usually due to facial scarring and are defined as areas where the scar tissue is hypertrophied or atrophied. In addition, the scar tissue may demonstrate a texture difference due to absence of follicular ostia and hair.

Facial scar recontouring is predicated on the fact that dark colors make protuberant surfaces appear to recede, while light colors make atrophic surfaces appear to project [9]. Thus lighter colors will minimize depressed areas of scarring, while darker colors will minimize protuberant areas of the scar. By using a variety of lighter and darker facial foundations, the scar can be painted to minimize the contour abnormalities.

Pigmentation Defects

Pigmentation defects are abnormalities solely in the color of the skin with no accompanying texture abnormalities; however, the color disparity between the defect and the surrounding skin is greater than can be covered by traditional facial foundations. Some pigmentation abnormalities arise from scarring post-cancer treatment, while others are due to systemic abnormalities or extrinsic effects, such as sun exposure [10, 11].

Pigmentation defects can be camouflaged by either applying an opaque cosmetic that allows none of the abnormal underlying skin tones to be appreciated or applying foundations of complementary colors. Using complementary colors allows the patient to wear a less-occlusive thinner facial foundation, since pigment blending is used to camouflage the color abnormality as opposed to a complete skin cover. For example, red pigmentation defects can be camouflaged by applying a green foundation, since green is the complementary color to red. The blending of the red skin with the green camouflage cream yields a brown tone, which can be more easily covered by a conventional nonsurgical facial foundation. Furthermore, yellow skin tones can be blended with a complementary colored purple foundation to also yield brown tones that can be covered with a nonsurgical facial foundation. If the pigmentation defect is simply lighter or darker than the surrounding skin, different shades of traditional facial foundations can be artistically applied to blend the colors and hide the pigmentation defect [12].

Camouflage Cosmetics

If the defect is too severe to cover with traditional facial foundations and cosmetics, it may be necessary to purchase cosmetic specifically designed to totally obscure the underlying skin. These corrective cosmetics are more difficult to apply and remove, but mastery will allow the patient with scarring to achieve a more normal and acceptable appearance [13].

Corrective cosmetic bases designed to achieve the desired skin color are available as hard grease paints, soft grease paints, pancakes, and liquids. The various products are discussed below:

- *Hard grease paints* come in stick form and consist of pigments in an anhydrous, waxy base. Application requires great skill and is more time consuming than other makeup bases. This product is extremely long-wearing, but mainly reserved for theatrical uses.
- *Soft grease paints* come in a jar or are squeezed from a tube and have a creamy texture due to the incorporation of low-viscosity oils in addition to waxes in the anhydrous preparation. They usually contain a high

proportion of titanium dioxide to provide superior coverage [14]. These products tend to have a high shine and do not survive body heat; thus some type of setting preparation is required to prolong wear.
- *Pancake products* are packaged in a flat, round container. The product is removed from the compact by stroking with a wet sponge. It is composed of talc, kaolin, zinc oxide, precipitated chalk, titanium dioxide, and iron oxide [15]. This product dries quickly and possesses a matte, or dull, finish. Unfortunately, it is easily removed with body warmth and perspiration, but is easy to retouch, if necessary.
- *Liquids* are the most popular camouflage facial foundations. They are creamy products, which are scooped from a jar or tin with a spatula and applied to the hand for warming. These products are the easiest to use since they exhibit a long playtime, good blending characteristics, minimal application skill, excellent coverage, and adequate wearability for most individuals [16].

Cosmetic Camouflage Application

Cosmetic camouflage application is an art, but any patient can master it. Mastery is essential to allow the patient to return to public life with confidence and dignity. All humans have the need to be accepted by their peers and perceived as beautiful in the eyes of those who matter to them. The basic steps for camouflaging are outlined below.

- *Corrective makeup color selection*: Selection of the makeup base is important. It is essential that the color selected be closest to the patient's natural skin color. It is possible that there will not be a color in the standard camouflaging facial foundation palette that is a perfect match. In this case, blending is necessary. However, no more than three colors should be combined. Combining more than three colors results in a muddy final color quality. If the patient has an underlying pigmentation problem, this abnormal skin color counts as one color, so only two colors of cosmetic can be mixed. For example, if the patient has a pink scar from wounding, the pink counts as one color. If there is a large congenital nevus on the face, the brown color of the lesion counts as one color.

- *Corrective color cosmetic blending*: Once the closest foundation color has been selected, it may be necessary to blend in colors that are dominant in the patient's complexion. For example, if the patient possesses solar elastosis and yellow skin undertones, yellow will need to be added to the corrective cosmetic. If the patient has rosacea with red skin undertones, red may be added. The blending of the corrective cosmetic to get exactly the right color can be done professionally by aestheticians that specialize in this type of work. In addition, there are some cosmetic lines (Dermablend, L'Oreal, New York) in department stores that will assist with this blending at the cosmetic counter.

  Blending is usually done by applying a small amount of the makeup to the back of the hand. This provides a good surface for blending which can be easily held up to the face to evaluate the color match and also warms the product which allows easier mixing and application.

- *Facial application*: The final blended corrective facial foundation can then be applied to the face. The foundation should be dabbed, not rubbed, and pressed into the skin over the scarred area or the area to be camouflaged initially. Rubbing will remove the cosmetic as it is applied. Since there are no appendageal structures in a scar, there is little to keep the facial foundation in place. Then, the makeup should be dabbed from the central face outward into the hairline for approximately 0.25 inches and blended over the ears and beneath the chin. The cosmetic should be feathered at the edges along the jawline to achieve a more natural appearance. The cosmetic should dry untouched for five minutes.

Following the drying period, the cosmetic must be set with an unpigmented finely ground talc-based powder to prevent smudging, improve wearability, provide waterproof characteristics, and impart a matte finish. The corrective facial foundation will not perform properly without this layer of powder. The powder should be dusted over the face with a large brush, followed by pressing the powder into the foundation with the fingers. Since the powder is not pigmented, pressing is important or the face will look like it was covered with flour.

At this point, the face will be one even color because the opaque product completely obscures the underlying skin. Normally, the central face (central forehead, nose, and chin) and upper cheeks are redder than the rest of the face due to increase blood flow in these areas. It is necessary to mimic natural color variations of the face to achieve a natural appearance with three-dimensionality as opposed to a flat uniformly colored face. Using a powdered or liquid blush can restore these red tones. Some of the newer blushes are liquids that contact light-reflective particles. These products are very effective when rubbed over the cheeks to reflect light and restore the high cheekbones characteristic of feminine beauty.

Finally, other colored facial cosmetics (eye shadow, eyeliner, mascara, eyebrow pencil, etc.) are usually necessary to give an attractive final appearance [17]. Without the use of other colored cosmetics the face will not appear natural. It is important for the patient to know that camouflage cosmetics will not mimic a clean washed face. The patient will need to redefine their look to a made-up face, which can take some adjustment in those who are not accustomed to wearing cosmetics. It is best for the patient to look at their face as a blank canvas to color and highlight, while camouflaging undesirable characteristics.

The camouflage cosmetics must be removed from the face at bedtime. This is very important. Camouflage cosmetics cannot be removed with traditional soap and water because they are waterproof, which is essential to their longwearing characteristics. The patient must purchase a special cleanser at the same location where the camouflage cosmetics was purchased. These cleansers are rubbed over the face to dissolve the cosmetic film. They are oil-based to solubilize the oil-based cosmetic film. Once the film has been loosened, the face must then be cleaned with soap and water rinsing. It is important to remove all cosmetics from the face and eyes [18].

There is a learning curve required to master corrective cosmetics. Fortunately, if a mistake is made or the final result is suboptimal, the face can be washed and the cosmetic application begun again. This can be repeated until the final result is satisfactory. It may take some time for the patient to achieve the look they desire and to gain social comfort with their new look. This is to be expected. Practice makes perfect is an important concept to remember. In time, the patient will pick up application speed and the artistry necessary for the successful use of corrective cosmetics.

Conducting a Cosmetic Product Consultation

There will be patients without facial scarring who simply desire to know which facial products are best. They may want advice on which cosmeceutical moisturizer to use or how to cleanse their face or which sunscreen is best. These are challenging questions for most aesthetic professionals because the diversity of products for selection is huge. Where do you start with your recommendations? Following the five outlined steps presented below may help in developing your own unique approach to the cosmetic consultation and providing cosmetic recommendations.

1) Identify the question.

The patient will need to frame their question before you can provide an answer. Ensure that the question is not vague, overly broad, or unrealistic. Patients who simply state their face looks awful and they need your help are not going to leave your office satisfied. Anyone seeking magical skin care products that offer surgical results has expectations that are unrealistic. It is critical that you tease this information out before recommending and/or selling consumer products that will not be able to achieve their desired outcomes. These patients may need help beyond product recommendations and might seek the help of a skin emotion specialist or a therapist with an interest in skin wellness. More concretely, you need to help the patient identify the area where they are seeking help. Do they want a sunscreen recommendation? Do they need a moisturizer recommendation? Are they having trouble with dry itchy skin and need a cleanser recommendation? The question needs to be directed to a single answer. There is not time in a traditional office visit to address more than one question. If your schedule permits, extended cosmetic product consultations can be useful to schedule for patients who wish to discuss product regimens in depth.

2) Determine where the patient purchases products.

There are many places where skin care products can be purchased, each with a different price point. There is no sense recommending a high-end moisturizer costing US$300 per bottle if the patient traditionally makes moisturizer purchases at the local chain drug store. Simply ask the patient where they like to shop for their skin care. This will help you to immediately hone in on what recommendations to make.

3) Have a sheet prepared of your favorite five to ten products in each category.

Any recommendations you make should be done in writing; otherwise the patient will not remember and will be calling your staff to reiterate the instructions. Prepare a list of recommendations in each category: facial moisturizer, body moisturizer, hand/foot moisturizer, sunscreen, cosmeceutical moisturizer for anti-aging, facial cleanser, body cleanser, etc. There should be five to ten product recommendations in each category, ranging from products you can purchase at the local chain drug store to cosmetic counter brands to boutique brands, some of which you may dispense in your office. You can then circle the products you think are most appropriate for the given patient based on their age and skin type. Be sure to include products for normal, oily, and dry skin. For this reason, a sheet with ten recommendations is better than five as it allows you to customize your suggestions better for each patient.

4) Discuss your product recommendations with the patient.

Once you have made your selections for the patient by circling your product recommendations, discuss with the patient why you have selected the product. You will need to familiarize yourself with the products and should know the basic important ingredients in each product recommended. For example, you may wish to recommend a certain sunscreen because it is water resistant, not greasy, and contains titanium dioxide, which is allergy free. You may wish to recommend a retinol-based cosmeceutical moisturizer because retinoids are the most widely studied cosmetic ingredient and can interact with retinoid receptors in the skin. It would be best if you developed a succinct rationale for each recommendation that you can rapidly share with the patient.

5) Advise the patient to try the products and if they are dissatisfied to return for another cosmetic consultation.

The patient may not like all of your recommendations. This is fine. No single skin care product fits all tastes. That is why there are so many to choose from, making the selection process challenging. Tell the patient that you are providing recommendations; they will need to try the products and make their final assessment. If they are not satisfied with your initial recommendations, they should return to the clinic for further discussion. They should return with their reasons as to why the product was suboptimal and you will then have a starting place for their next cosmetic consultation.

Conclusions

This chapter has examined topical, non-prescription cosmetic medicine – from basic human needs to the evolution of adornment procedures and skin products used today. The need to feel and be perceived as beautiful is psychologically important to humans; thus an understanding of corrective cosmetics and their use is necessary to help our patients improve their self-confidence and quality of life. Finally, the ability to efficiently conduct a cosmetic product consultation will enhance your practice and your patient's satisfaction with your aesthetic care.

References

1 Panati, C. (1987). Extraordinary Origins of Everyday Things, 225–226. Harper & Row, New York: Perennial Library.

2 Schlossman, M.L. and Feldman, A.J. (1988). Fluid foundations and blush make-up. In: The Chemistry and Manufacture of Cosmetics, 2e (ed. M.G. de Navarre), 741–765. Wheaton, IL: Allured Publishing Corporation.

3 Wells, F.V. and Lubowe, I.I. (1964). Cosmetics and the Skin, 141–149. New York: Reinhold Publishing Corporation.

4 Rutkin, P. (1988). Eye make-up. In: The Chemistry and Manufacture of Cosmetics, 2e (ed. M.G. de Navarre), 712–717. Wheaton, IL: Allured Publishing Corporation.

5 de Navarre, M.G. (1975). Lipstick. In: The Chemistry and Manufacture of Cosmetics, 2e, vol. IV, 767–769. Wheaton, IL: Allured Publishing Corporation.

6 Cunningham, J. (1992). Color cosmetics. In: Chemistry and Technology of the Cosmetics and Toiletries Industry (eds. D.F. Williams and

W.H. Schmitt), 143–149. London: Blackie Academic & Professional.

7 Wimmer, E.P. and Scholssman, M.L. (1992). The history of nail polish. Cosmet. Toilet. 107: 115–120.

8 Stewart, T.W. and Savage, D. (1972). Cosmetic camouflage in dermatology. Br. J. Dermatol. 86: 530–532.

9 Helland, J.R. and Schneider, M.F. (1985). Special Features, 41–46. New York: M Evans and Company.

10 Draelos, Z.K. (1993). Cosmetic camouflaging techniques. *Cutis* 52: 362–364.

11 Benmaman, O. and Sanchez, J.L. (1988). Treatment and camouflaging of pigmentary disorders. Clin. *Dermatol.* 6: 50–61.

12 Draelos, Z.D. (1989). Use of cover cosmetics for pigmentation abnormalities. Cosmet. *Dermatol.* 2: 14–16.

13 Rayner, V. (1993). Clinical Cosmetology: A Medical Approach to Esthetics Procedures, 116–122. Albany, New York: Milady Publishing Company.

14 Schlossman, M.L. and Feldman, A.J. (1988). Fluid foundation and blush makeup. In: The Chemistry and Manufacture of Cosmetics, vol. 2 (ed. M.G. de Navarre), 748–751. Wheaton, Illinois: Allured Publishing Corporation.

15 Wilkinson, J.B. and Moore, R.J. (1982). Harry's Cosmeticology, 7e, 304–307. New York: Chemical Publishing.

16 Reisch, M. (1961). Masking agents as adjunct therapy in cutaneous disorders. *Clin. Med.* 8 (5).

17 Draelos, Z.D. (1991). Cosmetics have a positive effect on the postsurgical patient. Cosmet. *Dermatol.* 4: 11–14.

18 Thomas, R.J. and Bluestein, J.L. (1989). Cosmetics and hairstyling as adjuvants to scar camouflage. In: Facial Scars (eds. R.J. Thomas and G. Richard), 349–351. St. Louis: CV Mosby.

4

An Approach to Cosmeceuticals

Emily C. Milam and Evan A. Rieder

The Ronald O. Perelman Department of Dermatology, New York University Grossman School of Medicine, New York, NY, USA

Introduction

The cosmeceutical industry is a vast, consumer-driven market with thriving sales since the early 2000s, reaching US$9.7 billion in 2011 and with projected sales of US$12.3 billion by 2025 [1, 2]. Demand for cosmeceuticals (dispensed by physicians, trichologists, and allied professionals) is driven by cultural and lifestyle factors, as well as societal salience placed on beauty and appearance. As importantly, with purchasing products from physicians and allied aesthetic practitioners comes the perception of safety and efficacy. Cosmeceuticals promise highly desirable skin improvements, including anti-aging, skin tightening, improved radiance, and more [3]. Such claims unsurprisingly invite both enthusiasm and suspicion.

The abundant cosmeceutical options and the validity of their assertions can be challenging to navigate for both consumers and physicians. Consumers place great value on products advertised as high performance and expect such products to fulfill their marketing claims. Moreover, patients expect aesthetic practitioners to have expert insight into which products are worth the cost and effort. As such, it is advisable that practitioners of all educational backgrounds, and particularly those who are dispensing products in their offices, be aware of the available clinical and basic science evidence describing cosmeceuticals' efficacy.

The quality of scientific evidence for cosmeceuticals and the active ingredients they contain varies widely, with some products demonstrating more substantial and convincing evidence than others [4]. This chapter will review the types of cosmeceuticals and provide insight into the available literature. For more detailed analysis of individual ingredients please see the References [3].

Case Study

Case 4.1   The Cosmeceutical Consultation
A 27-year-old woman presents to your aesthetic spa reporting that she is unhappy with the quality of her skin. She has tried many over-the-counter (OTC) topical creams and serums, ranging from products that are found in the drug store to luxury products that she purchased from medical spas and offices of plastic surgeons. While she initially did not want to spend much money on skin care, she decided that it was "worth it" after consulting with several aestheticians and physicians who explained to her the benefits of products being dispensed in their offices. How should you proceed?

Clinical Relevance and Implications

This is a particularly challenging case that raises questions concerning product definitions and product efficacy, as well as potential ethical issues regarding sales of products in aesthetic offices. While interesting to contemplate, the ethics of product sales are out of the scope of this chapter. The topics of product definitions and efficacy as well as an approach to the patient will be discussed below.

Definitions

"Cosmeceutical," uniting the words cosmetic and pharmaceutical, is a term that was originally popularized by Dr. Albert Kligman in the 1980s [5]. Cosmeceuticals are topical products that combine desirable features of cosmetics – which beautify or enhance appearance – with drugs – which therapeutically improve the skin's physiology and/or address a disease process. Cosmeceuticals typically contain at least one distinctive ingredient and promise beneficial effects beyond what a pure cosmetic product could offer. Claims include improved skin function, texture, tone, radiance, or firmness [3].

Cosmeceuticals are additionally appealing given their accessibility as OTC agents and widely held perception that natural or organic ingredients are healthy, holistic, restorative, and safe. "Natural" products are colloquially defined as having botanical, mineral, or animal origins. While cosmeceutical labels often describe products as "natural" or "organic," these terms are not recognized or regulated by the United States (US) Food and Drug Administration (FDA) [6]. In fact, the FDA does not recognize the cosmeceutical category, declaring that "a product can be a drug, a cosmetic, or a combination of both, but the term 'cosmeceutical' has no meaning under the law." [7] This is in contrast to products such as antidandruff shampoo, which is considered by the FDA to be both a cosmetic (a cleanser) and a drug verified to treat dandruff. Such products

must adhere to a drug monograph, or guidelines that stipulate the acceptable ingredients, formulations, doses, and labeling of an OTC product category, be it fluoride toothpastes or antiperspirants. The FDA permits the sale of these OTC products without formal drug applications because "they are generally recognized as safe and effective" (GRASE) and not mis-marketed.

In contrast, any cosmeceutical product that claims to significantly alter the skin's appearance or function but does not meet criteria for preexisting monographs would fall under the legislative purview of a pharmaceutical drug. Drugs must demonstrate premarket proof of efficacy and safety and must adhere to rigorous testing, marketing, and regulatory standards. This typically requires large, double-blind, and controlled clinical trials, which are costly and time intensive.

As such, it behooves cosmeceutical manufacturers to maintain some degree of ambiguity to health claims and marketing, straddling the imprecise line between cosmetic and drug. While an FDA-approved drug can claim to "decrease wrinkles," a cosmeceutical can only claim that it "decreases the appearance of wrinkles," [8] a looser assertion that sidesteps FDA regulation. As per Pandey et al. [9], another way to conceptualize cosmeceuticals is to confirm that the product has met three criteria:

1) Pharmaceutical activity and is usable on normal or near-normal skin
2) A defined benefit for minor cosmetic skin concerns
3) A very low risk profile

At present, the FDA does not have the resources or authority to conduct premarket approval of cosmeceutical product labeling. Instead, "it is the manufacturer's and/or distributor's responsibility to ensure that products are labeled properly." [10] Cosmeceuticals undergo investigation by regulatory bodies only in the event of safety issues – in effect a form of passive, postmarket surveillance. The Safe

Cosmetics and Personal Care Products Act of 2018 seeks to greatly expand FDA oversight of chemicals in cosmetic products. If passed, this legislation would require companies to disclose all toxic ingredients, report adverse events, and demonstrate that cosmetics meet safety standards prior to marketing [11].

While the majority of cosmeceutical products offer a benign safety profile, this category is not without potential adverse effects. Adverse skin reactions to cosmeceuticals may include irritant or allergic contact dermatitis, photosensitive reactions, unwanted pigmentary changes, comedogenicity, infections, hair and nail damage, and even systemic effects such as heavy metal toxicity [12].

Active Ingredients and Indications

Cosmeceuticals' therapeutic benefits are attributed to their active ingredients, which are often derived from botanicals (i.e. plant extracts), marine extracts, vitamins, or minerals [13]. Ingredients purportedly target a variety of skin conditions including acne vulgaris, rosacea, striae, cellulite, hair loss, aging skin and photodamage, xerosis, wrinkles, and dyspigmentation, typically via anti-inflammatory, antioxidant, and/or barrier-enhancing mechanisms [3].

Examples of active ingredients found in cosmeceuticals include hydroxy acids for superficial pigmentary and textural abnormalities and kojic acid for skin lightening [3].

Botanicals represent the largest category of cosmeceutical ingredients, and are overall regarded as safe by the FDA. They have numerous indications and include active ingredients such as chamomile, green tea, feverfew, witch hazel, soybean, milk thistle, tea tree oil, aloe vera, sandalwood, oatmeal, and licorice, among numerous others. Frequently used vitamins include vitamin A derivatives (retinoids), nicotinamide (vitamin B3), vitamin C, and vitamin E. Commonly advertised minerals include copper and selenium. Marine extracts include algae, seaweed, cyanobacteria, and coral and sponge-derived compounds. Most vitamins, minerals, and marine extracts are touted for their antioxidant and anti-aging properties [3].

Emerging categories such as peptides and stem cell extracts can help facilitate skin turnover and regeneration and may increase the production of collagen and elastin.

Of note, sunscreens – which either absorb, scatter, or reflect light to protect from ultraviolet A and/or B radiation – have historically been considered a cosmeceutical exempt from premarket FDA approval; however, recently proposed legislation may change this. In the proposed rule, chemical sunscreen ingredients such as oxybenzone and sunscreen vehicles such as towelettes will no longer be considered GRASE and may require additional testing in order to meet OTC monograph eligibility standards [14]. This could be a harbinger that other OTC products within the cosmeceutical category may increasingly become subject to renewed FDA scrutiny.

Approaching the Evidence

Despite their widespread use, most cosmeceuticals lack sufficient scientific evidence to support their therapeutic and safety claims. Rather, alleged efficacy and safety is often extrapolated from *in vitro* studies of active ingredients. An ingredient may demonstrate research success *in vitro* or in isolation, but lack efficacy in its marketed form due to an ineffective drug delivery vehicle, compound instability, poor penetration, or inadequate dosing, which are details examined in FDA-approved drug studies [3]. Therefore, the aesthetic practitioner and consumer must be wary of marketing claims that exaggerate the evidence, even if the hypothesized mechanism of action seems reasonable. Available data may hide behind the guise of "research," yet not adhere to the rigor or quality of standard drug data. Many cosmeceuticals are tested among a small cohort of participants and against inactive placebos. This is in contrast to the more robust trials required by the FDA, which include hundreds (or even thousands) of diverse study participants and head-to-head comparisons between a study drug and gold standard treatments [9]. As such, any available research should be assessed for its participant size, study methodologies, outcome data, and statistical tests. Kligman suggested asking three questions to assess the efficacy of a cosmeceutical product [15]:

1) Can the active ingredient penetrate the stratum corneum and be delivered in sufficient concentrations to its intended target over a time course consistent with its mechanism of action?
2) Is there a plausible mechanism of action in the target cell or tissue in human skin?
3) Are there published, double-blind, peer-reviewed, placebo-controlled, statistically significant clinical trials to substantiate the efficacy claims?

The Evidence Base is Limited

Few cosmeceuticals contain active ingredients with evidence-based proof of efficacy. Some ingredients, like vitamin A derivatives (retinoic acid precursors such as retinoids and retinol) for photodamage and wrinkle prevention, are accepted by both medical practitioners and the lay public [16]. Likewise, topical preparations of other select vitamins (e.g. vitamin C) can offer meaningful antioxidant and anti-aging properties [17]. Products such as cleansers and moisturizers form the backbone of all skin care and cosmeceuticals regimens [18]. Toners, scrubs, cloths, and mechanized devices all use a combination of surfactant-based cleansing with exfoliation to improve skin smoothness and increase light reflection. However, the majority of other products provide a greater challenge to assess. Even topical products with broad support from the lay public and many aesthetic practitioners, such as vitamin E and B3, may not contain a sufficient quantity of active ingredients to achieve or retain efficacy. Formulations of L-ascorbic acid (the active form of vitamin C), a notoriously light- and oxygen-sensitive molecule, may not be prepared in a way that retains stability and efficacy. Newer cosmeceuticals that utilize peptides, other topical vitamins, and stem cells to support their claims have a relatively poor evidence base with little data in human studies [13, 19]. Though working closely with aesthetic practitioners, the beauty and cosmeceutical industry innovates at a speed with which the scientific literature cannot keep pace.

Psychology, Skin Care, and Self-Care

The cosmeceutical industry employs extensive marketing and branding strategies to target the psychology of the average consumer. Advertisements often pathologize the aging process and highlight appearance-related vulnerabilities. This may be further exacerbated by the media's obsession with youth and beauty. Enchanting and emotive imagery – such as hour glasses connoting the passing of time or reflecting pools that conjure the fountain of youth – prey on the psyches of women, and increasingly men [20]. Catch-all phrases such as "clinically proven" or "dermatologist recommended" are emblazoned on marketing material, but often with limited to no supporting evidence. Celebrities or trusted experts such as dermatologists, plastic surgeons, aestheticians, and scientists are often hired to promote the cosmeceuticals and legitimize the claims of efficacy, or are offered free products in exchange for airtime on personal social media accounts.

For many, use of a cosmeceutical is a proactive step in the struggle against inevitable aging, garnering a sense of control. While more difficult to quantify, anecdotal evidence indicates that skin care through the use of cosmeceuticals and related skin care products is able to offer consumers a rewarding "self-care" experience. By allowing consumers to focus on precise, fine-motor movements used in the application of topical products, cosmeceuticals allow for the creation of a mindfulness experience. Mindfulness, a common psychological concept, is the experience of the moment. By freeing the mind of the average worries of the day, skin care and the use of cosmeceuticals can offer a respite from the stresses of daily life. While cosmeceuticals may provide patients with the comfort of using a product that they believe is safe and natural, in reality they may be expensive, largely untested, and often minimally effective.

Practical Solutions for Patient Consultation

Given the sheer number of products on the marketplace, it behooves the practitioner to approach the cosmeceutical consultation systematically. The following set of guidelines, modified from Pandey et al., may be useful and can be modified to suit your needs [9].

1) *Inform your patients that cosmeceuticals are not drugs.* Efficacy will be much slower and treatment is likely to be adjunctive, not monotherapy. Be realistic about expectations.
2) *Be a source of factual information.* In this era of social media influencers with minimal-to-no scientific training and the devaluation of truth, it is incumbent upon the aesthetic practitioner to be a source of reliable information for the consumer. Dispel myths and explain the evidence of products to your patients.
3) *Examine ingredients of products.* If the patient is already using cosmeceutical products, examine the ingredients to verify their contents and assess whether it is safe and/or recommended to continue using such products.

4) *Ensure patient adherence.* Be specific about the questions you ask to determine if the products are being used at the appropriate time of day and appropriate frequency. Likewise, ask about any other products being used. It is essential to know every topical that is being applied.
5) *Ensure that the patient is aware of the presence of fake and counterfeit products.* Buying from reputable sources can ensure product quality and minimize the potential for adverse events.
6) *Have a low threshold to refer patients to a board-certified dermatologist* if there is concern about topical side effects to a cosmeceutical.
7) *Consider the relative cost of products.* Some patients may desire or insist on using expensive cosmeceutical products. Others may be more cost conscious. Know and understand several products at different price points.

Conclusions

The idea that nature-derived ingredients can be therapeutic or even reverse disease processes is by no means a new or untrue concept. Many FDA-approved pharmaceutical medications, including antibiotics, opiates, and chemotherapy agents, were initially derived from nature, which we know offers great medicinal potential, much of which remains untapped. Though most cosmeceuticals have relied on empiric evidence, folk medicine, or word-of-mouth support, some have earned more scientific validation. Many others, however, lack credible supportive evidence.

Although most natural products are benign or offer acceptable safety profiles, this should not preclude them from scientific review. Presently, cosmeceuticals have minimal regulatory oversight and their quality assurance is nominal. Akin to the vitamin and mineral industry, the content and concentration of active ingredients can vary widely and claims often overstep available evidence. Cosmeceuticals can often propagate their claims unbridled by the authority or threat of supervising regulatory bodies

As consumers become more critical of product claims, astute and informed aesthetic practitioners are in a prime position to demystify the available evidence for cosmeceuticals.

By delineating between the products that seem too good to be true and those with more valid safety and efficacy data, we can effectively utilize our expertise in aesthetics, skin care, and the aging process to advocate for our patients.

References

1 GlobeNewswire. *Global physician dispensed cosmeceuticals industry*. Available from: https://www.globenewswire.com/news-release/2020/03/04/1994784/0/en/global-physician-dispensed-cosmeceuticals-industry.html (accessed 10 June 2020).

2 Packaged Facts. *Cosmeceuticals in the U.S., 6th Edition*. Available from: https://www.packagedfacts.com/cosmeceuticals-edition-6281775 (accessed 10 June 2020).

3 Milam, E.C. and Rieder, E.A. (2016). An approach to cosmeceuticals. *Journal of Drugs in Dermatology* 15 (4): 452–456.

4 Griffiths, T.W. and Griffiths, C.E. (2012). Cosmeceuticals. *Skinmed* 10 (5): 272–274.

5 Kligman, A. (2005). The future of cosmeceuticals: an interview with Albert Kligman, MD, PhD. Interview by Zoe Diana Draelos. *Dermatologic Surgery: Official Publication for American Society for Dermatologic Surgery [et al.]* 31 (7 Pt 2): 890–891.

6 Food and Drug Administration. *"Organic" cosmetics*. Available from: https://www.fda.gov/cosmetics/cosmetics-labeling-claims/organic-cosmetics (accessed 10 June 2020).

7 Food and Drug Administration. *Is it a cosmetic, a drug, or both? (Or is it soap?)*. Available from: https://www.fda.gov/cosmetics/cosmetics-laws-regulations/it-cosmetic-drug-or-both-or-it-soap (accessed 10 June 2020).

8 Draelos, Z.D. (2008). The cosmeceutical realm. *Clinics in Dermatology* 26 (6): 627–632.

9 Pandey, A., Jatana, G.K., and Sonthalia, S. (2020). Cosmeceuticals. StatPearls. Treasure Island, FL: StatPearls Publishing LLC.

10 Food and Drug Administration. *Does FDA pre-approve cosmetic product labeling?* Available from: https://www.fda.gov/industry/fda-basics-industry/does-fda-pre-approve-cosmetic-product-labeling (accessed 10 June 2020).

11 GovTrack.us. *H.R. 6903 – 115th Congress: Safe Cosmetics and Personal Care Products Act of 2018*. Available from: https://www.govtrack.us/congress/bills/115/hr6903 (accessed 10 June 2020).

12 Gao, X.H., Zhang, L., Wei, H., and Chen, H.D. (2008). Efficacy and safety of innovative cosmeceuticals. *Clinics in Dermatology* 26 (4): 367–374.

13 Draelos, Z.D. (2012). Cosmetics, categories, and the future. *Dermatologic Therapy* 25 (3): 223–228.

14 Food and Drug Administration. *FDA advances new proposed regulation to make sure that sunscreens are safe and effective*. Available from: https://www.fda.gov/news-events/press-announcements/fda-advances-new-proposed-regulation-make-sure-sunscreens-are-safe-and-effective (accessed 10 June 2020).

15 Kligman, D. (2000). Cosmeceuticals. *Dermatologic Clinics* 18 (4): 609–615.

16 Riahi, R.R., Bush, A.E., and Cohen, P.R. (2016). Topical retinoids: therapeutic mechanisms in the treatment of photodamaged skin. *American Journal of Clinical Dermatology* 17 (3): 265–276.

17 Draelos, Z.D. and Pachuk, C.J. (2020). Demonstration of the antioxidant capabilities of a product formulated with

antioxidants stabilized in their reduced form. *Journal of Drugs in Dermatology* 19 (1): 46–49.

18 Draelos, Z.D. (2018). The science behind skin care: moisturizers. *Journal of Cosmetic Dermatology* 17 (2): 138–144.

19 Draelos, Z.D. (2019). Cosmeceuticals: What's real, what's not. *Dermatologic Clinics* 37 (1): 107–115.

20 Smirnova, M.H. (2012). A will to youth: the woman's anti-aging elixir. *Social Science & Medicine* 75 (7): 1236–1243.

Part II

Assessment

5

Aesthetic Assessment and Theories of Beauty

Michael Abrouk[1], Leslie Harris[2], Evan A. Rieder[3], and Jill S. Waibel[4]

[1] *Dr. Phillip Frost Department of Dermatology & Cutaneous Surgery, University of Miami Miller School of Medicine, Miami, FL, USA*
[2] *Cosmetics and Fragrance Marketing and Management, Fashion Institute of Technology, New York, NY, USA*
[3] *The Ronald O. Perelman Department of Dermatology, New York University Grossman School of Medicine, New York, NY, USA*
[4] *Miami Dermatology & Laser Institute, Miami, FL, USA*

Introduction

Throughout history, civilizations have admired the beauty in the world. Beauty can be used to describe people, places, animals, objects, and even ideas. The focus of this chapter will be human beauty, starting with historical perspectives, then discussing mathematical and assessment beauty tools, and ending with case studies. Because the perception of beauty differs from person to person, different ideas of beauty have developed throughout history, which in turn have formed standards for human beauty. These standards have had a profound impact on today's society.

Beauty has long since been an important part of history. Beauty has been fought for, envied, and reshaped over the years. The Greeks found beauty fascinating; philosophers of the Classical Age dedicated their time attempting to define what made a person beautiful. Plato devised "golden proportions" which stated that in order for someone to be considered to have beauty, the width of an ideal face would be two-thirds its length and a nose should not be longer than the distance between the eyes [1]. The Greeks were very close to finding the answer that symmetry is inherently what attracts the human eye.

Though Plato attempted to use proportions, contemporary science proved that it is the symmetry between the left and right side of the face that shapes our perception of someone's appearance. If Cleopatra's nose had been half an inch longer, perhaps neither Caesar nor Mark Antony would have fallen in love with her. Throughout history, beauty has demonstrated that physical attractiveness is an important quality or possession, comparable to power, intelligence, strength, wealth, education, or family. Attractive physical features and their perception by the observer's brain inform the process of natural selection to optimize reproductive success. Throughout the world, attractive people show greater acquisition of resources. Both historically and in current times, beauty in men and women has opened opportunities to its possessors not available to the ordinary appearing [2].

In the late twentieth century, several groups, including Slater et al., reported that infants have the ability to recognize beauty [3]. Slater's work observed the preference of infants for attractive faces and found that newborns were able to process facial differences and tended to prefer attractive faces. When presented with two photographs, both similar in brightness and contrast, but portraying people measured differently on the attractiveness scale, babies fixated on the faces that were rated as more attractive. Beyond experientially gained knowledge, humans, even at an early age, have certain instinctual mechanisms to perceive their surroundings and understand facial differences.

Much time, currency, and emotional energy are spent in improving our appearance to reach the goal of beauty. Long coveted by women as a boost to self-confidence, psychological well-being, and attractiveness to potential mates, beauty is also important for men.

Although Plato could be considered the true originator of aesthetics, he also believed that beauty possessed a meaning deeper than skin and bone. Plato thought of beauty as an ideal beyond human perception, such as truth or goodness. For Plato, beauty was eternal and made manifest as even wonders of nature and fine art [4].

Beauty in our World

Beauty is one of the most enduring themes of western philosophy, dating back to Vitruvius's three laws of architecture: *firmitas*, *utilitas*, *venustas* (solidity, utility, beauty) [5]. In Plato's day, beauty was considered objective and there were rules and orders governing it. In the nineteenth century American philosopher Ralph Waldo Emerson posited that the beauty of nature can have a profound effect upon our senses: "those gateways from the outer world to the inner, and engender feelings such as awe, wonder, or amazement" [6]. When we think of beauty in nature, we might most immediately think of images that dazzle the senses – the prominence of a mountain, the expanse of the sea, or the blooming of a flower. Often it is merely the perception of these things itself which gives us pleasure, and this emotional or affective response on our part seems to be crucial to our experience of beauty. For Emerson, beauty in the natural world was not limited to certain parts of nature to the exclusion of others. He wrote that every landscape lies under "the necessity of being beautiful" and that "beauty breaks in everywhere" [6]. For Emerson, nature is beautiful because it is alive, moving, and reproductive. In nature we observe growth and development in living things, which can be contrasted with the static or deteriorating state of the vast majority of that which is man-made.

Our tastes and definitions of beauty change in response to other cultural influences, but they also change over time in response to shifts in our own society. These shifts in societal preferences in beauty can be seen in a variety of areas including architecture, fashion, and fine art, as well as body shape and facial features. German art historian Wilhelm Worringer suggested that over the span of human history, societies have oscillated between a preference for abstract and realistic art, and that those preferences have changed based on what the societies themselves were lacking [7]:

> Abstract art, infused as it was with harmony, stillness and rhythm, would appeal chiefly to societies yearning for calm – societies in which law and order were fraying, ideologies were shifting and a sense of physical danger was compounded by moral and spiritual confusion. Against such a turbulent background, humans would experience "an immense need for tranquility," and so would turn to the abstract, to patterned baskets or the minimalist art galleries [7].

Charles Darwin reviewed over one-hundred years of literature detailing facial expression in nonhuman primates. His work of 1872 is still the most encompassing work on this subject. Darwin's central hypotheses stated that facial expressions of nonhuman primates and man are similar and that the face is used to convey emotions and showcase beauty [8]. Darwin studied great masters in painting and sculpture and concluded that "in works of art, beauty is the chief object" (Figures 5.1 and 5.2).

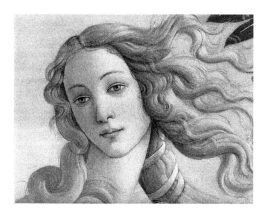

Figure 5.1 *The Birth of Venus* by Sandro Botticelli (1482–1485). Analysis of beauty of Venus: defined jawline, high cheekbones, angular nose, full lips, green eyes, gold thick, flowing hair. Symmetric and youthful. *Source*: Sandro Botticelli: The Birth of Venus (1445–1510).

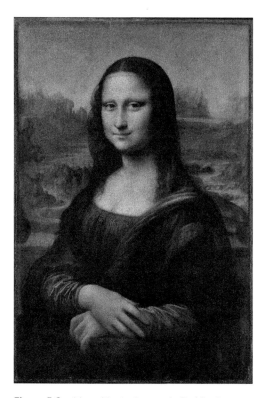

Figure 5.2 *Mona Lisa* by Leonardo Da Vinci (1503–1506). Analysis of beauty of Mona Lisa: elegantly dressed without jewelry. It is as if the artist wanted nothing to distract attention from her face, which is the epitome of Renaissance masterwork representing period female beauty. *Source*: Leonardo da Vinci.

Darwin also stated that "strongly contracted facial muscles destroy beauty." In a way, Darwin foreshadowed the much later development of neurotoxins by writing that if a drug could minimize an angry countenance, people would have more pleasant, beautiful expressions and hide their negative emotions [9].

The Link between Beauty and Mathematics: From Phi to the Golden Triangle

For many, beauty has a currency. While attractive features may arrive as a result of the luck of good genetics, psychological studies have also shown that beauty confers status. Beautiful people are perceived to be more intelligent, trustworthy, and altruistic. They are more likely to win arguments and avoid punishment for crimes [10]. Quite simply, society perceives the good-looking as morally and spiritually superior. These perceived attributes are then redirected onto the self in concepts of self-worth and self-esteem. As such, the desire to apply a scientific method to identify ideal beauty is no surprise, nor is the desire to seek out medical and professional providers to help achieve this defined beauty aesthetic.

Anthropological studies indicate that across cultures and geographies, people often agree on what constitutes a beautiful face [10]. A meta-analysis covering 919 studies and over 15 000 observers reported that people agree both within and across culture about who is attractive and who is not [11].

While this consensus has roots in biology, it has also been heavily influenced by the field of mathematics, most notably the theory of phi (also known as the "golden ratio," the "golden section," or the "divine ratio"). Phi is named for Phidias, a Greek architect and sculptor who famously applied the golden ratio to his design of the Parthenon [5]. The concept's credit, however, continues to be a source of debate. Though it is predominantly attributed to the Greek mathematician Pythagoras, other sources give credit to the Ancient Egyptians for first introducing the concept, or Euclid, who discussed phi in his mathematical treatise, *The Elements* [12].

In laypersons' terms, the golden ratio (or golden section) describes the most aesthetically pleasing point at which to segment a line: the point at which the longer segment, L, when divided by the shorter segment of the line, S, is equal to the ratio of the entire line, L+S, divided by L (L/S = (L+S)/L, where L+S = 1). This ratio is 1.618 [13] (Figure 5.3).

As a matter of geometry, the golden section of a line extends to the golden rectangle, triangle, and pentagon, and, as such, guided Classical Greek aesthetics at the time of its discovery [14]. It is important to note that the golden ratio was founded during a western philosophical period heavily influenced by rationalism, an approach that grounded knowledge in reasoning and logic. This philosophy naturally extended to concepts of aesthetics and beauty, and the notion of proportion, order, symmetry, and harmony.

Ever since its birth in Classical Greece, the golden ratio has persisted as an underlying benchmark for beauty, influencing a variety of aesthetic disciplines as well as deepening the understanding of beauty in the natural world. In art and architecture, famous examples of the golden ratio are found in works varying from Leonardi da Vinci's fifteenth-century masterpiece *The Last Supper* to the

design of the Taj Mahal and Notre Dame Cathedral, and even the United Nations building in New York [15]. In the world of music, Bach has been cited as a composer who incorporated the golden ratio in his Fugue in D minor [10]. In the natural sciences, the Fibonacci sequence, a thirteenth-century mathematical discovery of growth and arrangement, was found to have the golden ratio of phi. The Fibonacci sequence guides the aesthetic outcome of many natural forms, including helical and color patterns of flowers, the inherent harmony in the shape of nautical shells, and the structural organization of the astronomical galaxy. Even DNA's double helix structure contains the golden ratio [15]. The golden ratio also appears extensively throughout the human body and in the human face. No matter its application, the golden ratio remains significant for its mathematical connection to harmony and proportion, bestowing upon it an important role in dermatology and aesthetic medicine, given the associations between beauty and the currencies of status, self-worth, and psychological well-being.

Neoclassical Canons and Aesthetics

The aforementioned classical proportions have been applied throughout the development of aesthetic and procedural medicine and can play a guiding role in cosmetic practice. Facial proportions according to neoclassical canons and facial golden ratios are most often referenced. These certain fixed parameters exist within facial features; in a harmonious face, the ratio of 1:1.618 is often seen in measurements between fixed anatomic landmarks (Figures 5.4 and 5.5). Human sculptures made in Greece were derived from proportions that followed established rules or canons [16–18]. These rules were incorporated into the neoclassical canons for the human face by Renaissance artists such as Leonardo di Vinci, Bergmüller, and

The Golden Ratio

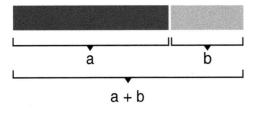

$$\frac{a}{b} = \frac{a+b}{a} = 1.618\ldots = \varphi$$

Figure 5.3 The golden ratio.

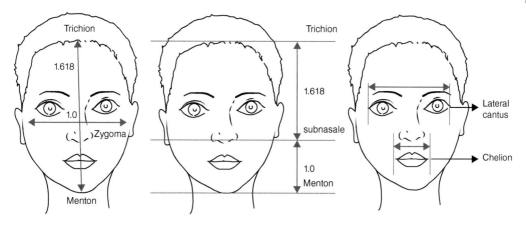

Figure 5.4 Phi (the golden ratio) in the human face.

Vitruvius [19, 20]. Subsequently these principles were adopted by aesthetic medical providers and are still in practice today.

The golden ratio has been used in the assessment of facial beauty and was popularized by American maxillofacial surgeon Dr. Steven Marquardt with the phi mask for the archetypical "ideal" facial ratios [16] (Figure 5.6). To generate this mask, Dr. Marquardt effectively overlayed a series of proportional ratios of 1 : 1.618 throughout the face.

While these ratios and neoclassical canons are theories guiding proportions and ratios of aesthetic assessment, they often do not adhere consistently to modern examples of beauty. Instead they can be useful in guiding aesthetic concepts; however, there are discrepancies between classical theories of beauty and contemporary aesthetic ideals. In comparing 16 Miss Universe modern facial proportions to neoclassical canons, several key divergences emerged. Most of the facial ratios of Miss Universe in the twenty-first century demonstrated a statistically significant difference from the facial golden ratios. Miss Universe winners showed a wider nasofacial angle and more nasal tip projection than neoclassical canons, among other facial differences. Thus a thorough understanding of both classical and contemporary beauty is critical in the aesthetic assessment and planning of cosmetic facial procedures [21].

Scales of Aesthetic Assessment

Since 1997 the number of cosmetic procedures performed in the United States has increased by more than several hundredfold. More specifically, nonsurgical cosmetic procedures have continued to increase, with a sustained increase of 17.8% from 2015 to 2019 [22]. The increased interest in nonsurgical cosmetic procedures has necessitated the development of scales to measure the degree of aging and the severity of facial wrinkles to objectively assess the degree of improvement from cosmetic procedures. The increase in treatment options and volume of patients pursuing these procedures parallels the efforts to measure the treatment effects using clinical means in the form of validated scales [23].

Multiple metrics have been developed for rhytides, including Likert five-point scales for brow positioning, static and dynamic forehead lines, marionette lines, and static and dynamic crow's feet [23]. There have even been efforts to develop validated composite assessment scales for the Global Face, as well as the upper face, mid face, lower face, and neck volume [23–27]. Many of these scales have been validated including the Glogau wrinkle scale which delineates facial rhytides into the following categories: type I, "no wrinkles;" type II, "wrinkles in motion;"

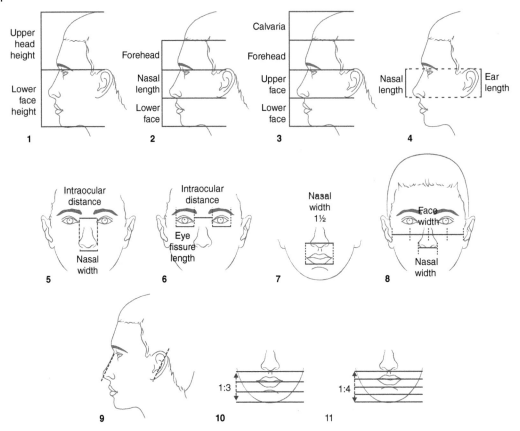

1. The head can be divided into equal halves at a horizontal line through the eyes. 2. The face can be divided into equal thirds, with the nose occupying the middle third. 3. The head can be divided into equal quarters, with the middle quarters being the forehead and nose. 4. The length of the ear is equal to the length of the nose. 5. The distance between the eyes is equal to the width of the nose. 6. The distance between the eyes is equal to the width of each eye (the face width can be divided into equal fifths). 7. The width of the mouth is 1½ times the width of the nose. 8. The width of the nose is one fourth the width of the face. 9. The nasal bridge inclination is the same as the ear inclination. 10. The lower face can be divided into equal thirds. 11. The lower face can be divided into equal quarters.

Figure 5.5 The neoclassical canons. *Source*: From ref. [3].

type III, "wrinkles at rest;" and type IV, "only wrinkles." The intent is to organize the discussion of therapies for photodamaged skin to permit rational comparisons of therapies and clinical results [26, 28].

Another often-used scale for cosmetic assessment is the Global Aesthetic Improvement Scale (GAIS). This metric is used to determine improvement after cosmetic procedures in comparison to baseline. The GAIS has a score of 1 (exceptional improvement), 2 (very improved patient), 3 (improved patient), 4 (unaltered patient), and 5 (worsened patient).

Aesthetic providers can also make use of validated scales for the assessment of scars.

These can be practically applied within an aesthetic practice taking into account surface changes such as pliability, firmness, color, thickness, perfusion, and three-dimensional topography [29]. Many scales have been validated for this assessment including the Vancouver Scar Scale (VSS), Manchester Scar Scale (MSS), Physician and Observer Scar Assessment Scale (POSAS), and Visual Analog Scale (VAS) [30]. One popular validated scale for rhytides often needed for FDA approval is the Lemperle Scale. This scale assesses wrinkles and was developed as a simple tool for use by plastic surgeons, dermatologists, and aesthetic surgeons who want to assess the changes

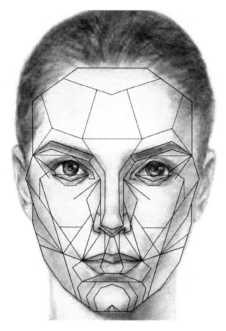

Figure 5.6 The phi mask of archetypical "ideal" facial ratios. Similar masks can be found at https://www.beautyanalysis.com/research/perfect-face/facial-masks/.

resulting from injecting filler materials in their patients. By correlating the grade of the wrinkle in the reference photographs with the wrinkle in a patient's face, a classification of 0–5 is assigned [31]. It has become widely used for clinical trials and FDA approvals.

How to Approach the Face

The goal of aesthetic treatments is comprehensive improvement, which, for most patients, will involve a combination of plastic surgery, lasers, and injectables. It is paramount as an aesthetic provider to understand the best treatment options for each anatomic region.

Facial aging is a multifactorial process that comes as a result of intrinsic and extrinsic factors. Signs of facial aging result from surface changes including solar elastosis and actinic damage as well as underlying structural change including fat atrophy, bone resorption, biometric volume loss, soft tissue loss, and skin laxity. These changes may result in various undesirable facial features, including thinning of the skin and increased skin laxity, rhytid formation, loss of facial volume, surface texture abnormalities, scarring, and pigmentary changes. Thus, during the consultation a provider must assess the patient's desire for treatment of an array of potential concerns. While it is paramount to carefully notice all changes resulting in facial aging, it is also important to assess the patient's willingness to accept your detailed findings. Sometimes patients present to the aesthetic practitioner with a simple cosmetic goal in mind and will be satisfied if that goal is achieved. Other patients may be willing to accept all findings and undergo any treatments that their provider recommends.

In an ideal situation, each patient should receive a customized treatment plan during the aesthetic consultation to return facial structures closer to the golden ratio. While the details remain outside the scope of this chapter, aesthetic practitioners should also be cognizant of variations in skin type by sex and race and how aesthetic approaches may change dramatically between patients of different sexes and skin types. Likewise, practitioners should know that beauty ideals and aesthetic goals may differ between patients of different age groups, genders, and cultures. Often different cultures have different norms and priorities of beauty. Asian patients tend to desire a light complexion that is devoid of brown spots and discoloration. Many Latina women like a fuller lip. Older white women tend to seek treatments to resurface wrinkles with laser and more invasive surgical approaches for lower facial laxity. Finally, the astute aesthetic practitioner must stay current with beauty trends and recognize that standards of beauty and the procedures that people are willing to undergo will vary over time.

Below are a few cases to illustrate the use of multiple modalities to yield pleasing aesthetic results for an aging face. For more on specific gender-based approaches to the aesthetic patient see Chapters 6–8.

Case Studies

Case 5.1   Sagging Skin and Surface Textural Abnormalities
A 75-year-old woman presents to your office reporting that "I look older than I feel." She has no history of cosmetic procedures but is open to your surgical and nonsurgical recommendations for treatment. You note substantial periocular aging as well as lower face laxity and sun damage (Table 5.1). 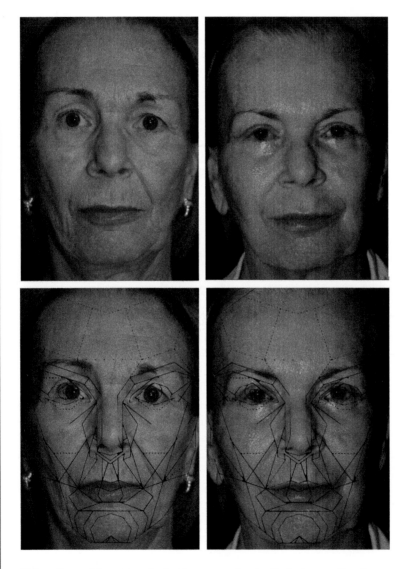   Using the golden triangle in the second set of photos, anti-aging procedures can take patients closer to the scientific angles of beauty

Case 5.1 (Continued)

Table 5.1 Sagging skin and surface textural abnormalities.

Aesthetic challenge	Aesthetic solution	Comments
Eyelid dermatochalasis Lower facial laxity and rhytides Lower eyelid redundancy	Upper brow blepharoplasty Perioral traditional Erbium resurfacingt	Photos are one week postoperative. Patient underwent upper lid blepharoplasty with oculoplastic surgeon and then same-day Erbium traditional laser resurfacing and CO_2 fractional resurfacing

Case 5.2 Dynamic and Static Rhytides with Volume Loss

A 55-year-old woman presents to your clinic for cosmetic consultation. She requests your expertise for rejuvenation but states that "I want to look like myself – but myself 10 years ago!" On examination, she has both static and dynamic rhytides, actinic damage, and evidence of temple, midface, and lower face volume loss (Table 5.2).

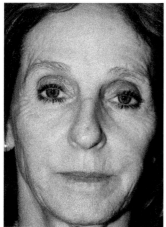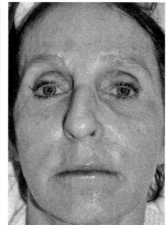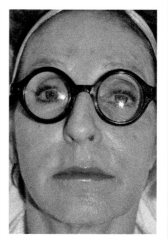

Table 5.2 Dynamic and static rhytides with volume loss.

Aesthetic challenge	Aesthetic solution
Fat atrophy, bone resorption, biometric volume loss, skin laxity, solar elastosis, and actinic damage	Laser resurfacing Neurotoxin to the glabella, forehead, and periorbital muscles Hyaluronic acid filler to lips and periorbital scaffolding Poly-L-lactic acid to lower face

Case 5.3 Lower Face Sun Damage, Fat Migration, and Skin Laxity

An 80-year-old woman presents for treatment of her mid and lower face. She has never had a cosmetic procedure before and would like to avoid plastic surgery. On examination she demonstrates evidence of substantial fat pad descent and atrophy, rhytides and laxity, and severe sun damage (Table 5.3).

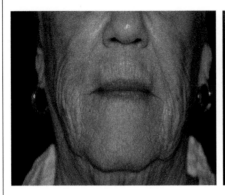 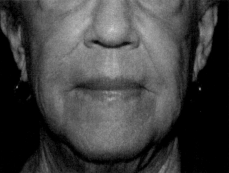

Table 5.3 Lower face sun damage, fat migration, and skin laxity.

Aesthetic challenge	Aesthetic solution
Fat atrophy, severe rhytides, skin laxity, solar elastosis, and actinic damage	Laser resurfacing Hyaluronic acid filler to lips and periorbital scaffolding

Case 5.4 Solar Damage on a Background of Inflammatory Skin Disease

A 43-year-old woman with chronic rosacea presents for evaluation of skin quality. Although her rosacea bumps have been controlled with prescription medications, she reports that her face is "constantly red" despite consistent use of broad-spectrum, high-SPF sunscreen. On examination she has diffuse sun damage on a background of erythema (Table 5.4).

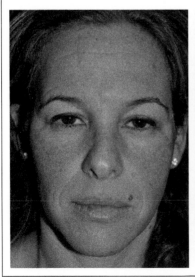 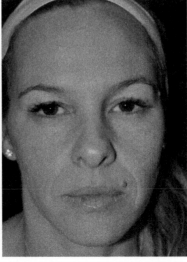

(Continued)

Case 5.4 (Continued)	

Table 5.4   Solar damage on a background of inflammatory skin disease.

Aesthetic challenge	Aesthetic solution
Dyschromia with solar lentigines	Alexandrite laser for larger brown lentigines
Diffuse sun damage	Pulsed dye laser for rosacea
Rosacea	Intense pulsed light with two passes for background sun damage
Moderate static forehead rhytides	Neurotoxin to upper face

Case 5.5 Overfiling	

A 39-year-old woman presents to your office after having seen a number of other aesthetic practitioners. She has had multiple fillers and neurotoxins but recently has begun to look at herself in the mirror and no longer recognizes who she sees. On examination her midface is overfilled, exaggerating the contours of her malar eminences, causing extensive medial cheek convexity, and obscuring the nasojugal and palpebomalar grooves (Table 5.5).

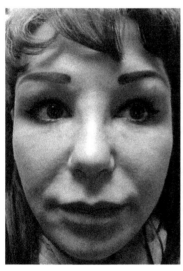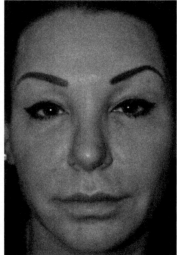

Table 5.5   Overfilling.

Aesthetic challenge	Aesthetic solution
Overfilled due to too much hyaluronic acid filler	Hyaluronidase

Conclusions

Beauty holds a special value in societies, both historical and contemporary. Much of the documented scientific history of beauty can be traced back to Classical Greece, where the standards of beauty were canonized throughout a scientific understanding of art, nature, architecture, and the human form. Twentieth- and twenty-first-century aesthetic practitioners have adopted and applied these concepts to today's world of minimally invasive and plastic surgical procedures. With this foundational knowledge, we will be able to adjust to a rapidly evolving global population as beauty preferences change and the concepts of race and gender gain more fluidity.

The authors of this chapter believe the pursuit of beauty should be an individual's decision. Discussing and modifying the beauty of another human comes with great responsibility. Our role as aesthetic providers is to help empower humans in their journeys to look and feel their best, so that their outward appearance reflects their inner state of being. Thanks to advances in aesthetic medicine, we are aging more gracefully than ever before. And with improved appearances come improved psychological well-being and quality of life. We finally may be uncovering the path to the elusive foundation of youth through mathematics and contemporary aesthetic procedures.

References

1 Griffin, G.R. and Kim, J.C. (2013). Ideal female brow aesthetics. *Clin. Plast. Surg* 40 (1): 147–155. https://doi.org/10.1016/j. cps.2012.07.003.

2 Marwick, A. (2004). It: A History of Human Beauty. London: Bloomsbury.

3 Slater, A., Bremner, G., Johnson, S.P. et al. (2000). Newborn infants' preference for attractive faces: the role of internal and external facial features. *Infancy* 1 (2): 265–274.

4 Hofstadter, A. and Kuhns, R. (1976). Philosophies of Art and Beauty: Selected Readings in Aesthetics from Plato to Heidegger. Chicago: University of Chicago Press.

5 Camerota, F.A. (2014). Scientific Concept of Beauty in Architecture: Vitruvius Meets Descartes, Galileo, and Newton, 215–241. Cham: Springer https://doi. org/10.1007/978-3-319-05998-3_10.

6 Emerson, R.W. (2009). Nature, Addresses and Lectures. Charleston: BiblioBazaar.

7 Worringer, W. (2014). Abstraction and Empathy: A Contribution to the Psychology of Style. Eastford, CT: Martino Fine Books.

8 Grammer, K., Fink, B., Møller, A.P., and Thornhill, R. (2003). Darwinian aesthetics: sexual selection and the biology of beauty. *Biol. Rev. Camb. Philos. Soc.* 78 (3): 385–407. https://doi.org/10.1017/S1464793102006085.

9 Chevalier-Skolnikoff, S. (2006). Facial expression of emotion in nonhuman primates. In: Darwin and Facial Expression: A Century of Research in Review, 273. Los Altos: Institute for the Study of Human Knowledge.

10 Etcoff, N.L. (2014). Survival of the Prettiest: The Science of Beauty. New York: Anchor Books.

11 Meisner, G. History of the Golden Ratio. https://www.goldennumber.net/golden-ratio/ (accessed 31 May 2020).

12 Naini, F.B., Moss, J.P., and Gill, D.S. (2006). The enigma of facial beauty: esthetics, proportions, deformity, and controversy. *Am. J. Orthod. Dentofac. Orthop.* 130 (3): 277–282. https://doi.org/10.1016/j. ajodo.2005.09.027.

13 Yalta, K., Ozturk, S., and Yetkin, E. (2016). Golden ratio and the heart: a review of divine aesthetics. *Int. J. Cardiol.* 214: 107–112. https://doi.org/10.1016/j. ijcard.2016.03.166.

14 Green, C.D. (1995). All that glitters: a review of psychological research on the aesthetics of the golden section. *Perception* 24 (8): 937–968. https://doi.org/10.1068/p240937.

15 Katyal, P., Gupta, P., Gulati, N., and Hemant, J. (2019). A compendium of Fibonacci ratio. *J. Clin. Diagn. Res.* 13 (11): AB03–AB10. https://doi.org/10.7860/ JCDR/2019/42772.13317.

16 Holland, E. (2008). Marquardt's phi mask: pitfalls of relying on fashion models and the golden ratio to describe a beautiful face. *Aesth. Plast. Surg.* 32: 200–208. https://doi. org/10.1007/s00266-007-9080-z.

17 Ricketts, R.M. (1982). Divine proportion in facial esthetics. *Clin. Plast. Surg.* 9 (4): 401–422.

18 Jayaratne, Y.S.N., Deutsch, C.K., McGrath, C.P.J., and Zwahlen, R.A. (2012). Are neoclassical canons valid for southern Chinese faces? *PLoS One* 7 https://doi.org/10.1371/journal.pone.0052593.

19 Edler, R.J. (2001). Background considerations to facial aesthetics. *J. Orthod.* 28 (2) https://doi.org/10.1093/ortho/28.2.159.

20 Le, T.T., Farkas, L.G., Ngim, R.C.K. et al. (2002). Proportionality in Asian and North American Caucasian faces using neoclassical facial canons as criteria. *Aesthet. Plast. Surg.* 26 https://doi.org/10.1007/s00266-001-0033-7.

21 Burusapat, C. and Lekdaeng, P. (2019). What is the most beautiful facial proportion in the 21st century? Comparative study among Miss Universe, Miss Universe Thailand, neoclassical canons, and facial golden ratios. *Plast. Reconstr. Surg. – Glob. Open* 7 (2): 1–10. https://doi.org/10.1097/GOX.0000000000002044.

22 The Aesthetic Society (2014). Aesthetic Plastic Surgery National Databank 2019. New York: The Aesthetic Society.

23 Rzany, B., Carruthers, A., Carruthers, J. et al. (2012). Validated composite assessment scales for the global face. *Dermatol. Surg.* 38 (2 Part 2): 294–308. https://doi.org/10.1111/j.1524-4725.2011.02252.x.

24 Flynn, T.C., Carruthers, A., Carruthers, J. et al. (2012). Validated assessment scales for the upper face. *Dermatol. Surg.* 38 (2 Part 2): 309–319. https://doi.org/10.1111/j.1524-4725.2011.02248.x.

25 Carruthers, A. and Carruthers, J. (2010). A validated facial grading scale: the future of facial ageing measurement tools? *J. Cosmet. Laser Ther.* 12 (5): 235–241. https://doi.org/10.3109/14764172.2010.514920.

26 Glogau, R.G. (1996). Aesthetic and anatomic analysis of the aging skin. *Semin. Cutan. Med. Surg.* 15 (3): 134–138. https://doi.org/10.1016/S1085-5629(96)80003-4.

27 Sattler, G., Carruthers, A., Carruthers, J. et al. (2012). Validated assessment scale for neck volume. *Dermatol. Surg.* 38 (2 Part 2): 343–350. https://doi.org/10.1111/j.1524-4725.2011.02253.x.

28 Narins, R.S., Carruthers, J., Flynn, T.C. et al. (2012). Validated assessment scales for the lower face. *Dermatol. Surg.* 38 (2 Part II): 333–342. https://doi.org/10.1111/j.1524-4725.2011.02247.x.

29 Perry, D.M., McGrouther, D.A., and Bayat, A. (2010). Current tools for noninvasive objective assessment of skin scars. *Plast. Reconstr. Surg.* 126 (3): 912–923. https://doi.org/10.1097/PRS.0b013e3181e6046b.

30 Fearmonti, R., Bond, J., Erdmann, D., and Levinson, H. (2010). A review of scar scales and scar measuring devices. *Eplasty* 10: e43.

31 Lemperle, G., Holmes, R.E., Cohen, S.R., and Lemperle, S.M. (2001). A classification of facial wrinkles. *Plast. Reconstr. Surg.* 108 (6): 1735–1750. https://doi.org/10.1097/00006534-200111000-00048.

6

The Cosmetic Consultation

Anatomy and Psychology   The Female Patient

Eagan Zettlemoyer[1] and Noëlle S. Sherber[2,3]

[1] *Drexel University College of Medicine, Philadelphia, PA, USA*
[2] *Sherber and Rad, Washington, DC, USA*
[3] *Department of Dermatology, George Washington University School of Medicine & Health Sciences, Washington, DC, USA*

Introduction

Historically, women have comprised the overwhelming majority of those considering cosmetic treatment. Despite the ongoing rise in the number of men undergoing cosmetic procedures, women account for approximately 92% of aesthetic nonsurgical and surgical treatments [1]. While each patient has individual goals, female patients will often approach their aesthetic specialist seeking a more youthful and optimized facial appearance. The initial consultation is an important opportunity to learn the patient's motivations for seeking care. In aesthetic medicine, it is key to appreciate that reasons for seeking cosmetic procedures can range from practical to emotional and psychological [2]. The consultation is also a chance to gain an understanding of the patient's goals, concerns, and self-perception. It is especially important in the case of the cosmetically naïve patient to assess and ensure realistic expectations such that the patient has a clear understanding of her potential results from cosmetic intervention [3]. Knowing how to both recognize and respond to psychiatric red flags in a patient's presentation will also help guide decision-making to determine whether the patient would benefit more from a cosmetic procedure or from an alternative intervention [4]. This chapter reviews the defining features of female facial anatomy and describes how to structure a consultation to favor arriving at the optimal course of treatment.

Female Facial Anatomy

Female facial anatomy differs from male facial anatomy in ways ranging from nuanced to dramatic, and an understanding of these differences is critical in aesthetic medicine. Given the many sex-based variations that exist in facial anatomy, it is not surprising that the aesthetic ideals typically sought by female patients differ from those of men (Figure 6.1). Factors beyond sex differences that affect female aesthetic ideals include race, ethnicity, age, and cultural influences such as current beauty trends [5]. For example, the standard facial shape of Caucasian women differs from that of East Asian women in that the latter exhibits an increase in bizygomatic, bitemporal, and bigonal width, with

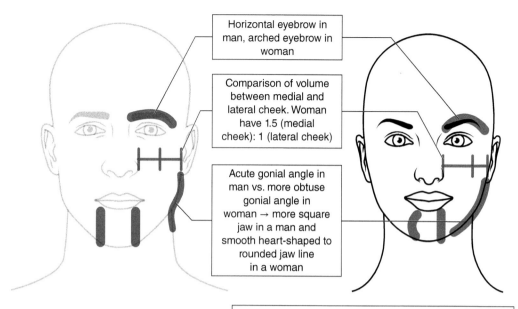

Horizontal eyebrow in man, arched eyebrow in woman

Comparison of volume between medial and lateral cheek. Woman have 1.5 (medial cheek): 1 (lateral cheek)

Acute gonial angle in man vs. more obtuse gonial angle in woman → more square jaw in a man and smooth heart-shaped to rounded jaw line in a woman

• Woman have a smaller forehead than men
• woman have a chin with less anterior protrusion than men
• woman have thinner skin at all anatomic levels than men

Figure 6.1 Gender dimorphism in the human face.

retrusion of the forehead, orbital rims, medial maxilla, pyriform margins, and chin; the nose exhibits a low bridge with lesser anterior projection [6]. Thus the conventional idea of "mathematical beauty" that suggests the existence of a single aesthetic ideal or golden ratio has long been controversial, in part due to the many interrelated factors that influence facial attractiveness. While there is not one universal standard, there are pertinent characteristics of female anatomy in the upper, middle, and lower face.

Upper Face: Standard Female Anatomy

The upper third of the face is defined as the features spanning from the hairline to the inferior borders of the lower eyelids. As compared to men, women have a skull that is approximately 80% as large and have variances in skeletal proportion and facial shape. The female forehead has a smaller surface area than the male forehead; it is shorter in width and height, with a notably less prominent supraorbital ridge. This gives women a softer and less angular upper facial appearance [7]. Notwithstanding

confounding variables such as brow height alteration via neurotoxin treatment, the average height of the female forehead as measured from the hairline to the peak of the brow has been shown to be about 5 cm [5].

Moving inferiorly, the standard female eyebrow begins medially at the level of or slightly inferior to the superior orbital rim; it tends to sit higher on the orbital rim than does the male eyebrow. The female eyebrow ascends laterally with an arch that peaks near the vertical plane of the lateral canthus or lateral limbus, or somewhere between these two planes. The lateral third of the brow then descends laterally. The lateral end of the female eyebrow is generally aligned 1–2 mm above the lowest portion of the medial brow [5].

The standard upper eyelid crease position in women is located superior to that seen in men, resting up to 12 mm above the upper eyelid margin. The female upper lid tends to exhibit more pretarsal show than does the male upper lid. As for eye shape, the canthal tilt is slightly more positive in women than in men [5]. Recent clinical evidence suggests that females' mean interpupillary distance is 59.2 mm [8]. There are fewer significant anatomical distinctions between the female and male lower eyelids; however, it should be noted that women generally have a shorter horizontal lid fissure [5].

Upper Face: Ideal Female Anatomy

While there is no universal definition of ideal female forehead anatomy, a feminine forehead is anatomically smaller than the male forehead and importantly exhibits minimal anterior projection at the glabella. Studies have shown a strong association between femininity and the upper third of the face, and some suggest that this anatomic area is the most significant contributor in determining overall female attractiveness. Along these lines, a feminizing forehead cranioplasty to reduce both supraorbital ridge projection at the glabella and posterior slope of the upper forehead is an increasingly popular procedure among male-to-female (MTF) transgender patients [9].

The female eyebrow plays a central role in the historical evolution of feminine aesthetic ideals. Dating back to the 1970s, the ideal brow was described as having medial and lateral ends on the same horizontal plane. During this time, the ideal apex was directly superior to the lateral limbus. By the end of the 1980s, among the most significant changes apparent in eyebrow aesthetics was the movement of the apex away from the lateral limbus more laterally to rest above the lateral canthus. There was also considerable debate over whether the medial brow should begin inferior or superior to the superior orbital rim. Clinical studies in the 1990s supported the notion that the medial brow should begin at the level of or slightly inferior to the superior orbital rim. More recent literature describes a gradual lateral migration of the ideal feminine brow arriving at a shape that is lower and less arched than before, rendering it less distinguishable from the male brow [5, 10, 11].

As for ideal eyelids, recent clinical evidence suggests that, while the mean attractive pretarsal show height is 4.5 mm in women, having a greater upper lid fold to pretarsal show ratio tends to be the more salient indicator of upper eyelid attractiveness. Ideal measurements of these ratios – which change gradually from the medial to the lateral portions of the lid – have not been defined [12]. A positive canthal tilt is also generally viewed as an attractive feminine feature [13]. Lastly, the female lower lid should have a shorter horizontal fissure than the male lower lid; however, attractive lower lid measurements have also not been defined [5].

Upper Face: Changes with Time

As skin loses elasticity over time, several key changes in the upper third of the face occur (Figure 6.2). The medial forehead undergoes flattening to an extent, and both dynamic and etched rhytides become increasingly apparent [14]. Additionally, the loss of elasticity

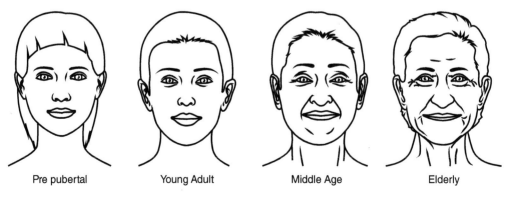

Pre pubertal   Young Adult   Middle Age   Elderly

Figure 6.2 Facial aging in women.

contributes to the descent of the brows toward the eyes. In both men and women, lateral brow ptosis is evident earlier in life as compared to medial ptosis; this is largely due to progressive loss of support from both the insertion of the frontalis muscle fibers as well as other deeper anatomical structures [5]. According to the American Society for Aesthetic Plastic Surgery, treatment with botulinum toxin continues to be the most sought-after nonsurgical cosmetic procedure among women, and treatment with Botox can simultaneously smooth forehead lines and improve eyebrow ptosis [1].

Over time, decreased eyelid elasticity is observed in combination with atrophy of the orbital fat pads. Additionally, a deeper and wider orbit develops due to downward displacement of intraorbital fat over a weakened orbital septum; this process also leads to a double convexity of the lower eyelid [14]. The horizontal eyelid fissure is described gradually to lengthen through young adulthood, before shortening in later years. There is an increase with age in the distance between the lower lash line and the center of the pupil by up to 0.5 mm in women [15]. Although not nonsurgical options, upper and lower blepharoplasties are increasingly popular procedures among our aging population as potential solutions to these changes in eyelid appearance [1].

Middle Face: Standard Female Anatomy

The middle third of the face includes the features spanning from the lid–cheek junction to the superior border of the upper lip. The female lower eyelid–cheek junction should transition smoothly from the concavity of the malar body, adjacent to the preseptal lid, to the convexity of the cheek. A clinical study developed a novel parameter called *WIZDOM* (Width of the Interzygomatic Distance of the Midface) to evaluate female midface position, as defined by a horizontal line connecting the right and left malar apexes and representing the most anterior point of malar body projection. While *WIZDOM* has been used to evaluate *ideal* female midface measurements, more research is needed to quantify *standard* female midface measurements [8].

The standard female nose has a dorsum that lies vertically on the midline of the face without deviating from the midline [16]. Standard dorsal curvature in women is either straight or slightly concave. From the anteroposterior view, the nasal dorsum forms a smooth curved line from the medial eyebrows to the alar base [17]. The mean nasolabial angle is greater in women than in men. In addition to sex-based differences, the literature includes reports of anthropologic variability in nasolabial angle measurements across ethnicities [18]. For example, the standard African-American nose has a greater alar width, nasal tip projection, and nasal bridge inclination than does the standard Caucasian nose [19]. Additionally, East Asian and Caucasian patients tend to display more obtuse nasolabial angles, whereas West African patients often display more acute nasolabial angles. Some ethnicities may exhibit fewer sex-based differences in nasal angle measurements [18].

Middle Face: Ideal Female Anatomy

Treating the midface has developed into a central tenet of aesthetic rejuvenation, and accordingly there are several objective means of measuring midface aesthetic ideals. The ideal location of the female malar apex – the most anterior point of projection of the malar body – has long been controversial. In a recent clinical study involving 55 "attractive" female participants, the mean distance between the right and left malar apex was found to be 108 mm. Another clinical study described the ideal distance between the malar apex and the ipsilateral medial canthus as approximately 1.618 times the distance between the left and right medial canthus. However, these descriptions have not yet been reproduced, as more study participants are needed and other topographical facial landmarks must be taken into account [8].

Moving medially to the nose, while there is not one universal ideal nasal shape that considers differing ethnic and sex norms, there is significant clinical evidence suggesting that female noses exuding mathematical averageness and symmetry are deemed most attractive [20]. The ideal nasal dorsum is either straight or slightly concave in women. The nasal dorsum should be parallel to a straight line drawn from the nasion to the nasal tip, and should lie 1–2 mm posterior. The attractive female nose also exhibits a supratip break in the nasal profile at the point where the nasal dorsum transitions to the nasal tip [17]. A recent clinical study found that the ideal nasolabial angle in women falls between 100.9 and 108.9° – greater than in men [18].

Middle Face: Changes with Time

Both volumetric and gravitational changes contribute to midface aging. As buccal hollowing and loss of subcutaneous fullness in the malar prominence occur, the appearance of the inferior border of the orbicularis oculi muscle becomes increasingly obvious, which causes the malar crescent over the zygomatic eminence and the nasojugal fold to deepen. Ptosis of cheek fat results in more prominent nasolabial folds, and loss of malar fullness occurs; both of these processes promote a subsequent increase in cheek concavity [14]. Hyaluronic acid filler treatments continue to be among the leading nonsurgical cosmetic procedures sought by female aesthetic patients, and these injectable treatments are increasingly used to address midfacial volume loss [1].

As for the nose, aging alters both the nasal cartilage and the soft tissue envelope. Most of the volumetric depletion occurs in the nasion, glabella, and upper dorsum. The nasofrontal angle is blunted with progressive flattening of the medial forehead, yielding the appearance of a longer nasal dorsum. Additionally, ptosis of the nasal tip results from weakening of the cartilaginous attachments between the superior and inferior lateral nasal cartilages.

Pyriform remodeling and resorption of the upper maxilla further exacerbate ptosis of the nasal tip; pyriform remodeling also affects the position of the alar base, promoting the development of a more acute nasolabial angle [14]. Women currently represent more than four out of five rhinoplasty patients, and rhinoplasty is often performed to attain a more ideal nasolabial angle, among other goals [1].

Lower Face: Standard Female Anatomy

The lips are a highly cosmetically significant feature of the lower third of the face. Both upper and lower lip height is smaller in women than in men. Despite this absolute height relationship, clinical evidence suggests that there is no significant sex-based difference in the ratio of lip surface area to total lower face surface area, although some studies cite that the female lip makes up a larger proportion of the lower face. A study of Caucasian subjects did not detect a gender difference in the vermilion height of the upper and lower lip, but found upper vermilion height to be typically shorter than lower vermilion height [21].

The jawline and chin are other salient features defining the lower third of the face. The jawbone, or mandible, is less prominent in women than in men, primarily due to the greater gonial angle and smaller mental protuberance [22]. The overall facial shape in women is more oval than square, and a well-defined jawline is a key part of maintaining this oval shape [23]. The female chin tends to exhibit underdeveloped lateral tubercles and less anterior protrusion in comparison to the male chin, contributing to the more oval-like facial shape observed in women [24]. Again, it is important to consider that the degree to which sex-based differences are observed may vary across cultures and ethnicities.

Lower Face: Ideal Female Anatomy

Similarly to the ideal eyebrow, the ideal lip shape is highly subject to beauty trends that may be present in one culture and nearly nonexistent in another. The controversial "golden ratio" defines the ideal height ratio of the midline-upper to midline-lower lip as 1 : 1.6, additionally specifying an upper lip projection of 3.5 mm and a lower lip projection of 2.2 mm. More recent studies have suggested that the ideal lip height ratio may actually be closer to 1 : 2. Overall, more generalizable features of the aesthetic female lip include fullness, symmetry, and well-demarcated vermilion borders. According to one clinical study, female lips should exhibit a surface area equal to approximately 10% of the lower third of the face, and more attractive lips have a greater ratio of lower vermillion height to chin–mouth distance. It should be noted, however, that beyond the subjective idea of fuller lips, there is currently no universal lip dimension deemed as most attractive in women [25].

One lower face aesthetic that is less dependent on ever-evolving trends is the general preference for symmetry and averageness in the jawline and chin. Evidence suggests that the attractive female jawline is straight and does not exhibit a mandibular angle that is excessively prominent. Recent studies in women across various cultures demonstrate a significant preference for a bimaxillary retrusive profile and a somewhat anteriorly projecting chin. Clinical evidence suggests that people of many racial backgrounds consider an oval facial shape most attractive and youthful in women [6]. Thus there are many different factors to consider when addressing cosmetic concerns of the lower third of the face in women.

Lower Face: Changes with Time

With age, the lips and perioral area undergo soft tissue lengthening, thinning, and volumetric depletion. Clinical evidence suggests that sagittal lip length increases by an average of nearly 20% in aging women. The thickness of the upper lip has been shown to decrease at all levels, with the most significant reduction in thickness occurring at the vermiliocutaneous junction. This process results in loss of anterior projection, or loss of pouting, of the upper lip. This lengthening and thinning is a culmination of both caudal redistribution of tissue and volumetric depletion [26]. Perioral wrinkling can result from loss of underlying support attributable to maxillary resorption [14]. Revolumizing treatments for aging lips are available and range from temporary injectable dermal fillers (i.e. hyaluronic acid) to more permanent structural fat grafting [25].

Volumetric and gravitational changes seen with age have a profound impact on the female jawline and chin. Loss of jawline definition is multifactorial and can relate to resorption of alveolar bone and diminishing malar and perioral fat deposits. A weakened masseteric ligament causes facial fat to move downward toward the mandible, resulting in the development of jowls; this process contributes to gradual squaring of the face and further loss of jawline definition. As for the chin, further anterior protrusion of the chin results from a decrease in lateral and inferior chin volume, while ptosis of the lateral chin develops from lateral mental atrophy. From the anteroposterior view, the combined effects often give the perception of a widened chin. Dermal fillers and energy-based devices offer effective nonsurgical cosmetic improvements in the proportions and overall aesthetic appearance of the aging jawline and chin in women [14].

Skin: Standard Female Anatomy

Adult female skin differs from adult male skin in thickness, hormone metabolism, hair pattern, sweat rate, and surface pH, among other characteristics [27]. While subcutaneous fat is more prominent in women than in men, female skin is thinner at all anatomic levels, including both the dermis and epidermis [7]. All dermal layers considered, the average ratio of female to male skin thickness is 1–1.2. Studies have shown that in women of reproductive potential thickness of the skin correlated positively with the level of sex hormones; this may reflect the consequence of hormone-induced water retention in the skin. Gender-based differences in skin's microflora can be partially attributed to variations in sebum, sweat, and epidermal pH. Clinical evidence suggests that Caucasian men, for example, average 3 μg of sebum per square centimeter of skin surface as compared to 0.7 μg/cm^2 in Caucasian women. This is indicative of women overall having less oily skin than men. Additionally, women perspire at a slower rate than men; adjusting for sex differences in body surface area, men sweat at a rate 30–40% greater than women [27].

Skin: Ideal Female Anatomy

Although there is no universally accepted quantifiable scale to determine female skin ideals, women often use subjective language such as smooth, soft, clean, and glowing when asked to describe attractive skin. Not only is ideal female skin highly subjective, but also it is for many women potentially unattainable. In a 2019 survey of over two-thousand US consumers, 34% of respondents reported "always [using] apps to modify or erase something on [their] face before posting a photo on social media" [28]. Findings such as this support the notion that many women feel unsatisfied with their skin's natural appearance. However, nonsurgical procedures that address these concerns – such as laser, light, and radiofrequency treatment – continue to boast over a 95% patient satisfaction rating according to the 2019 American Society of Dermatologic Surgery (ASDS) Consumer Survey [29].

Skin: Changes with Time

Several studies cite that men's skin thickness steadily declines throughout the aging process, whereas skin thickness in women remains fairly constant until around the fifth decade of life, when it begins to gradually decrease. As compared to premenopause, postmenopausal skin is 10% thinner. This decrease in skin thickness has been shown to be a result of hormonal changes [27]. In addition to epidermal thinning, loss of collagen in the dermal layer reduces skin's elasticity. Although sebaceous glands increase in size with age, their net secretory output decreases, resulting in drier skin in postmenopausal women [30]. Net secretory output of sweat glands also decreases with age, yielding reduced perspiration in older women [27]. The hormonal changes associated with pregnancy are associated with various other changes in skin appearance and physiology. In addition to the numerous dermatoses of pregnancy, common skin alterations that occur include hyperpigmentation, blood vessel dilation (increased formation of spider angiomas), hyperhidrosis, and acne [31].

Structuring the Consult

A thoughtful approach to the initial consultation is essential for the aesthetic specialist to establish a positive relationship with the patient. Obtaining high-quality new patient photographs is a key step to set the stage for a successful consultation (Table 6.1). Photography in aesthetic medicine serves several purposes including medicolegal photo-documentation, patient education, expectation setting, preprocedural planning, and postprocedural evaluation of results [32]. If obtaining postprocedural photographs, they should ideally be taken with the same setup and settings and by the same individual who took the patient's preprocedural photographs to ensure consistency [33]. Accurate and detailed photographs can also act as important documentation in identifying dysmorphic patients, who comprise a considerable subset of the cosmetic patient population. Reliable photographic equipment, and even lighting and proper patient positioning are

Table 6.1 Structuring the consult: photography.

Equipment	• High-quality, digital camera (iPads and digital single-lens reflex [DSLR] cameras are readily available) for immediate photo review • Use the same camera for pre- and postprocedural photographs
Lighting	• Optimal lighting involves using more than one light source • Even lighting helps prevent exaggeration, distortion, or elimination of certain facial features • Use the same lighting for pre- and postprocedural photographs

Positioning	• Patient should typically look straight forward and be void of facial expression
	• Conventional photographer views include:
	  – left lateral
	  – left oblique
	  – frontal
	  – right oblique
	  – right lateral
	• Some patients may require additional angles

Consent	• Informed consent must be obtained if the specialist wishes to use any of the patient's photographs for purposes extending beyond the patient's direct care

all necessary in obtaining useful photographs. The convention is to take these initial photos from five views: left lateral, left oblique, frontal, right oblique, and right lateral. Depending on the procedures that the patient is considering, the aesthetic provider may want to take additional photos from other angles and positioning as well, such as the worm's eye view for rhinoplasty [32].

In addition to review of the new patient photographs, the aesthetic specialist will want to go over intake information such as medical history gathered prior to the visit. Effective intake forms should include the patient's current medications, prior medical history (including history of cosmetic procedures, skin cancer, or other medical conditions), and any specific concerns that the patient would like to address. This key intake step will make the initial consultation more efficient, help the specialist determine which approaches may or may not work for the patient, and provide the specialist with more insight into the patient's perspective [34]. The aesthetic specialist may want to approach the initial consultation utilizing the LEAP (Listen, Educate and Empower, Align, Perform) technique. This technique was created to help foster good communication and realistic expectation setting, which have been shown to lead to more positive patient outcomes. It is discussed in depth in Chapter 16. Clinical studies have unsurprisingly shown that patients seeking cosmetic enhancement are most often motivated by a desire to have a more attractive, youthful appearance or to achieve beautiful skin. In a 2018 prospective multicenter observational study, over 80% of cosmetic patients reported being motivated by the desire to appear more youthful and rejuvenated, with nearly 90% of patients saying they wanted to look better for themselves, not for others. Procedure-specific variations in drivers have also been investigated. The same observational study found that patients pursuing skin-tightening treatments, laser treatments for pigmentation, neurotoxins, and other injectable treatments were similarly motivated largely by the innate desire to enhance their physical appearance [2]. Patients often report wanting to look more attractive not only in person but also in photographs. In a recent clinical study, almost all patients divulged that they sought out cosmetic intervention to correct undesirable features that they had noticed in photographs even more so than in person [35]. While the motivation simply to look more attractive is a key factor, motivations for seeking cosmetic intervention extend far beyond the desire to enhance one's physical appearance [2].

Common reasons for pursuing nonsurgical cosmetic procedures can range from practical to emotional and psychological motivations. These motivations can relate to physical health, success in the workplace, quality of social life, and emotional well-being. Preventing a condition or symptom from worsening is a commonly cited motive found in clinical studies on patient motivations, as is proactively protecting their long-term health. Since confidence plays a crucial role in the professional setting, patients also report being motivated by the desire to increase their confidence in school or in the workplace. Clinical evidence suggests that career-oriented patients are motivated not only by the desire to look better in a professional setting but also by the desire to remain competitive in their careers [2].

As for motivations related to social well-being, published literature reflects that patients often want to: improve their romantic lives, look better for upcoming social events, look good when running into people, and/or feel less self-conscious [2, 35]. A 2015 prospective cohort study found that approximately one-third of cosmetic patients had experienced a "major life event" within the year prior to cosmetic intervention. The study suggests an external motivation creating the hope that cosmetic intervention will help resolve the stress associated with these events; this may set up a scenario in which post-procedural results can be unlikely to meet expectations [3]. Finally, as for motivations related to emotional well-being, clinical evidence demonstrates that an overwhelming majority of patients want to: improve self-confidence, feel happier with themselves, treat themselves or feel rewarded, and feel less self-consciousness, anxiety, frustration, or other negative feelings [2]. Cosmetic patients are evidently motivated by numerous factors extending well beyond vanity, and understanding the interplay of these motivations as well as patients' self-perceptions will help the aesthetic specialist better counsel patients on cosmetic procedures and thus improve patient outcomes.

After listening to the patient, the provider should paraphrase their understanding of the patient's concerns and goals. It is also crucial to directly elicit the patient's motivations during the aesthetic consultation [36]. This is an opportunity to educate the patient on the relevant cosmetic procedures, making sure to cover the benefits, risks, alternatives, and realistic outcomes of such intervention [37]. At this point in the consultation, the new patient photographs may prove helpful in illustrating the provider's descriptions of what are the realistic outcomes. The mirror is another highly effective tool that, when given to the patient in consultation, may help bring to the surface their more specific goals and concerns [34]. Physicians have found that investing time in educating the patient can improve the patient experience by empowering them to more actively participate in treatment-related decisions. Patient education and expectation-setting enable the patient to make a more informed decision about their treatment [37]. Another notable finding highlighting the importance of the physician–patient relationship is that "patients frequently report higher satisfaction based not on the technical aptitude of their treating physician but on the quality of the interactions with their treating physician" [3]. Now, the goal is to align the plan with that of the patient in order to create an optimal treatment plan. The literature has shown that authentic agreement between a provider and the patient on the best course of treatment promotes more patient trust in the provider and ultimately a better patient outcome [37].

Case Studies

Case 6.1   The Cosmetically Naïve Patient

AF is a 27-year-old Caucasian woman with no significant past medical history who presents for cosmetic consultation. She found the practice through an online search of local board-certified dermatologists. Beyond the occasional at-home chemical peel and spa facial, she has never undergone a cosmetic treatment. She is looking to be more proactive about skin care and to explore minimally invasive cosmetic treatments with the aim of improving her appearance and preventing age-related changes. She first mentions that she is interested in laser treatments for uneven skin tone, enlarged pores, and acne, and explains that she is apprehensive after seeing images of patients bleeding from the face after "Vampire facials" on reality television. Despite this, she wants to "try something new" since she feels that the results from her subscription skin care and makeup boxes have disappointed her recently. She then pulls out her phone and shows you several selfies taken with a Snapchat filter that magnified the appearance of her lips. She flips back and forth between this and a picture of a young Instagram influencer who evidently has had lip augmentation, and she voices that she wants lips like hers. She goes on to divulge that every time she takes a picture with her girlfriends, she feels that she has the thinnest lips of everyone in the photo, which has bothered her for several years. On review of her social history, you learn that she and her longtime boyfriend recently broke up. She also just moved to the city to start a new job in the coming weeks.

Clinical Relevance and Implications

This case presentation highlights several salient possible characteristics of the millennial patient and of the cosmetically naïve patient. The ASDS survey data show that millennials are increasingly turning to nonsurgical cosmetic procedures, with a 50% increase in neuromodulator treatment among patients aged 30 and younger between 2012 and 2016; use of soft-tissue fillers doubled in this age group between 2015 and 2016 [38]. Millennials are digital natives, the first generation born into the internet world, and accordingly social media plays a central role in influencing their decisions on seeking cosmetic intervention. This is reflected in the 2019 ASDS consumer survey, where 43% of all patients reported that the provider's social media presence influenced their decision to schedule a consultation [29]. Millennials are the largest generation in American history and are rapidly on track to become the largest patient cohort in aesthetics [39].

In this case, the patient showed heavily edited selfies on the Snapchat app as well as a picture of an Instagram influencer and expressed her desire to look more like these photos. A 2019 analysis of the relevant medical literature shows that the increasingly widespread use of social media has given rise to forms of body dysmorphic disorder (BDD) such as "snapchat dysmorphia" and "selfie dysmorphia." Patients presenting with symptoms of these dysmorphias often dedicate a significant amount of time to taking and editing pictures of themselves, creating an inaccurate and unrealistic self-image. If presented with a substantially edited or filtered photograph in consultation, it is important for the aesthetic specialist to assess the patient for indicators of unrealistic expectations. According to the same 2019 commentary, "although most users of social media filters lead normal lives and are able to maintain reasonable expectations about their appearances," it may not be advisable to perform cosmetic procedures on those who are not able to make rational judgments either on their facial features or on possible outcomes of cosmetic intervention [40].

On review of the patient's social history, she reveals that she and her longtime boyfriend recently broke up and that she is preparing for a new job. In a 2015 prospective cohort study of 72 cosmetic patients, nearly one-third of patients had undergone a "major life event" within the year preceding their cosmetic consultation. Almost half of these patients had also sought therapy or counseling at least in part due to such events. Examples of major life events may include divorce, death of a loved one, or change in employment. The study suggested that "such events are considered major life stressors and can be associated with a level of psychosocial stress that could contraindicate surgery" [3]. While the patient may still be a suitable candidate for cosmetic intervention, it is important to be cognizant of both the patient's demeanor when discussing significant personal events and of how this event may be influencing their self-perceptions and decision-making.

The cosmetically naïve patient may express a combination of realistic and unrealistic treatment goals. Educating the above patient on proactive skin care measures and counseling her on the benefits of laser treatments will likely prove less challenging than achieving her desired lip aesthetic. While it may be feasible for the patient to achieve the Instagram influencer's lip fullness and shape, the aesthetic specialist may determine that immediately using the amount of filler required for that transformation is not advisable given the differences in facial anatomy between the patient and the influencer, and given that this will be the patient's first ever cosmetic procedure. With proper patient education, the patient can make the informed decision together with the specialist to start slowly with the filler treatment, and to add more filler over time if needed. If the specialist can successfully convey the relevant information to the patient while expressing an understanding of her perspective, the patient may be more inclined to align her thoughts with those of the specialist on the safest and best treatment plan moving forward. Use of a hyaluronic acid filler, which is dissolvable with hyaluronidase, is advisable in this case since the effect of the treatment can be reversed if the patient ends up feeling differently than she imagined about having augmented lips.

Case 6.2 The Cosmetically Experienced Patient

HM is a 59-year-old Asian-American woman with no relevant past medical history who presents for cosmetic consultation. She was referred by her good friend who frequents the practice. She has seen numerous dermatologists previously and has been on a regular schedule of Botox treatment every three months, as well as occasional under eye and lower face dermal filler treatments. She also infrequently undergoes chemical peels. She says that she is happy that Botox softens her lines and wrinkles, adding that she has a big birthday coming up in a few months and wants to ensure that she looks her best in photos and when seeing friends. On review of her social history, you learn that she and her husband of 30 years live together and their two children are currently away at college. You also learn that she is an executive in the fashion industry and more recently has felt increasingly older relative to her colleagues. She reiterates her desire to appear youthful but natural. She volunteers that she has not been completely happy with her aesthetic improvements achieved previously and is hopeful that you can offer other approaches.

Clinical Relevance and Implications

This case presentation brings to light numerous potential characteristics of the cosmetically experienced patient. The above patient reports that she occasionally incorporates filler treatments into her Botox regimen. A comprehensive panfacial approach confers greatest benefit to the cosmetic patient, which is a best practice of aesthetic treatment and is borne out in clinical research [41]. The HARMONY study was the first of its kind – a clinical trial to investigate the impact of a global approach to aesthetic facial rejuvenation. A global (or multimodal) approach involves using various minimally invasive treatment modalities to address multiple facial areas in the context of the entire face's anatomy and age-related change. The HARMONY study showed that a multimodal approach helps patients achieve an optimal aesthetic outcome [42]. Further analysis of the HARMONY study suggests that a multimodal approach to facial rejuvenation also confers greater psychosocial benefits to the patient [41].

In the initial consultation, the patient volunteers that she "has felt increasingly older relative to her colleagues." Since the patient is in a leadership position at work, she likely gives presentations, heads meetings, and is seen in many other ways by her coworkers; therefore it is plausible that she may be seeking aesthetic enhancement at least in part due to career-related concerns. Clinical evidence suggests that the desire to increase confidence and competitiveness in the workplace is a common motivation for seeking aesthetic enhancement. Thus the patient's mentioning of her workplace concern likely reflects a reasonable practical motivation for seeking nonsurgical cosmetic procedures [2].

The patient expresses that she has not been content with her previous aesthetic treatments and has seen many other dermatologists in the past. This may or may not be a sign of unrealistic expectations and BDD. A 2016 clinical study of female aesthetic patients found that patients with BDD have a greater tendency to feel dissatisfied with the results of their cosmetic procedures. While many female aesthetic patients report higher self-esteem, greater quality of life, and other positive psychological outcomes postaesthetic treatment, those suffering from BDD typically do not show similar improvements in psychological outcomes. The use of targeted questionnaires or other intake forms may aid in identification of patients exhibiting underlying body image disorders [43]. If the aesthetic specialist is able to learn the specific reasons for the patient's unhappiness with previous treatments, this information may help the specialist determine the patient's likelihood of a successful outcome through further cosmetic intervention. Clinically, a patient who has already been under the care of multiple other aesthetic specialists may present as a more complex technical treatment challenge due to either poorly executed previous treatments that left fibrosis or sub-par results, or the patient's own personal grievances [4]. However, the patient may be well suited for cosmetic intervention if her history of treatment by many other dermatologists relates to circumstances such as relocating or other personal preferences; she also may never have had a multimodality treatment approach suitable to her needs and a concrete rationale for dissatisfaction. In this situation, the patient's expectations may be perfectly reasonable, suggesting likelihood of a positive outcome.

Conclusions

A thoughtfully structured cosmetic consultation builds relationship and rapport with a patient, and also provides invaluable insights into motivations and expectations. Create a consistent system for collecting intake information and obtaining photo-documentation. Give the interaction sufficient time to foster an understanding of why the patient is presenting now and why the patient would like to pursue aesthetic treatment. A foundational understanding of anatomy, and its variances by age and by cultural norms, is critical for treatment safety as well as for creating a suitable treatment plan. Inasmuch as assessing medical history and baseline anatomy is integral to a cosmetic consultation, assessing psychological fitness is paramount. A successful consultation educates the patient and creates doctor–patient convergence with a safe and effective plan and aligned expectations. The best outcome is the establishment of trust and, of course, a happy patient.

References

1 American Society for Aesthetic Plastic Surgery. Cosmetic (Aesthetic) Surgery National Data Bank Statistics 2018. Available at: https://www.surgery.org/sites/default/files/ASAPS-Stats2018.pdf (accessed 21 October2020).

2 Maisel, A., Waldman, A., Furlan, K. et al. (2018). Self-reported patient motivations for seeking cosmetic procedures. *JAMA Dermatology* 154 (10): 1167–1174.

3 Sobanko, J.F., Taglienti, A.J., Wilson, A.J. et al. (2015). Motivations for seeking minimally invasive cosmetic procedures in an academic outpatient setting. *Aesthetic Surgery Journal* 35 (8): 1014–1020.

4 Gorney, M. (2007). Recognition of the patient unsuitable for aesthetic surgery. *Aesthetic Surgery Journal* 27 (6): 626–629.

5 Sedgh, J. (2018). The aesthetics of the upper face and brow: male and female differences. *Facial Plastic Surgery* 34 (2): 114–118.

6 Samizadeh, S. and Wu, W. (2018). Ideals of facial beauty amongst the Chinese population: results from a large national survey. *Aesthetic Plastic Surgery* 42 (6): 1540–1550.

7 Rossi, A.M., Fitzgerald, R., and Humphrey, S. (2017). Facial soft tissue augmentation in males: an anatomical and practical approach. *Dermatologic Surgery* 43 (2): 131–139.

8 Linkov, G., Mally, P., Czyz, C.N. et al. (2018). Quantification of the aesthetically desirable female midface position. *Aesthetic Surgery Journal* 38 (3): 231–240.

9 Spiegel, J.H. (2011). Facial determinants of female gender and feminizing forehead cranioplasty. *The Laryngoscope* 121 (2): 250–261.

10 Griffin, G.R. and Kim, J.C. (2013). Ideal female brow aesthetics. *Clinics in Plastic Surgery* 40 (1): 147–155.

11 Roth, J.M. and Metzinger, S.E. (2003). Quantifying the arch position of the female eyebrow. *Archives of Facial Plastic Surgery* 5 (3): 235–239.

12 Vaca, E.E., Bricker, J.T., Helenowski, I. et al. (2019). Identifying aesthetically appealing upper eyelid topographic proportions. *Aesthetic Surgery Journal* 39 (8): 824–834.

13 Tepper, O.M., Steinbrech, D., Howell, M.H. et al. (2015). A retrospective review of patients undergoing lateral canthoplasty techniques to manage existing or potential lower eyelid malposition: identification of seven key preoperative findings. *Plastic and Reconstructive Surgery* 136 (1): 40–49.

14 Coleman, S.R. and Grover, R. (2006). The anatomy of the aging face: volume loss and changes in 3-dimensional topography. *Aesthetic Surgery Journal* 26 (1): 4–9.

15 Van den Bosch, W.A., Leenders, I., and Mulder, P. (1999). Topographic anatomy of the eyelids, and the effects of sex and age. *British Journal of Ophthalmology* 83 (3): 347–352.

16 Kienstra, M.A., Gassner, H.G., Sherris, D.A. et al. (2003). A grading system for nasal dorsal deformities. *Archives of Facial Plastic Surgery* 5 (2): 138–143.

17 Sykes, J.M., Tapias, V., and Kim, J.E. (2011). Management of the nasal dorsum. *Facial Plastic Surgery* 27 (2): 192–202.

18 Sinno, H.H., Markarian, M.K., Ibrahim, A.M. et al. (2014). The ideal nasolabial angle in

rhinoplasty: a preference analysis of the general population. *Plastic and Reconstructive Surgery* 134 (2): 201–210.

19 Porter, J.P. and Olson, K.L. (2003). Analysis of the African American female nose. *Plastic and Reconstructive Surgery* 111 (2): 620–626; discussion 627–8.

20 Van Zijl, F.V.W.J., Perrett, D.I., Lohuis, P.J.F.M. et al. (2020). The value of averageness in aesthetic rhinoplasty: humans like average noses. *Aesthetic Surgery Journal*; sjaa010.

21 Anic-Milosevic, S., Mestrovic, S., Prlic, A. et al. (2010). Proportions in the upper lip-lower lip-chin area of the lower face as determined by photogrammetric method. *Journal of Cranio-Maxillofacial Surgery* 38 (2): 90–95.

22 Breeland, G. and Patel, B.C. Anatomy, head and neck, mandible. In: StatPearls [Internet], 2020. Treasure Island, FL: StatPearls Publishing.

23 Goodman, G.J. (2015). The oval female facial shape – a study in beauty. *Dermatologic Surgery* 41 (12): 1375–1383.

24 Thayer, Z.M. and Dobson, S.D. (2010). Sexual dimorphism in chin shape: implications for adaptive hypotheses. *American Journal of Physical Anthropology* 143 (3): 417–425.

25 Popenko, N.A., Tripathi, P.B., Devcic, Z. et al. (2017). A quantitative approach to determining the ideal female lip aesthetic and its effect on facial attractiveness. *JAMA Facial Plastic Surgery* 19 (4): 261–267.

26 Ramaut, L., Tonnard, P., Verpaele, A. et al. (2019). Aging of the upper lip: part I: a retrospective analysis of metric changes in soft tissue on magnetic resonance imaging. *Plastic and Reconstructive Surgery* 143 (2): 440–446.

27 Giacomoni, P.U., Mammone, T., and Teri, M. (2009 Sep). Gender-linked differences in human skin. *Journal of Dermatological Science* 55 (3): 144–149.

28 Allergan 360° Aesthetics Report™, 2019 Edition – Beyond Beauty. Available at https://www.allergan.com/

medical-aesthetics/allergan-360-aesthetics-report (accessed 23 May 2020).

29 ASDS Consumer Survey on Cosmetic Dermatologic Procedures, 2019. Available at https://www.asds.net/medical-professionals/practice-resources/asds-consumer-survey-on-cosmetic-dermatologic-procedures (accessed 23 May 2020).

30 Fenske, N.A. and Lober, C.W. (1986). Structural and functional changes of normal aging skin. *Journal of the American Academy of Dermatology* 15 (4 Pt 1): 571–585.

31 Geraghty, L.N. and Pomeranz, M.K. (2011). Physiologic changes and dermatoses of pregnancy. *International Journal of Dermatology* 50 (7): 771–782.

32 Zhang, C., Guo, X., Han, X. et al. (2018). Six-position, frontal view photography in blepharoplasty: a simple method. *Aesthetic Plastic Surgery* 42 (5): 1312–1319.

33 Archibald, D.J., Carlson, M.L., and Friedman, O. (2010). Pitfalls of nonstandardized photography. *Facial Plastic Surgery Clinics of North America* 18 (2): 253–266.

34 Werschler, W.P., Calkin, J.M., Laub, D.A. et al. (2015). Aesthetic dermatologic treatments: consensus from the experts. *Journal of Clinical and Aesthetic Dermatology* 8 (10): S2–S7.

35 Waldman, A., Maisel, A., Weil, A. et al. (2019). Patients believe that cosmetic procedures affect their quality of life: an interview study of patient-reported motivations. *Journal of the American Academy of Dermatology* 80 (6): 1671–1681.

36 Lista, F., Mistry, B.D., Singh, Y. et al. (2015). The safety of aesthetic labiaplasty: a plastic surgery experience. *Aesthetic Surgery Journal* 35 (6): 689–695.

37 Watchmaker, J., Kandula, P., and Kaminer, M.S. (2020). L.E.A.P.ing into the cosmetic consult. *Journal of Cosmetic Dermatology* 19 (6): 1499–1500.

38 ASDS Survey: Nearly 10.5 Million Treatments Performed in 2016. Published 30 May 2017. Available at: https://www.asds.

net/skin-experts/news-room/press-releases/
asds-survey-nearly-105-million-treatments-
performed-in-2016 (accessed 23 May 2020).

39 Sherber, N. (2018). The millennial mindset.
Journal of Drugs in Dermatology 17 (12):
1340–1342.

40 Wang, J.V., Rieder, E.A., Schoenberg, E. et al.
(2020). Patient perception of beauty on social
media: professional and bioethical
obligations in esthetics. *Journal of Cosmetic
Dermatology* 19 (5): 1129–1130.

41 Dayan, S., Rivkin, A., Sykes, J.M. et al.
(2019). Aesthetic treatment positively
impacts social perception: analysis of
subjects from the HARMONY study.
Aesthetic Surgery Journal 39 (12): 1380–1389.

42 Narurkar, V.A., Cohen, J.L., Dayan, S. et al.
(2016). A comprehensive approach to
multimodal facial aesthetic treatment:
injection techniques and treatment
characteristics from the HARMONY study.
Dermatologic Surgery 42 (2): S177–S191.

43 Wang, Q., Cao, C., Guo, R. et al. (2016).
Avoiding psychological pitfalls in aesthetic
medical procedures. *Aesthetic Plastic Surgery*
40 (6): 954–961.

7

The Cosmetic Consultation

Anatomy and Psychology – The Male Patient

Kalee Shah[1], Nathaniel Lampley III[2], and Anthony Rossi[1,3]

[1] Department of Dermatology, Weill Cornell Medicine, New York, NY, USA
[2] University of Cincinnati College of Medicine, Cincinnati, OH, USA
[3] Dermatology Service, Department of Medicine, Memorial Sloan Kettering Cancer Center, New York, NY, USA

Funding source: This research is funded in part by a grant from the National Cancer Institute/National Institutes of Health (P30-CA008748) made to the Memorial Sloan Kettering Cancer Center.

Conflict of interest: Dr. Rossi has no relevant conflicts of interest related to this manuscript but has received grant funding from LeoiLab, Regen Pharmaceuticals, Society of MSKCC, ASDS/A, The Skin Cancer Foundation, and the A. Ward Ford Memorial Grant. He has also served on the advisory board, as a consultant, or has given educational presentations for Allergan, Inc.; Galderma Inc.; Evolus Inc.; Elekta; Biofrontera, Quantia; Merz Inc.; Dynamed; Skinuvia, Perf-Action, Cutera, Canfield, and LAM therapeutics.

Introduction

The field of aesthetic medicine has traditionally focused on improving the physical attractiveness of women. As both society and the medical community normalize the male beauty conscience, the discipline of aesthetic medicine has become more appreciative and accommodating to the male gender. The male face and its contributions to masculinity and attractiveness are increasingly being studied. Because of this relatively recent public shift, male patients often present for a cosmetic consultation without knowing exactly what they wish to achieve and how they wish to achieve it. In order to conduct a successful consultation, providers must have an adequate understanding of male facial anatomy and the key differences between female and male anatomy. Appreciating facial dimorphism not only allows the provider to tailor treatments and techniques to the male patient, but also provides insight into the underlying reasons the patient presents for treatment. Self-perceived attractiveness and masculinity have a propensity to significantly impact the patient's psychological well-being, performance, and achievement [1]. If a man's facial features can be altered to a point where they are perceived as more attractive, then it follows logically that such physical alterations would have a positive impact on his mental and emotional health. However, for the cosmetic patient the

Table 7.1 Key differences between male and female facial anatomy.

Feature	Female	Male
Skull	Smaller bony structure	Larger bony structure (1.25×)
Glabella	Narrow	Wider and protruding
Forehead	Average 5 cm length	Average 6–8 cm length
	Flat angle between hairline and supraorbital ridge	Anterior projection from hairline to supraorbital ridge
Eyebrow	High set	Horizontal
	Arched	Overhangs supraorbital ridge
Nose	Straight or concave dorsum	Straight or convex dorsum
	Supratip accentuation	Wide nasal root and ala
Cheek	Malar to zygomatic ratio 1.5 : 1	Malar to zygomatic ratio 1 : 1
Lips	Shorter philtrum	Longer philtrum
	Greater vermillion lip height	Greater cutaneous lip height
Mandible	Narrower	Wider
	Obtuse gonial angle	Acute gonial angle
Chin	Narrower	Wider
	Rounded/trapezoid shape	Square shape
Skin	Thinner epidermis and dermis	Increased epidermal and dermal thickness
	Smaller muscle mass	Larger muscle mass
	Lower sebaceous gland activity	Increased sebaceous gland activity
	More subcutaneous fat	Less subcutaneous fat

aforementioned logic may not always be true, particularly for patients with unreasonable expectations or underlying body dysmorphia. The most frequently reported reasons for male patients to seek aesthetic procedures are dating success, career success, and general sense of youth and attractiveness [2]. This chapter reviews male anatomy and provides a framework for approaching a cosmetic consultation with a male patient, specifically highlighting differences between men and women (Table 7.1). It is important to note that most research to date is conducted through a heteronormative lens, assuming an alignment of biological sex, sexuality, and gender identity. In addition, a Caucasian/European ideal has historically been put forth on beauty. As societal norms regarding gender and sexuality expand, and ethnic variations are embraced, aesthetic providers may encounter patients that desire a middle ground between a classically masculine and classically feminine aesthetic.

Male Facial Anatomy

Facial sexual dimorphism is the foundation for perception of attractiveness (Figure 7.1). Facial dimorphism is seen during the first year of life and becomes amplified during puberty when secondary sex characteristics develop [3, 4]. The male growth period extends beyond the female growth period, allowing males to develop more prominent facial features such as jawline and cheekbones. It is widely accepted that masculine facial features are considered physically attractive by individuals who prefer a masculine phenotype [4]. From an evolutionary

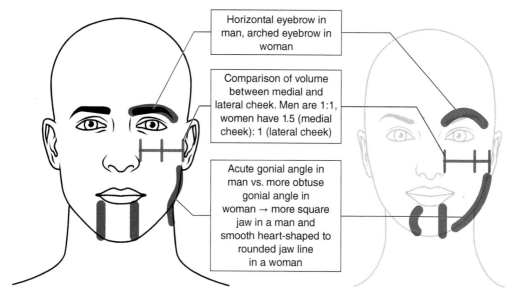

Figure 7.1 Gender dimorphism in the human face.

standpoint, masculine facial features are considered attractive because they are perceived to be reflective of the man's fitness. Evolutionary support for this theory includes findings that higher levels of testosterone correlate with greater immunity [5]. Further affirmation of the association between masculine facial features and attractiveness is evidence demonstrating a linear relationship between facial masculinity and mate preference in subjects who prefer a masculine phenotype [6]. While the standards and ideals of masculinity vary greatly depending on race and ethnicity, pertinent anatomical patterns are detailed below.

Upper Face: Standard Male Anatomy

The upper third of the face includes the forehead encompassing the male hairline, as well as the temporal fossa, and upper periorbital regions. The male skull is 1.25 times larger than the female skull and varies in proportion and overall shape. A prominent difference between men and women in the upper face is the size and shape of the forehead. In men the

forehead is longer and wider; it slopes backwards at a sharp angle toward the hairline [7]. In contrast, women typically have a flat angle between the supraorbital ridge and the hairline, giving a softer appearance. The height of the forehead measured from the eyebrows to the hairline is typically 1–2 cm longer in males, about 6 cm, but may be influenced by receding hairlines [8]. The glabella is wider and projects more anteriorly in men. The corrugator supercilli, the key muscles that create frown lines or "the 11s," extends further laterally onto the frontalis in men. Glabellar muscle mass is also higher in men, as evidenced by increasing doses of neurotoxin required to treat glabellar wrinkles [9].With regards to eyebrows, men tend to have thicker and straighter eyebrows that are positioned horizontally straight across the orbital rim, without the pronounced arch seen in female eyebrows [9]. The male upper eyelid crease is positioned lower, situated at a minimum of 8 mm above the lid margin, compared to 12 mm in women. The eyelid appears fuller and has a less pretarsal show [7, 8]. Lower eyelid and lateral canthal anatomical features are similar between men and women [8].

Upper Face: Ideal Male Anatomy

The eyes and eyebrows are major points of emphasis in aesthetic enhancement of the male upper face. The ideal eyebrow varies with face shape but is related to the proportionality of various periorbital features. The intercanthal axis should have a slight medial to lateral tilt and the upper lid crease should be even with the lash line. The medial part of the upper lid margin should be positioned slightly more superior than the lateral part of the upper lid margin. The medial and lateral extensions of the supratarsal upper skin folds should not exceed the inner medial canthus and lateral orbital rim, respectively [10]. Men often prefer to maintain a linear, horizontal placement of their brow that sits lower on the orbital ridge. However, a brow that overhangs the ridge significantly can give a perception of aggression [11]. Determining a patient's personal preferences with regards to eyebrow shape and placement is imperative before proceeding with neurotoxin injections for forehead and glabellar lines. These preferences can significantly impact injection technique as well as patient satisfaction.

Upper Face: Changes with Time

The aging process creates a disparity between the superficial and the deep structures of the upper face. The decrease in subcutaneous mass withdraws support from many of the superficial structures and makes the underlying anatomical structures appear more prominent. Specifically, the brow begins to droop caudally, as a combination of intrinsic and extrinsic photoaging occurs. Muscles of facial expression begin to lose their tone, while blood vessels and the skull's bony outline become more apparent with the loss of volume and descent of superficial and deep fat compartments [12].

Middle Face: Standard Male Anatomy

The middle third of the face includes the lower periorbital regions, nose, and cheeks. Key distinctions between the masculine and feminine are as follows. The orbital height is actually greater in males than in females. However, due to proportions of facial mass, women's eyes appear larger and higher than men's eyes. As previously mentioned, the upper eyelids in men are fuller and positioned lower, with a less pronounced canthal tilt. There are no noteworthy differences in the lower eyelids of men and women [13].

The anatomy of the male nose clearly demonstrates the angular and size differences between the male and female face. Increased volume of cartilage and bone contributes to the larger size of the male nose. The nasal bones meet at a sharper angle, forming a more defined nasal aperture. The angle between the nose and glabella is also more acute, contributing to appearance of prominent glabellar projection [13]. Finally, the nasal root and alar widths are wider, particularly in East Asian and men of Sub-Saharan African descent [14].

While male cheekbones are fuller with larger malar volume, male cheeks appear less prominent than female cheeks due to a decreased concentration of underlying soft tissue and fat. Similarly, the interzygomatic distance is larger in men but appears more conspicuous in females. The ratio of maxillary to mandibular fullness is lower in males, which contributes to a more defined jawline and hardened face [13].

Middle Face: Ideal Male Anatomy

The nose is the focal point for aesthetic enhancement of the male face. The nose's size, curvature, and angular relationship with the surrounding facial structures are its greatest contributions to facial attractiveness. The ideal nasal length is one-third of the vertical height of the mid-facial area and the nasal tip projection should be a few millimeters higher than the nasion [15]. It should also have little-to-no supratip accentuation, a feature commonly thought to be attractive in female nasal anatomy. The ideal male nose has a superiorly positioned nasion with a straight profile that lacks a dorsal hump [16]. The ideal nasofrontal angle is approximately 115° and the ideal nasolabial angle is approximately 95° [16, 17]. In the model male face, the medial and lateral cheek projection is in a ratio of 1.1 : 1, in comparison to the female ratio of 1.5 : 1 [11].

Middle Face: Changes with Time

The age-associated changes in the middle third of the face contribute to an overall loss in structural and functional proportionality (Figure 7.2). A loss in infraorbital subcutaneous tissue permits orbicularis oculi muscle overexpression and infraorbital fat pad exposure. This creates the appearance of periocular wrinkles, or "crow's feet," and palpebral bags, respectively. The periocular region also develops a "tired" appearance because of red, blue, or brown discoloration seen as a result of decreased distance between the orbicularis oculi muscle and the overlying infraorbital skin. This is further compounded by extrinsic photodamage [12].

Lower Face: Standard Male Anatomy

The lower third of the face includes the perioral, chin, and mandibular regions. The length of the philtrum, between the base of the columella and cupid's bow, is greater in men than in women. The upper lip is longer and narrower in males, with a greater ratio of upper cutaneous lip height to upper vermillion lip height. For this reason, male lips appear less defined than female lips [13].

Facial dimorphism of the jawline and chin plays a significant role in the perception of gender. The mandible is larger and thicker in men, which produces a wider lower face compared to women [7, 13, 18]. This is partially due to a broader ascending ramus, larger condyles, and orientation of the mandibular attachments. The gonial angle is typically less than 125° in both sexes, but men tend to have a more acute, or sharp, gonial angle by approximately 2.7°. A softer, or more obtuse, gonial angle is generally considered a feminizing feature.

The male chin is wider and taller and exhibits greater anterior projection. The chin and lower jaw are as much as 20% longer in men [13]. The anatomy of the canines contributes significantly to facial dimorphism of the chin. The male chin contains bilateral mental eminences, while the female chin has a single medial mental eminence [13]. This produces a square chin shape in men, as compared to a rounded or trapezoid shape in women.

Lower Face: Ideal Male Anatomy

The jawline is the focal point in the enhancement of the lower third of the face. The ideal jawline is both youthful and masculine in appearance. A paucity of lax tissue around the lower mandible permits a visual delineation

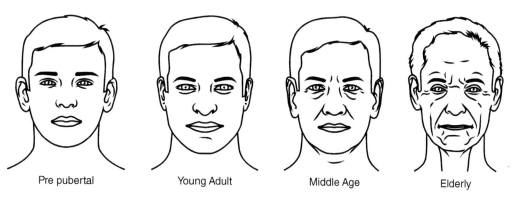

Pre pubertal   Young Adult   Middle Age   Elderly

Figure 7.2 Facial aging in men.

between the face and neck. Ideally, the vertical position of the angle of the jaw should be at the level of the oral commissure. The ideal angle is parallel to a line from the lateral canthus to the ipsilateral nasal ala. The radius of the gonial curvature should be wider than it is pointy. The ideal intergonial width is equal to the interzygomatic width; however, normal width is about 10% less. Males tend to prefer procedures that accentuate the angle of the jaw, as they believe it is more visually attractive and masculine [19].

Lower Face: Changes with Time

Aging creates an appearance of excess skin in the lower third of the face. A decrease in subcutaneous perioral and malar fat coupled with the resorption of alveolar bone causes the jawline to appear less sharply defined. The weakening of the masseteric ligament and lack of subcutaneous fullness forms facial jowls, contributing to the "turkey neck" deformity. The descent of the hyoid bone and larynx blunt the cervicomental angle, furthering the appearance of excess skin [12].

Skin: Standard Male Anatomy

Many facets of adult male skin are different than female skin, such as consistency, tone, hormone metabolism, hair distribution, sweat, and pH. Like other internal organs, the skin is considered a steroidogenic tissue; it metabolizes and is influenced by sex hormones. In women, testosterone is converted to estradiol in the skin by the enzyme aromatase. An excess of testosterone in women can lead to female-pattern hair loss or hirsutism. Similarly, in men, testosterone leads to beard growth and male-pattern hair loss. Men also have higher levels of nonsex hormones, which may contribute to delayed wound healing and increased ultraviolet (UV)-related cancers [20].

Male skin is thicker than female skin but has less subcutaneous fat [7]. It is between 30 and 175 μm thicker than female skin, depending on the location being measured [13]. The total hydroxyproline content, a major component of collagen, is overall lower in women than men [20]. While not technically a component of skin, muscle mass and facial muscle movement are also greater in men. These likely account for the observation that men tend to have an increased number and depth of rhytides. Men also have greater sebum production. The average Caucasian man has 3 μg of sebum per square centimeter as compared to 0.7 μg/cm^2 in Caucasian women [20]. Excess sebum is related to increased pore size and acne, which are both considered to be aesthetically undesirable.

Skin color and tone varies between genders. It is determined by the quantity and quality of melanin, as well as cutaneous vasculature. Men and women have the same melanocyte distribution, but men demonstrate a stronger response to sun-induced pigmentation and retain pigmentation longer than their female counterparts. This perceived darker complexion with less reflective properties has been attributed to men having a more vascularized upper dermis, as well as the presence of facial hair [20].

Skin: Ideal Male Anatomy

Men historically practice less sun-protective behavior than women, as evidenced by the increased rate of skin cancer. Ideally, male cutaneous anatomy would be devoid of pigmentary alterations, sebaceous hyperplasia, and benign epidermal growths. It would retain elasticity and exhibit decreased ptosis. Interestingly, certain male demographics tolerate more signs of cutaneous aging compared to their female counterparts.

Skin: Changes with Time

Male skin undergoes a constant decrease in thickness over time after the age of 20, whereas female skin thickness starts decreasing rapidly

Table 7.2 Cosmetic preferences among men.

Top cosmetic concerns in men	Male treatment priorities[a]
1) Hair loss	1) Crow's feet and tear troughs
2) Tear trough deformity	2) Forehead lines
3) Double chin	3) Double chin
4) Crow's feet	4) Glabellar lines
5) Forehead lines	5) Oral commissures and chin

[a] Does not include hair loss.
Source: Adapted from ref. [2].

after menopause, around age 50. Soft tissue loss in men has been linked to age-related decreases in testosterone (gradual andropause), volume loss, and photoaging [7, 20]. These factors contribute to the ptotic appearance of the aging male face. Deep expression wrinkles are more common in aging men than in aging women due to differences in subcutaneous adipose tissue composition [20]. A study to quantify soft tissue loss in men with magnetic resonance imaging (MRI) found that there was a decline in soft tissue thickness at all measured anatomical sites over time. The anatomical sites with the greatest percentage change between the young age group and elderly age group were the infraorbital area (40% reduction), temples (23% reduction), medial cheeks (22% reduction), and lateral cheeks (15% reduction) [21]. These data correlate well with reported cosmetic preferences among men to prioritize correction of tear trough deformities and crow's feet [2] (Table 7.2).

Genitalia: Standard Male Anatomy

There are no established standards for penile or scrotum anatomy, but there have been several studies that report average phallus sizes in a particular population. A study of over 15 000 Caucasian men reported that the average penis is 9.16 cm in flaccid length and 13.23 cm in flaccid stretch length. Flaccid stretch length is considered a rough estimate of erect penile size [22]. Phallus size differs within ethnic and racial groups, as well as by height, weight, and body mass index [23]. A micropenis is defined as length and girth 2.5 standard deviations or lower than the mean; less than 0.14% of the male population meets this criteria. Educating patients on clinical averages and statistics about micropenis may aid in reassuring their anxieties related to phallus size.

Genitalia: Ideal Male Anatomy

There is no true ideal phallus, but men who worry about the appearance of their penis are usually focused on the length and girth of the penis. Furthermore, it has been shown that there is a discrepancy between what men perceive the size of their penis to be and its actual size. This discrepancy is most notable in patients with body dysmorphic disorder (BDD) [24]. In contrast, women rate different aspects of penile anatomy as aesthetically important. In fact, a study of heterosexual women found that penile length was the sixth most important feature out of eight features. The most important features to women were the general cosmetic appearance, skin appearance, and pubic hair appearance [25].

Structuring the Consult, Considering Patient Motivations and Psychology

A comprehensive understanding of patient motivations and gender-specific preferences, as well as facial dimorphism is paramount in providing successful aesthetic care to men. While male patients represent a growing demographic in the aesthetics industry, the majority of research, education, and marketing efforts are still oriented toward women. A cross-sectional study of 600 aesthetically oriented but injectable-naïve men in the United States found that awareness of available noninvasive facial aesthetic procedures was low – with 69% of participants aware of laser skin resurfacing and only 39% of patients aware of dermal fillers. The trial rates for all facial aesthetic procedures were even lower (2–6%) [2]. As men are less likely to have experience with aesthetics in general, education of efficacious noninvasive procedures including expected outcomes, downtime, and risks should be at the center of the initial cosmetic consultation for male patients.

Prior to engaging in the consultation and planning treatment, the aesthetic provider should familiarize themselves with gender-specific motivations for seeking cosmetic treatments. Similar to women, men are primarily motivated by an intrinsically driven desire to appear youthful, rejuvenated, and less tired. About one-third of single men surveyed in a cross-sectional online survey study reported that improving dating prospects was a factor contributing to their desire to pursue facial injectable treatments. Notably, increasing workplace competitiveness and job performance were important extrinsic motivating factors reported by men [2]. Men may feel that they are subject to discrimination in the workplace due to age or attractiveness and therefore are likely to pursue procedures with minimal downtime to maintain their "market value" [26]. The reasons for pursuing aesthetic procedures were generally consistent among age groups, with the exception that more men aged 55–59 wanted to "look good for their age" than respondents aged 30–44. Additional male-specific motivations that may influence aesthetic treatment are the desire to appear more masculine and the desire to compensate for ongoing hair loss [27].

Male patients presenting for cosmetic procedures tend to be less savvy in regards to skin health and skin care in comparison to their female counterparts. Therefore the cosmetic consultation provides an opportunity to educate male patients on the nature of photoaging, skin cancer carcinogenesis, and sun-protective behaviors. In general, male patients are less likely to receive outpatient dermatologic care (whether medical or cosmetic) compared to women [28]. Alarmingly, a majority of men do not wear sunscreen, do not follow recommended sunscreen usage guidelines, and are not aware of skin cancer warning signs [29, 30]. After reviewing these important topics, the aesthetic provider can continue to discuss personal skin care. The most mature segment of the male cosmetics market is comprised of products that address facial hair, such as razors and shaving creams [31]. Significant education may be necessary with regards to personal care products and anti-aging products. Since men have thicker and oiler skin than women, they tend to choose personal care products that are harsher on the skin [32]. With regards to cleansing products, men consider translucent products that do not leave a residue as more masculine and more desired. In contrast, women tend to prefer opaque, creamier products [32]. For topical medications men prefer gel formulations to all others, and notably dislike ointments. The majority also favors packaging in tubes [33]. The anti-aging product sector is a slow-growing slice of the male cosmetics market. Barriers to adoption include the perceived poor immediate efficacy in topical anti-aging products as well as lack of need. Many men desire the "rugged, coarse" look, as it indicates masculinity and maturity [34]. The aesthetic provider should recognize these preferences and recommend products accordingly, to improve patient adherence and ensure desired outcomes.

Cosmetic procedures have become more socially acceptable among men. Social media, the internet, and television, as well as fluidity in gender identity and expansion of gender roles have contributed to this rise [26]. Between invasive and less-invasive cosmetic procedures, men gravitate to minimally invasive procedures because of the ability to achieve results without extended downtime. They also tend to prefer to undergo multiple treatments in a single day, rather than spreading out treatments over multiple sessions [35]. A survey of aesthetically oriented but cosmetically naïve men revealed that men were most concerned with treating tear troughs, crow's feet, forehead lines, and double chin (Table 7.2). An over-whelming majority (79%) of men that were concerned about hair loss would prioritize treating hair loss above any of the aforementioned aesthetic concerns. While this study provides invaluable insight to the aesthetic provider, it is important to note that most men surveyed were Caucasian. A subsequent large multinational survey-based study of facial aging found that regardless of racial/ethnic group, the first signs of aging reported were forehead lines and nasolabial folds, followed by crow's feet, under-eye puffiness, and tear trough deformities. However, the onset of advanced aging was delayed in black and Asian men as compared to their Caucasian and Hispanic counterparts [29]. Unique concerns of men with Fitzpatrick skin types IV–VI include pigmentary alterations such as melasma and hair disorders such as acne keloidalis nuchae and pseudofolliculitis barbae. These conditions may be targeted with topical medications and laser treatments. Asian men may particularly desire to have a more open eyelid, which may be achieved by neurotoxin injections [36]. There is limited published literature regarding aesthetic preferences in patients who identify outside of the heterosexual, cis-gender identity. Further research is needed to investigate these preferences. An important exception is aesthetic preferences in transgender patients. This topic is well studied and covered extensively in Chapter 8.

In Chapter 6, authors Zettlemoyer and Sherber provide a detailed framework for the successful cosmetic consultation in female patients, which includes reviewing the intake form, taking detailed baseline photographs, and noting the use of the LEAP method to communicate effectively. The male cosmetic consultation should largely be structured the same, with several important caveats. As men are less familiar with available aesthetic interventions and have more misconceptions about safety and expected outcomes, a large portion of the consultation may be spent on patient education [2, 27]. During the course of the

consultation, the aesthetic provider should proactively address the concerns men frequently report that limit their comfort in cosmetic procedures – namely safety, cost, and the fear of unnatural results [2]. By anticipating these questions, the provider will build trust with the patient and increase the patient's confidence that the practitioner is able to tailor historically female-oriented procedures to fit their needs. Due to the anticipated time requirements for a thorough consultation, consider performing the consultation without anticipation of a cosmetic procedure on the same visit. According to the American Society of Plastic Surgeons annual survey, the top five male cosmetic surgical procedures in 2019 were nose reshaping, eyelid surgery, liposuction, breast reduction, and hair transplantation. The top five minimally invasive procedures in men that year were botulinum toxin type A, laser hair removal, microdermabrasion, soft tissue fillers, and chemical peels [37].

Case Studies

Case 7.1 The Cosmetically Naïve Patient
AG is a 52-year-old African-American man with a history of hypertension who presents to your practice for a cosmetic consultation. He recently read an article in a men's health magazine about noninvasive cosmetic procedures and saw that you were quoted in the piece. He has never seen a dermatologist, let alone an aesthetic provider before. When you ask about his general skin care regimen, he says he washes his face and body daily with Irish Spring bar soap and hair with Head and Shoulders 2-in-1 shampoo and conditioner. He also recently started using an eye cream that his wife bought for him. He does not use moisturizer and stopped wearing sunscreen because he disliked the white film it

(Continued)

Case 7.1 (Continued)

left behind. His goal for treatment is to look and feel younger, but he does not know specifically how this can be accomplished. He is very worried about looking more feminine because of the commercials of cosmetic procedures that he sees on TV. When reviewing his general medical history, he mentions his fear of needles and says he always faints when he gets his blood drawn at the doctor's office. Through your conversation you also learn that he is retired and smokes cigars on the weekend while he plays golf.

Clinical Relevance and Implications

This patient is an African-American man who is presenting for cosmetic consultation for facial rejuvenation. In general, men tend to be less healthy compared to women and tend to have engaged in activities that accelerate photoaging such as smoking or working/relaxing outside without sun protection [29, 38]. The patient in this case has limited understanding of skin health – using abrasive bar soaps to cleanse his face and products purchased by his spouse. He regularly engages in golfing, an outdoor activity tied to substantial sun exposure, but does not wear sunscreen. Therefore the first step for improving his cosmetic outcome is to implement a simple, yet effective skin care regimen. Recommend a facial cleanser and anti-aging moisturizer that are gentle on the skin but are formulated as gels or creams and that appear translucent in color, in keeping with male consumer preferences [32]. Next, counsel the patient on the deleterious effects of ultraviolet radiation (UVR) on the skin, highlighting the role of UVR in skin photoaging and hyperpigmentation in all skin types. Finally, share a list of sheer sunscreens that will be more acceptable to the patient.

This patient desires to "look and feel younger" but cannot pinpoint specific problem areas that he is interested in targeting. While an open-ended approach to consultation is ideal for most cosmetic patients, some male patients may require additional coaching when choosing treatment modalities for their specific goals. Understanding facial aging and male anatomy is therefore essential to providing guidance to male cosmetic patients. In a large multinational study of over 800 men, black men reported the first signs of facial aging starting in their 40s, nearly 10–20 years after surveyed Caucasian patients. The first signs of advanced facial aging were forehead lines and prominent nasolabial folds, followed by crow's feet, under-eye puffiness, glabellar lines, tear trough deformity, and finally oral commissure lines. Few surveyed black men complained of mid-face volume loss, even those that were well into their 70s [29]. With this knowledge, the aesthetic provider may suggest neurotoxin injections to the forehead and glabellar lines and dermal fillers for prominent nasolabial folds as a starting point. The provider should review specific techniques that will be used to prevent feminizing the face, a concern that the patient expressed during the consultation.

After deciding on therapy, the provider should counsel the patient about postprocedure complications in detail, specifically highlighting differences between men and women. Men have a higher risk of bruising, skin infections, and poor wound healing after cosmetic procedures compared to their female counterparts [35]. The provider should also caution that he may require more units of neurotoxin and more syringes of fillers than a woman would because men have more robust facial musculature and thicker skin [39]. This may have cost implications based on the practice's fee structure and the patient may need return visits.

Finally, this patient reveals that he is fearful of needles and has had vasovagal episodes in the past. This is critical to keep in mind in order to maintain patient and physician safety during treatment. Men may be less tolerant of pain than women, so proactive pain control is key. Consider giving the patient topical anesthetic agents, nerve blocks, or even a mild anxiolytic prior to the procedure. Additionally, always be prepared to manage vasovagal episodes – have water, juice, or snacks readily available if necessary. Finally, consider the adjuvant use of one of the psychological tools discussed in the latter chapters of this textbook.

Case 7.2   The Aesthetically Oriented Patient

KF is a 29-year-old Korean-American man with a history of rhinoplasty who presents for cosmetic consultation. He works as a social media director and has been saving up money for the last year to see you. He tells you that you recently treated one of his female coworkers with neurotoxins and fillers and is hoping you can achieve a similar cosmetic result with him. In particular, he is looking to make his lips more full and soften his square jawline. He visits an aesthetician monthly for facials and chemical peels and says he has had multiple sessions of neurotoxin injections in his forehead, as well as hyaluronic acid filler in his cheeks and tear troughs. He states that he is overall satisfied with the result but knows that improvements can be made. As you are discussing treatment options he mentions that he has to attend a large wedding with his boyfriend in two weeks and wants to make sure he has no bruising for that event.

Clinical Relevance and Implications

This patient is an aesthetically oriented and cosmetically experienced patient. He works as a social media director and visits an aesthetician regularly for light chemical peels and has had successful minimally invasive surgical procedures in the past. An open-ended cosmetic consultation employing the LEAP method (see Chapter 16) would be effective in this case as the patient has specific thoughts and concerns he would like to address. The patient expresses a desire to soften his jawline

and augment the size of his lips modeled after the cosmetic result in one of his female colleagues. Classically masculine features include a prominent, sharp jawline and chin, thinner lips, and horizontal eyebrows, which this patient is looking to correct with cosmetic procedures [35]. Within a solely heteronormative construct this may be mistaken for BDD or gender dysphoria because the patient is looking for a feminized look. However, cosmetic providers should recall that aesthetic ideals reported in the literature are largely based on studies of heterosexual men and women. There is a growing movement of both male and female patients that desire an androgynous or gender-neutral appearance. Women want to have stronger jaw lines that are characteristically considered masculine, while men look to soften features with lip and chin augmentation [40, 41]. This new trend is likely driven by shifts in pop culture and a greater acceptance of all forms of gender expression. According to a 2017 Harris Poll, 35% of Generation Z and 12% of millennials identify as transgender or gender nonconforming [40]. In order to make their offices more inclusive, providers may consider expanding the typical medical intake form to include options for other gender identities outside of male and female, as well as preferred pronouns [42].

Case 7.3   The Patient Desiring Genital Augmentation

MS is a 42-year-old Caucasian man with history of high cholesterol, diabetes, and basal cell carcinoma who presents for cosmetic consultation. He sees a female dermatologist in your practice for annual skin examinations and androgenic alopecia, but he asked to be referred to you, a male provider, for his next cosmetic appointment. After some hesitation, he opens up and tells you that he is interested in exploring ways to improve the appearance of his

(Continued)

Case 7.3 (Continued)

genitals. For many years he has been worried that his penis is too small and that his scrotum has many wrinkles. He denies urologic or sexual dysfunction, but states that his ex-wife did not enjoy sexual intercourse. He would like to discuss some nonsurgical options that he read about on the Internet. On review of his social history, you find out that he was married to his high-school girlfriend for the last 20 years but got divorced 1 year ago. He has recently started dating again. Physical examination does not reveal micropenis.

Clinical Relevance and Implications

Genital enhancement and rejuvenation is an emerging field within cosmetic medicine. Dissatisfaction with penis size is quite prevalent in the heterosexual male population – with 45% of men reporting displeasure with their size compared to 15% of their female partners expressing dissatisfaction with their partner's size [22]. With the advent of dermal fillers and neurotoxins, aesthetic providers may be approached to perform penile or scrotal augmentation – procedures that were previously exclusively done by urologists or surgeons due to the invasive nature of traditional treatment options.

The overwhelming majority of patients that complain of small penis have normal length and girth, as well as normal physiologic function [43]. Patients with micropenis, defined as a penis that is less than 7.5 cm in length in erect length and less than 4 cm in flaccid length, should be referred to experienced urological reconstructive surgeons for evaluation of complex surgical management [43]. While penile augmentation is associated with high patient satisfaction [44], increasing the length and girth of penis size for cosmetic purposes remains highly controversial. Neurotoxin injections into the scrotum, colloquially referred to as "Scrotox," are used to reduce wrinkles, decrease sweating, and make the scrotum appear larger. Risks include intravascular injection and potential effect on sperm viability [45].

When a patient presents for consultation for penile or scrotal enhancement, a comprehensive medical and psychiatric history should be taken. Throughout the consultation, practitioners should remain vigilant for signs of pathologic psychological distress and frank BDD. Some general signs of BDD include mirror checking or avoidance, reassurance seeking, touching disliked areas, excessive exercise, comparing appearance with that of others, excessive tanning, and seeking multiple cosmetic procedures. These patients often have poor insight into the condition and will seek cosmetic or dermatological treatments to treat the perceived "defects" rather than confront the underlying dysmorphia. They are often hard to satisfy, and cosmetic procedures rarely improve their bodily perception. One in 50 men meet the criteria for BDD, which typically starts during teenage years and without proper intervention continues throughout adulthood The patient in the above case presentation displays several concerning signs of body dysmorphia. First, he describes preoccupation with penile size for many years despite objective clinical evidence of normal size and functioning. He is recently divorced and interested in starting to date again, which may indicate underlying insecurities of sexual performance and masculinity. In this case, the aesthetic provider may consider screening the patient for penile dysmorphic disorder (PDD) with the Cosmetic Procedure Screening Scale for PDD (COPS-P). This nine-point questionnaire has been validated to differentiate patients with small penis anxiety with PDD from those without PDD [22, 46]. If results are concerning, referral to a sexual health psychologist may be beneficial. BDD is covered in further detail in Chapter 15.

Conclusions

The cosmetic consultation is arguably more important when treating male patients compared to female patients. A clear, concise, but thorough consultation that covers the various treatment approaches, individual risks and benefits, expected outcomes, and anticipated costs will strengthen the patient–provider relationship and result in higher likelihood of treatment satisfaction. Provide sample before and after photos to further make these points concrete. Identify motivations and gender-specific behavioral patterns

that may inform the treatment plan. Male patients require specialized approaches and altered techniques for neurotoxin injections, soft tissue fillers, and chemical peels, among other procedures. It is critical that aesthetic providers familiarize themselves with ideal male anatomy, as it varies across a spectrum of different gender identities and cultural backgrounds.

References

1 Umberson, D. and Hughes, M. (1987). The impact of physical attractiveness on achievement and psychological well-being. *Soc. Psychol. Q* 60: 227–236.

2 Jagdeo, J., Keaney, T., Narurkar, V. et al. (2016). Facial treatment preferences among aesthetically oriented men. *Dermatol. Surg.* 42 (10): 1155–1163.

3 Bulygina, E., Mitteroecker, P., and Aiello, L. (2006). Ontogeny of facial dimorphism and patterns of individual development within one human population. *Am. J. Phys. Anthropol.* 131 (3): 432–443.

4 Hu, Y., Abbasi, N.U.H., Zhang, Y., and Chen, H. (2018). The effect of target sex, sexual dimorphism, and facial attractiveness on perceptions of target attractiveness and trustworthiness. *Front. Psychol.* 9: 942.

5 Little, A.C., Jones, B.C., and DeBruine, L.M. (2011). Facial attractiveness: evolutionary based research. *Philos. Trans. R. Soc. Lond. B Biol. Sci.* 366 (1571): 1638–1659.

6 DeBruine, L.M., Jones, B.C., Little, A.C. et al. (2006). Correlated preferences for facial masculinity and ideal or actual partner's masculinity. *Proc. Biol. Sci.* 273 (1592): 1355–1360.

7 Rossi, A.M., Fitzgerald, R., and Humphrey, S. (2017). Facial soft tissue augmentation in males: an anatomical and practical approach. *Dermatol. Surg.* 43 (2): 131–139.

8 Sedgh, J. (2018). The aesthetics of the upper face and brow: male and female differences. *Facial Plast. Surg.* 34 (2): 114–118.

9 Jones, I.T. and Fabi, S.G. (2018). The use of neurotoxins in the male face. *Dermatol. Clin.* 36 (1): 29–42.

10 Yalçınkaya, E., Cingi, C., Söken, H. et al. (2016). Aesthetic analysis of the ideal eyebrow shape and position. *Eur. Arch. Otorhinolaryngol* 273 (2): 305–310.

11 Rossi, A.M. (2014). Men's aesthetic dermatology. *Semin. Cutan. Med. Surg* 33 (4): 188–197.

12 Coleman, S.R. and Grover, R. (2006). The anatomy of the aging face: volume loss and changes in 3-dimensional topography. *Aesthet. Surg. J.* 26 (1): 4–9.

13 Somenek, M. (2018). Gender-related facial surgical goals. *Facial Plast. Surg.* 34 (5): 474–479.

14 Vashi, N.A., de Castro Maymone, M.B., and Kundu, R.V. (2016). Aging differences in ethnic skin. *J. Clin. Aesthet. Dermatol.* 9 (1): 31–38.

15 Choi, J.Y., Park, J.H., Javidnia, H., and Sykes, J.M. (2013). Effect of various facial angles and measurements on the ideal position of the nasal tip in the Asian patient population. *JAMA Facial Plast. Surg.* 15 (6): 417–421.

16 Naini, F.B., Cobourne, M.T., Garagiola, U. et al. (2016). Nasofrontal angle and nasal dorsal aesthetics: a quantitative investigation of idealized and normative values. *Facial Plast. Surg.* 32 (4): 444–451.

17 Guyuron, B. (2014). Discussion: the ideal nasolabial angle in rhinoplasty: a preference analysis of the general population. *Plast. Reconstr. Surg.* 134 (2): 211–213.

18 Mydlova, M., Dupej, J., Koudelova, J., and Veleminska, J. (2015). Sexual dimorphism of facial appearance in ageing human adults: a cross-sectional study. *Forensic Sci. Int.* 257: 519.e1–519.e9.

19 Mommaerts, M.Y. (2016). The ideal male jaw angle – an internet survey. *J. Craniomaxillofac. Surg.* 44 (4): 381–391.

20 Giacomoni, P.U., Mammone, T., and Teri, M. (2009). Gender-linked differences in human skin. *J. Dermatol. Sci.* 55 (3): 144–149.

21 Wysong, A., Kim, D., Joseph, T. et al. (2014). Quantifying soft tissue loss in the aging male face using magnetic resonance imaging. *Dermatol. Surg.* 40 (7): 786–793.

22 Choi, E.J. and Yafi, F.A. (2020). What is normal and who qualifies? Validated questionnaires for penile size assessment and body dysmorphic disorder. *J. Sex. Med.* 17 (7): 1242–1245.

23 Littara, A., Melone, R., Morales-Medina, J.C. et al. (2019). Cosmetic penile enhancement surgery: a 3-year single-centre retrospective clinical evaluation of 355 cases. *Sci. Rep.* 9 (1): 6323.

24 Veale, D., Miles, S., Read, J. et al. (2016). Relationship between self-discrepancy and worries about penis size in men with body dysmorphic disorder. *Body Image* 17: 48–56.

25 Ruppen-Greeff, N.K., Weber, D.M., Gobet, R., and Landolt, M.A. (2015). What is a good looking penis? How women rate the penile appearance of men with surgically corrected hypospadias. *J. Sex. Med.* 12 (8): 1737–1745.

26 Rieder, E.A., Mu, E.W., and Brauer, J.A. (2015). Men and cosmetics: social and psychological trends of an emerging demographic. *J. Drugs Dermatol.* 14 (9): 1023–1026.

27 Handler, M.Z. and Goldberg, D.J. (2018). Cosmetic concerns among men. *Dermatol. Clin.* 36 (1): 5–10.

28 Tripathi, R., Knusel, K.D., Ezaldein, H.H. et al. (2018). Association of demographic and socioeconomic characteristics with differences in use of outpatient dermatology services in the United States. *JAMA Dermatol.* 154 (11): 1286–1291.

29 Rossi, A.M., Eviatar, J., Green, J.B. et al. (2017). Signs of facial aging in men in a diverse, multinational study: timing and preventive behaviors. *Dermatol. Surg.* 43 (2): 210–220.

30 Skin Cancer Foundation (2012). New Survey Reveals Gender Divide Surrounding Skin Cancer Awareness and Prevention. Available from: https://www.prnewswire.com/ news-releases/new-survey-reveals-gender-divide-surrounding-skin-cancer-awareness-and-prevention-159696285.html (accessed 12 October 2020).

31 Elsner, P. (2012). Overview and trends in male grooming. *Br. J. Dermatol.* 166 (1): 2–5.

32 Crudele, J., Kim, E., Murray, K., and Regan, J. (2019). The importance of understanding consumer preferences for dermatologist recommended skin cleansing and care products. *J. Drugs Dermatol.* 18 (1): 75–79.

33 Girdwichai, N., Chanprapaph, K., and Vachiramon, V. (2018). Behaviors and attitudes toward cosmetic treatments among men. *J. Clin. Aesthet. Dermatol.* 11 (3): 42–48.

34 Draelos, Z.D. (2018). Cosmeceuticals for male skin. *Dermatol. Clin.* 36 (1): 17–20.

35 Cohen, B.E., Bashey, S., and Wysong, A. (2017). Literature review of cosmetic procedures in men: approaches and techniques are gender specific. *Am. J. Clin. Dermatol.* 18 (1): 87–96.

36 Henry, M. (2018). Cosmetic concerns among ethnic men. *Dermatol. Clin.* 36 (1): 11–16.

37 American Society of Plastic Surgeons (2019). New Survey Reveals Gender Divide Surrounding Skin Cancer Awareness and Prevention. Plastic Surgery Statistics Report. Available from: https://www.plasticsurgery. org/documents/news/statistics/2019/ plastic-surgery-statistics-full-report-2019.pdf (accessed 18 October 2020).

38 Chatham, D.R. (2005). Special considerations for the male patient: things I wish I knew when I started practice. *Facial Plast. Surg.* 21 (4): 232–239.

39 Keaney, T.C., Anolik, R., Braz, A. et al. (2018). The male aesthetic patient: facial anatomy, concepts of attractiveness, and treatment patterns. *J. Drugs Dermatol.* 17 (1): 19–28.

40 Hope, A. (2019, 3 Dec.). Inside the rise of gender-neutral cosmetic procedures. Men's Health. Available from: https://www.menshealth.com/grooming/a30085911/gender-neutral-cosmetic-procedures.

41 Oranges, C.M., Gohritz, A., Tremp, M., and Schaefer, D.J. (2016). Body contouring: the success of the androgynous model. *Plast. Reconstr. Surg. Glob. Open* 4 (4): e668.

42 Maragh-Bass, A.C., Torain, M., Adler, R. et al. (2017). Risks, benefits, and importance of collecting sexual orientation and gender identity data in healthcare settings: a multi-method analysis of patient and provider perspectives. *LGBT Health* 4 (2): 141–152.

43 Vardi, Y., Har-Shai, Y., Gil, T., and Gruenwald, I. (2008). A critical analysis of penile enhancement procedures for patients with normal penile size: surgical techniques, success, and complications. *Eur. Urol.* 54 (5): 1042–1050.

44 Yang, D.Y., Jeong, H.C., Ko, K. et al. (2020). Comparison of clinical outcomes between hyaluronic and polylactic acid filler injections for penile augmentation in men reporting a small penis: a multicenter, patient-blinded/evaluator-blinded, non-inferiority, randomized comparative trial with 18 months of follow-up. *J. Clin. Med.* 9 (4): 1024.

45 Ramelli, E., Brault, N., Tierny, C. et al. (2020). Intrascrotal injection of botulinum toxin a, a male genital aesthetic demand: technique and limits. *Prog. Urol.* 30 (6): 312–317.

46 Veale, D., Miles, S., Read, J. et al. (2015). Penile dysmorphic disorder: development of a screening scale. *Arch. Sex. Behav.* 44 (8): 2311–2321.

8

The Cosmetic Consultation

Anatomy and Psychology – The Transgender Patient

Brian Ginsberg

Chelsea Skin & Laser, New York, NY, USA
Department of Dermatology, Icahn School of Medicine at Mount Sinai, New York, NY, USA

Introduction

With aesthetic injectables available and advancing since the 1980s and the continued development of other cosmetic technologies and procedures, physicians have been able to finesse their skills at providing optimal rejuvenation and enhancements for their patients. However, the use of these products for the gender affirmation of transgender individuals has only recently begun to become established. With approximately 700 000 transgender individuals in the United States, and their presence becoming more exposed and accepted in our culture, the proper care for them as patients – both practically and compassionately – is of growing importance.

Transgender individuals are those whose gender identity does not match their sex assigned at birth (of note, the term cisgender signifies concordance of identity and assigned sex) [1]. This term is irrespective of appearance, medications taken, or procedures undergone. For those physically transitioning, having an appearance that matches one's identity can be of great significance. In one cross-sectional study looking at priorities for transformation, most transwomen (transgender women, assigned male at birth) preferred procedures for their face, as compared to transmen (transgender men, assigned female at birth) who preferred their chests [2]. This likely in part reflects what they feel has the greatest impact on self and public perception. Of note, genital procedures were chosen last by both. Perhaps most importantly, gender affirmation procedures have been shown to have a significantly positive psychological impact, improving quality of life measurements across many fields [3, 4].

Anatomy

To help a patient affirm their gender, it is imperative to understand the key differences between the standard phenotypic presentations of cisgender men and women [5]. Certain facial features are so nuanced between men and women that often a person can identify somebody's gender by one feature alone (Table 8.1). There is also significant sexual dimorphism between a masculine and feminine body, beyond the chest and genitalia [6]. On average, women have a smaller waist when compared to their hips, and their hips are also customarily larger than in men. Body fat percentage is generally higher in women than in men. Men are

Essential Psychiatry for the Aesthetic Practitioner, First Edition. Edited by Evan A. Rieder and Richard G. Fried.
© 2021 John Wiley & Sons Ltd. Published 2021 by John Wiley & Sons Ltd.

Table 8.1 Facial differences between traditionally masculine and feminine faces.

Feature	Masculine	Feminine
Forehead	Wide with prominent supraorbital ridge	Large and smooth
Eyebrow	Flat	Arched
Eyes	Deeper-set	Open-appearing
Nose	Larger, wider	Smaller and upturned
Cheeks	Flat, broad	Full, angled
Jaw	Square-shaped	Heart-shaped
Lips	Thin	Full
Chin	Long and square	Thin and pointed

also more visibly hairy, with more terminal hairs on the face, chest, abdomen, and back (women have more vellus hair, comparatively).

Hormones used for medical transitioning may have already started the process of masculinizing or feminizing a patient's face, scalp, and body [2]. Muscle and fat redistribution is fairly universal. Testosterone may induce male-pattern hair loss yet increased facial and body hair, and many transmen report changes to their facial contours, especially their jaw, cheeks, and chin. Estrogen reduces facial hair, although not always completely, and many transwomen report significant structural changes to their cheeks and lips. Changes often take up to two years of being on therapy to fully achieve, and often take longer. For this reason, many patients may be looking for only temporary enhancements, especially early in their treatment, as they wait for their natural changes to plateau.

Structuring the Consult

Language

It is important to recognize that a patient's visit starts long before they meet the provider. Transgender patients are especially more likely to have experienced a negative healthcare experience in the past, and may come bearing feelings of reservation, anxiety, anger, or guilt, and care should be taken to respect and understand this [7]. The visit can become an opportunity to show your patient that care can be provided with optimal cultural competence. All staff members, especially those with direct patient interaction, should be fully trained on the proper way to address and care for transgender patients. Additionally, the office itself should be welcoming, including having gender neutral restrooms or a trans-affirming restroom policy. Other ways of showing immediate trans-inclusivity include having transgender individuals on your website and in-office literature (Table 8.2) [8].

The patient intake form should include both legal and gender-affirming options for patients. They should be able to write their legal name as well as their preferred name. Many cisgender patients who also do not go by their legal name will appreciate the opportunity to write a preferred name. A patient should be given sufficient options for documenting gender (note: the form should say "gender" not "sex", as sex denotes chromosomes rather than identity). One way to do this is to have the gender option as a write-in rather than having things to circle, especially as patients may identify outside of the gender binary, including identities such as agender, genderqueer, and gender nonconforming. It is equally important to ask a patient for their preferred pronouns. Again, this may

Table 8.2 Checklist to make your office more trans-friendly.

- Staff education, including pronoun use
- Inclusive intake forms
- Unisex restrooms or inclusive restroom policy
- LGBT magazines, books, and/or pamphlets
- Post a visible nondiscrimination policy

Table 8.3 Common terminology.

Term	Definition	Examples
Sex	Biological trait assigned at birth based on chromosomes and/or genitalia	Male, female, intersex
Gender (gender identity)	Self-identified trait reflecting attitudes, feelings, and behaviors culturally associated with it	Man, woman, transgender man (transman), transgender woman (transwoman), agender, genderqueer, genderfluid, gender nonconforming, nonbinary, and more
Gender expression	Physical appearance or behaviors that express gender identity (though may not reflect it)	Masculine, feminine, androgynous
Cisgender	One's gender identity aligns with one's sex assigned at birth	
Transgender	One's gender identity does not align with one's sex at birth	
Transsexual	Historical medical term that was used for transgender individuals who have undergone medical or surgical transitioning	
Cross dresser	One who dresses as the opposite gender but does not identity as it	Note: a "Drag Queen" or "Drag King" is a cross dresser who does so for entertainment
		Note: a "Transvestite" is a cross dresser who does so for pleasure
Gender dysphoria	Discomfort with the incongruence of one's gender and sex assigned at birth (has DSM-5 full definition)	
Preferred pronouns	The pronoun a person chooses to refer to themself	She/her/hers, they/them/their, zie/hir/hirs, and others
Sexual orientation	Identity based on attraction	Gay, lesbian, bisexual, queer, pansexual
Sexual behavior	Reflects with whom somebody has sexual activity	Has sex with men, women, or both

fall outside the gender binary, with pronoun sets including (but not limited to) they/them/theirs, zie/hir/hirs, and ze/zir/zirs. Proper gender and pronoun identifiers should be clearly documented so that all staff members know how to communicate with and about the patient appropriately so as to create a maximally comfortable and inclusive environment. (See Table 8.3.)

Medical and Surgical History

There are also unique aspects of the medical and surgical history that may be notably relevant during the intake. It is important to know which hormones/medications are being taken and for how long [9]. This may make it easier to predict where in the natural transformation process the patient is, and perhaps also to predict where it may go. Feminizing individuals often take estrogen with or without an antiandrogen, such as spironolactone or a 5-alpha reductase inhibitor. Masculinizing individuals often take one of many forms of testosterone. It is also important to ask about gender affirmation surgery, including facial surgeries, "top surgery" (chest/breast surgery) and "bottom surgery" (the creation of neogenitalia), and, if relevant, the patient's plans to do so [10]. For masculinizing individuals, it may be relevant to ask about if they have had a hysterectomy or oophorectomy. This procedure may or may not accompany bottom surgery, and is sometimes done on its own regardless of bottom surgery. This issue has implications regarding pregnancy potential (individuals who have their uterus and ovaries can still get pregnant while taking testosterone, even after bottom surgery, as the vagina is often maintained) [11]. Such a line of inquiry has come to be known as taking an "organ inventory." It is essential to remember that many transgender individuals have no desire to have any hormonal or surgical interventions, so it should never be assumed that they have done or are planning to do so. In general, when caring for any patient, in particular transgender individuals, it is best to never make assumptions about history, practices, or desires.

Nonsurgical Interventions

Another aspect of relevant history to ascertain is prior nonsurgical interventions. It is important to ask, in an unassuming manner, what products were injected and by whom. The rates of illicit filler use (including use of products from nonmedical silicone to cement) have been reported to be between 20 and 50% among transgender individuals in the United States, and even higher in some other countries [12–15]. Patients may come in for correction of prior work, treatment of consequences of illicit use (i.e. granulomas, infections), or treatment overlying prior work. With a history of illicit use, it may be warranted to assume potential presence of an underlying infection or inactive biofilm.

Treatment Step 1: Skin Care Principles and Preferences

Hormones have lasting effects on skin quality, mostly through sebum stimulation or reduction [16]. Within months of use, estrogens dramatically reduce sebum production. For many individuals, this improves skin quality, reduces acne, and even stimulates neocollagenesis. Some transgender women, however, may present with complaints of dryness or sensitivity as a consequence. There are also reports of nail fragility. Gentle and hydrating products should be encouraged for such patients if applicable.

More significant is testosterone's effect on increasing sebum production. While the effect is more gradual, many transmen experience severe oiliness and consequently acne. This escalation may last two years or more [17]. Elevated body mass index (BMI) has been shown to worsen this severity. This can be further intensified by smoking. Both areas – BMI and smoking – can be addressed with good patient counseling [18]. Treatment of elevated skin sebum and severe acne is identical to that in cisgender men, with the only exception being with the use of iPledge for isotretinoin prescriptions. At the time of publication of this book, transgender men who have a uterus and ovaries, even if on testosterone, must still be registered as females of reproductive potential [19–22]. Therefore a considerate and thorough conversation must be had with the patient without allowing iPledge to be a barrier to a potentially necessary medication. It is imperative to balance such a discussion with a clear understanding of patients' potential frustrations and hesitations.

Treatment Step 2: Minimal-Risk Procedural Options

Above all, it is always most important to understand what the patient truly desires. Do they want a specific feature modified? Do they simply want to look more feminine or masculine? Are they nonbinary and hope to find an aesthetic somewhere in between?

For many facial differences, injectable neurotoxins and soft tissue fillers can be utilized effectively to achieve the desired outcome (Figure 8.1) [23, 24]. Neurotoxins can affect forehead texture, eyebrow shape, apparent eye size, and jaw contour (via masseter injections). Fillers can affect the shape of the brows, nose, cheeks, lips, chin, and gonial angle. Some of these features can also be enhanced with fat transfer, liposuction, or chemical lipolysis.

Another common concern for many transgender individuals is their hair [25]. Transwomen may have male-pattern hair loss from their innate hormones, especially if they

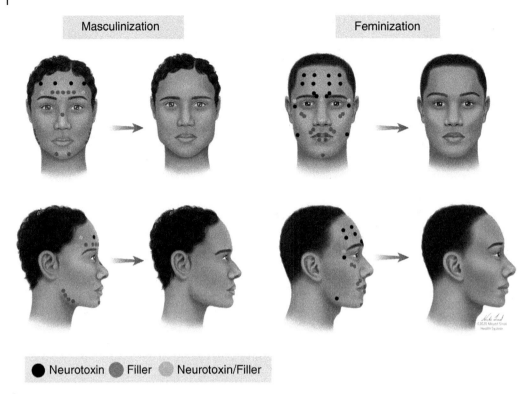

Figure 8.1 Applications of cosmetic injectables for facial masculinization and feminization. *Source:* ©2020 Mount Sinai Health System.

started their medical transition after the loss had already begun. Medical options for these patients include minoxidil, finasteride/dutasteride, and/or spironolactone [26]. However, for those who have lost substantial hair, transplantation may ultimately be the only option. For those aesthetic practitioners performing hair transplantation, it is essential to recognize that a feminine hairline is different from a masculine one in that it is lower and more rounded [27]. For transmen, testosterone causes androgenetic alopecia in two-thirds of individuals. Nonetheless, many consider this a desired or more masculine trait. While both minoxidil and finasteride remain suitable options in the same manner that they are used for cisgender men, it is unclear as to finasteride's effects on interfering with testosterone's development of wanted secondary sex characteristics; it may be in one's best interest to avoid use until such characteristics are fully developed. One study did show

that such characteristics were not reversed once starting finasteride [28]. Additionally, while some do desire to have a more full scalp, some transmen instead seek hair transplants for their beards or eyebrows.

Hair reduction is perhaps the most sought-out procedure by transgender individuals. In one study, it was the most common facial procedure done by transgender women, above both surgery and injectables [2]. Estrogens do reduce facial and body hair, but often not sufficiently [16]. Permanent facial hair removal could have a significant psychological benefit for a transwoman who otherwise has to live with the burden and reminder of having to shave her beard daily.

Individuals may also come for hair removal preoperatively for gender-affirming bottom surgery [29]. For vaginoplasty (the creation of the neovagina from penile or scrotal skin), hair removal is necessary to reduce intravaginal hair-induced bezoars, infection, and inflammation.

For phalloplasty (the creation of a penis from a flap or graft, usually from the arm or leg), hair removal is important as to not have hair run the full length of the neophallus or within the neourethra. Patients are often familiar with the area that needs to be epilated, but becoming familiar with these procedures would be helpful for consultation and treatment planning. Depending on the patient's skin and hair color, either laser or electrolysis may be a preferred option.

Both bottom and top surgery, especially mastectomies, may lead to scars. Often a mastectomy scar can be quite obvious – whether hypertrophic, dyspigmented, or both – making it uncomfortable for someone to take their shirt off. Many scars can be improved with techniques ranging from simple injections to lasers.

Finally, body contouring may be sought for a more complete physical transformation. Liposuction and fat-grafting, with or without implants, are the best methods of obtaining these outcomes. Radiofrequency, cryolipolysis, or ultrasound procedures can be added for more subtle enhancements, with realistic expectations set.

Setting Expectations

There are many benefits to nonsurgical approaches to facial gender affirmation. Patients may not wish to seek a permanent change, either because their hormones have not fully induced natural modification or because they are still understanding their own self-perception. They may not be candidates for surgery for medical or financial reasons. They may not have the time to recover from a more invasive approach. It is important to have the discussion with your patients that, while excellent outcomes are achievable with nonsurgical interventions, there are limitations. For certain outcomes, surgery may be the preferred, and sometimes the only, option for obtaining the desired results.

Treating Minors

Individuals are starting the transitioning process earlier and earlier every year, with many taking medications to alter puberty to maximize their adult gender-affirmed appearance. Due to the extreme changes in facial and body structure during adolescence, facial surgery is often not ideal or advised. Someone in their late-teens may desire a specific modification to help them feel more comfortable in their own skin, especially in an already difficult time in their lives. Nonsurgical procedures provide the benefit of being generally safe, reversible, and short-lived. For an adolescent presenting to your office for such a procedure, parental consent must be obtained if the patient is under the age of 18. Some medical ethicists feel that aesthetic procedures are only appropriate if there has first been a mental health evaluation [30].

Case Studies

Case 8.1   Acne and Hair Loss in a Transgender Man

A 25-year-old transgender man presents with acne and hair loss. He has always had moderate acne of the face, chest, and back that he was able to keep under control with topical medications and the occasional oral antibiotic for acne flares, but he states that this is unlike anything he has ever had. He says that it started to get bad four months after he started "T" and is only getting worse. He currently uses an over-the-counter benzoyl peroxide 4% wash in the morning and prescription tazarotene 0.1% cream at night.

(Continued)

Case 8.1 (Continued)

His last dermatologist most recently also prescribed him oral doxycycline. However, he stopped after two months because he didn't think it was working and he didn't feel comfortable at the other doctor's office. Around the same time he also noticed hair loss that has been progressing. His medical history is notable for depression. He takes testosterone and fluoxetine daily. He started testosterone eight months ago. His surgical history is negative. His social history is notable for smoking, gay sexual orientation, and sexual activity with men as the receptive partner in both his genitals and anus. His gender identity is male. Pronouns are he/him/his. Physical examination shows severe nodulocystic facial acne with scarring and male-pattern hair loss. His chest examination reveals an elastic bandage tightly wrapped around the chest and back, which the patient was reluctant to remove, but upon your understanding discussion revealed similarly severe acne and scarring.

Clinical Relevance and Implications

This case represents the most common transition-related visit encountered by this author with transgender patients. This patient is coming due to poor experiences with prior clinicians. In fact, one-third of transgender individuals report having had a negative healthcare experience due to their gender identity, and almost a quarter of individuals have subsequently avoided healthcare when needed. For these patients it is especially important to create a welcoming atmosphere, with well-educated staff, affirming restroom policies, inclusive forms, and appropriate use of pronouns. His reluctance to undo his chest binding may also be reflective of negative experiences in the past, or rather personal discomfort with his body. Acne is one of the most common conditions treated by dermatologists in all patients, and this is especially true in trans men, who may refer to their testosterone therapy as "T." This patient would be a good candidate for isotretinoin. Even though he takes testosterone, his surgical history is negative, which implies that he is still capable of getting pregnant, especially as he has receptive sex with men. Of note, even without bottom surgery, many trans men prefer not to refer to their genitalia as a vagina. He would have to be registered on iPledge as a female of reproductive potential. Even if he did not have receptive sex, he would still have to be classified this way, just as a celibate nun would. Depression, as noted in this patient, is much more common in transgender individuals than in the general population, and should be properly managed and monitored during treatment [31]. Smoking has been linked to worsening the acneigenic effects of testosterone, so cessation counseling would be relevant as part of the discussion. Also relevant would be a discussion about chest binding – that he should consider a better-fitted binding device that more evenly distributes the compression and is more breathable [32, 33]. If he is planning on getting top surgery he should speak with his surgeon about isotretinoin. Some surgeons prefer that patients are off this medication for a certain period of time before having the surgery. As for his hair loss, treatment would be analogous to medications available to a cisgender male: topical minoxidil, finasteride, and transplant surgery. The one caveat is that, being on testosterone for only eight months, it is likely that the development of desired secondary sex characteristics (voice change, body hair, body shape) is not complete, and it is not clear the degree that finasteride has on those continued changes. Therefore the current recommendation would be to consider delaying the initiation of finasteride until those changes have plateaued.

Case 8.2 Aesthetic Consultation with a Nonbinary Patient

A 40-year-old individual presents for aesthetic consultation. They say they have had many aesthetic consultations and procedures. They are looking for more feminine lips and eyes, but otherwise do not want to change the shape of their face. They said that the last time they had their lips injected was six months ago in Thailand. They are concerned that there is still a nodule that they can feel in their lower lip which sometimes can hurt. They do not take any hormones or have had any surgeries. Physical examination reveals a masculine-appearing patient with a full beard and a traditionally male wardrobe. Examination of the mouth reveals a 2-mm, red, tender nodule within the mucosal aspect of the lower lip.

soften crow's feet and arch the brows may help create this desired effect. Before starting these procedures, a more detailed history about their prior filler use should be obtained. Thailand, for example, has one of the highest rates of illicit product use, approaching 68% in some reports. The presence of a red, tender nodule is highly concerning for illicit use. All inflammatory nodules should be treated for infection unless one is otherwise confident of an alternative cause. This is especially important to consider before any injection of intralesional glucocorticoids to reduce the nodule or additional filler for augmentation. Treatment should include mycobacterial coverage, with a sample regimen including four to six weeks of minocycline [34]. One may also consider tissue sampling of the nodule for culture. After any infection has been treated or excluded, management of the residual nodule and going forward with lip volumization can be considered.

Clinical Relevance and Implications

As with all patients, the aesthetic consultation of a transgender patient should be geared toward a patient's desired outcomes. While some patients come in and say things such as "make me look younger" or ". . . more beautiful," the statement from transgender individuals may be closer to "I would like to look more feminine." Nevertheless, it should never be assumed that a patient desires to look more feminine or masculine, especially if they identify somewhere on the nonbinary aspect of the gender spectrum. For this patient, they may prefer a predominantly masculine appearance with some feminine attributes, such as their mouth and eyes. Simple lip volumization with soft tissue fillers along with periorbital neurotoxin to

Conclusions

Aesthetic practitioners of a range of educational backgrounds can play a large role in the physical transformation of transgender individuals. Understanding basic anatomical differences between masculine and feminine features and the medical and surgical interventions available to the transgender population allows any provider to utilize their core knowledge to aid in the transitioning process. As important is the understanding of the psychological implications of a transgender individual's medical experience, both prior to and during their appointment, and providing a culturally competent approach to meeting their medical and personal needs.

References

1 GLAAD (2020). Transgender FAQ. Available from: https://www.glaad.org/transgender/transfaq.

2 Ginsberg, B., Calderon, M., Seminara, N., and Day, D. (2016). A potential role for the dermatologist in the physical transformation

of transgender people: a survey of attitudes and practices within the transgender community. *Journal of the American Academy of Dermatology* 74 (2): 303–308.

3 Wernick, J., Busa, S., Matouk, K. et al. (2019). A systematic review of the psychological benefits of gender-affirming surgery. *Urologic Clinics of North America* 46 (4): 475–486.

4 Owen-Smith, A., Gerth, J., Sineath, R. et al. (2018). Association between gender confirmation treatments and perceived gender congruence, body image satisfaction, and mental health in a cohort of transgender individuals. *Journal of Sexual Medicine.* 15 (4): 591–600.

5 Deschamps-Braly, J. (2018). Facial gender confirmation surgery. *Clinics in Plastic Surgery.* 45 (3): 323–331.

6 Bredella, M. (2017). Sex differences in body composition. *Advances in Experimental Medicine and Biology* 1043: 9–27.

7 Bradford, J., Reisner, S., Honnold, J., and Xavier, J. (2013). Experiences of transgender-related discrimination and implications for health: results from the Virginia transgender health initiative study. *American Journal of Public Health* 103 (10): 1820–1829.

8 Coren, J., Coren, C., Pagliaro, S., and Weiss, L. (2011). Assessing your office for care of lesbian, gay, bisexual, and transgender patients. *The Health Care Manager* 30 (1): 66–70.

9 T'Sjoen, G., Arcelus, J., Gooren, L. et al. (2018). Endocrinology of transgender medicine. *Endocrine Reviews* 40 (1): 97–117.

10 Selvaggi, G. and Bellringer, J. (2011). Gender reassignment surgery: an overview. *Nature Reviews Urology* 8 (5): 274–282.

11 Light, A., Obedin-Maliver, J., Sevelius, J., and Kerns, J. (2014). Transgender men who experienced pregnancy after female-to-male gender transitioning. *Obstetrics & Gynecology* 124 (6): 1120–1127.

12 Xavier, J., Bobbin, M., Singer, B., and Budd, E. (2005). A needs assessment of transgendered people of color living in Washington, DC. *International Journal of Transgenderism* 8 (2–3): 31–47.

13 Nemoto, T., Operario, D., and Keatley, J. (2005). Health and social services for male-to-female transgender persons of color in San Francisco. *International Journal of Transgenderism* 8 (2–3): 5–19.

14 Silva-Santisteban, A., Raymond, H., Salazar, X. et al. (2011). Understanding the HIV/AIDS epidemic in transgender women of Lima, Peru: results from a sero-epidemiologic study using respondent driven sampling. *AIDS and Behavior* 16 (4): 872–881.

15 Guadamuz, T., Wimonsate, W., Varangrat, A. et al. (2010). HIV prevalence, risk behavior, hormone use and surgical history among transgender persons in Thailand. *AIDS and Behavior* 15 (3): 650–658.

16 Giltay, E. and Gooren, L. (2000). Effects of sex steroid deprivation/administration on hair growth and skin sebum production in transsexual males and females. *Journal of Clinical Endocrinology & Metabolism* 85 (8): 2913–2921.

17 Motosko, C., Zakhem, G., Pomeranz, M., and Hazen, A. (2018). Acne: a side-effect of masculinizing hormonal therapy in transgender patients. *British Journal of Dermatology* 180 (1): 26–30.

18 Park, J., Carter, E., and Larson, A. (2019). Risk factors for acne development in the first 2 years after initiating masculinizing testosterone therapy among transgender men. *Journal of the American Academy of Dermatology* 81 (2): 617–618.

19 Katz, K. (2016). Transgender patients, isotretinoin, and US Food and Drug Administration-mandated risk evaluation and mitigation strategies. *JAMA Dermatology* 152 (5): 513.

20 Rieder, E., Nagler, A., and Leger, M. (2016). In response to Ginsberg et al.: "A potential role for the dermatologist in the physical transformation of transgender people: a survey of attitudes and practices within the transgender community".

Journal of the American Academy of Dermatology 75 (2): e73.

21 Watchmaker, J., Watchmaker, L., and Abbott, J. (2019). Pink or blue? Unpacking the packaging of iPLEDGE. *Journal of the American Academy of Dermatology* 80 (6): e167.

22 Yeung, H., Chen, S., Katz, K., and Stoff, B. (2016). Prescribing isotretinoin in the United States for transgender individuals: ethical considerations. *Journal of the American Academy of Dermatology* 75 (3): 648–651.

23 Ascha, M., Swanson, M., Massie, J. et al. (2018). Nonsurgical management of facial masculinization and feminization. *Aesthetic Surgery Journal* 39 (5): NP123–NP137.

24 Dhingra, N., Bonati, L., Wang, E. et al. (2019). Medical and aesthetic procedural dermatology recommendations for transgender patients undergoing transition. *Journal of the American Academy of Dermatology* 80 (6): 1712–1721.

25 Gao, Y., Maurer, T., and Mirmirani, P. (2018). Understanding and addressing hair disorders in transgender individuals. *American Journal of Clinical Dermatology* 19 (4): 517–527.

26 Stevenson, M., Wixon, N., and Safer, J. (2016). Scalp hair regrowth in hormone-treated transgender woman. *Transgender Health.* 1 (1): 202–204.

27 Bared, A. and Epstein, J. (2019). Hair transplantation techniques for the transgender patient. *Facial Plastic Surgery Clinics of North America* 27 (2): 227–232.

28 Moreno-Arrones, O., Becerra, A., and Vano-Galvan, S. (2017). Therapeutic

experience with oral finasteride for androgenetic alopecia in female-to-male transgender patients. *Clinical and Experimental Dermatology* 42 (7): 743–748.

29 Zhang, W., Garrett, G., Arron, S., and Garcia, M. (2016). Laser hair removal for genital gender affirming surgery. *Translational Andrology and Urology* 5 (3): 381–387.

30 Waldman, R., Waldman, S., and Grant-Kels, J. (2018). The ethics of performing noninvasive, reversible gender-affirming procedures on transgender adolescents. *Journal of the American Academy of Dermatology* 79 (6): 1166–1168.

31 Campos-Muñoz, L., López-De Lara, D., Conde-Taboada, A. et al. (2020). Depression in transgender adolescents under treatment with isotretinoin. *Clinical and Experimental Dermatology* 45 (5): 615–616.

32 Jarrett, B., Corbet, A., Gardner, I. et al. (2018). Chest binding and care seeking among transmasculine adults: a cross-sectional study. *Transgender Health* 3 (1): 170–178.

33 Peitzmeier, S., Gardner, I., Weinand, J. et al. (2016). Health impact of chest binding among transgender adults: a community-engaged, cross-sectional study. *Culture, Health & Sexuality* 19 (1): 64–75.

34 Styperek, A., Bayers, S., Beer, M., and Beer, K. (2013). Nonmedical-grade injections of permanent fillers: medical and medicolegal considerations. *Journal of Clinical and Aesthetic Dermatology* 6 (4): 22–29.

Part III

Perception

9

Aesthetic Interventions and the Perception of the Self

Quality of Life and Patient Reported Outcomes

Danielle Weitzer[1] and Richard G. Fried[2]

[1] *Department of Psychiatry, Rowan University School of Osteopathic Medicine, Stratford, NJ, USA*
[2] *Yardley Dermatology Associates, Yardley, PA, USA*

Introduction

The human attribute of facial and body attractiveness has long been portrayed as a genetic gift, allowing potential access to fame and fortune. Contemporary societies purvey strong messages and images via innumerable media sources, providing us with coveted ideals for beauty. These pervasive and overwhelming messages serve as the "ordained governance" of beauty, thus ultimately directing and orchestrating the fantasized outcomes of the ideal cosmetic intervention. From these portrayals, our patients can be motivated to pursue appropriate and truly therapeutic cosmetic interventions that can improve their cognitive, emotional, and functional status. The intrapsychic and psychosocial improvements can be liberating and life changing. Traditionally, the term "cosmetic" suggests that the procedure is not necessary, elective in nature, and without medical or functional implications. We suggest that the designation of such a procedure as purely cosmetic may diminish its importance and functional benefits.

The positive emotional changes that result from cosmetic interventions are often much deeper than the objective appearance itself. Sadly, many individuals believe that they are not entitled to such "superficial indulgences" and that their genetic appearance lies too far from societal ideals of beauty to warrant or justify any attempt at enhancement. This is a sad and incorrect assumption since the real-world experience of cosmetic clinicians and the scientific data suggest that well-chosen cosmetic interventions can profoundly enhance the feelings and functioning of people. Demonstrated consistently through patient-reported outcomes (PROs), aesthetic procedures have substantial impact on metrics beyond anatomic improvement and aesthetic correction [1].

As one's appearance changes, the perception of the self and others may change, which often does influence our cognitive dialogs, intrapsychic world, functional status, and many of our lifestyle choices. In many populations, these interventions can even improve functional status and be ultimately lifesaving. This chapter utilizes over 30 years of clinical experience to adopt a narrative approach in exploring how cosmetic procedures can change these factors, with a real-life case example and a discussion on how functionality and quality of life may, in fact, be the most significant outcomes following aesthetic treatment. Though undeniably important measurements of patient satisfaction, PROs will not be discussed in granular detail. For additional information on PROs see the References list.

Perception of Self

Self-perception is a very individualized process which can, in and of itself, shape a person's entire identity and influence how one experiences all aspects of their life. It has long been recognized that facial and body appearance has a direct link to self-perception [2]. In addition, facial expressions serve as cues to an individual's underlying mood and personality style, thus influencing how others perceive them. People who are happy with their facial appearance are often more confident, outgoing, and energetic [3]. Outward signs of aging and "wear and tear" can also impact one's self-perception when consciously or subconsciously interpreted as stigmata of deterioration and decline. Restoration of a younger facial appearance can diminish some of the distress and anxiety associated with the visible signs of aging, leading to more positive perceptions and expectations.

When considering a youthful appearance, light-reflective patterns can strongly affect our perceptions. For example, the full and elevated malar eminence of the young face easily reflects light, thus brightening the upper cheeks and the eyes, creating a "bright eyed," well-rested, and energetic appearance. With age, there is often deflation and downward descent of the upper cheeks, resulting in a flatter, duller, and less-reflective architecture. This may give the appearance of being tired and "drained." In addition, there is often an elongation of the cheeks secondary to the upper cheek deflation, causing redundancy of the nasolabial folds and accentuation of the pre-jowl sulcus. Colloquial expressions such as "Why the long face?" illustrate the perceived association of sadness and lackluster emotional states with these facial architectural changes. Numerous soft tissue fillers have been shown to be effective in restoring a younger appearance, both by observers and as reported by patients themselves [4, 5].

Almost inevitably for all of us, the aging process at some point will remind us that we are "not what we used to be." For some, this can precipitate the proverbial "midlife crisis" [6]. The "crisis" reflects a realization that there will be deterioration and decline to come and that the "best years" may be behind us, with a limited time ahead of us to pursue our goals and pleasures. As the signs of aging become more evident, an internal dialogue of "gloom and doom" can evolve. For most, this is mildly intrusive, but for some it can become dominant obsession and perseveration. Cosmetic intervention can be helpful in "talking back" to the negative ideation and providing visible "proof" of preserved youthfulness; this can be liberating both emotionally and functionally. For the smaller population with persistent perseveration and depressive symptoms, treatment with a psychiatrist or psychologist may be necessary.

Beyond architecture, perception of self is also influenced by neoplasms and functional change. Dyspigmentation, scars, ectasias, poikiloderma, sebaceous hyperplasia, seborrheic keratoses, and textural abnormalities all can negatively affect self-perception, based on their cosmetic appearance and symbolic significance. The arrival of the first seborrheic keratosis may elicit memories of an encrusted parent or grandparent, thus arousing the fear that they will follow suit. Years of clinical experience dictates that though such lesions are often dismissed by healthcare providers as benign or insignificant, they can in fact be associated with significant feelings of anxiety and depression. Affected individuals' self-perceptions often include descriptors such as ugly, dirty, old, repulsive, and disgusting. Persistent scars may serve as perpetual reminders of trauma and/or ridicule and rejection that occurred as a result.

Clearly, cosmetic interventions including lasers and lights, soft tissue fillers, neurotoxins, chemical peels, surgical intervention, and beyond can have profoundly meaningful benefits for our patients. As with all cosmetic interventions, it is essential to assess that expectations are realistic, appropriate, and attainable. If they are not, both the patient and clinician may bear the burden of that dissatisfaction for an extended period of time [7].

Perception by Others

Ideally, we wish that our facial appearance sends accurate emotional messages that convey to others only what we wish to share. Unfortunately, anatomy, physiology, and aging can prohibit or distort these messages. By way of example, dynamic wrinkling in the glabellar region can make us look angry, judgmental, disapproving, stressed, and distressed. Similarly, downturned angulation of the oral commissures can be interpreted as sadness, anger, or disapproval. Injection of neurotoxins and fillers can be extremely effective in reducing or eliminating unintended conveyance of negative emotions. Specifically, a softer glabella and neutral oral commissures allow for a more neutral, kind, and positive appearance. This kinder and gentler appearance decreases the likelihood that others with whom the person interacts will erect a defensive posture in anticipation of negativity. As the interaction with the other person proceeds, the treated glabella remains largely relaxed, while other voluntary facial expressions such as upward or lateral movement of the oral commissures, smiles, soft nonjudgmental eyes, and kind words can be helpful in enhancing our likability. In essence, neurotoxins and fillers can give patients more control over the outcomes of their interactions with others.

In contrast to the above "accurate conveyance of emotional states," neurotoxins and fillers can be helpful in hiding negative thoughts and emotional reactions. It can be difficult or impossible to consciously or willfully inhibit glabellar contractions in the face of frustration or disgust. With well-placed neurotoxins on board, the lack of evident "glabellar disgust" can avert negative social or business interactions.

Facial scarring can significantly affect how others perceive us. Individuals with facial scarring are frequently judged by others as less attractive, less confident, less happy, less healthy, and less successful [8]. In addition, they are more likely to be perceived as insecure and shy [8]. Given these data, it is likely that the amelioration of facial scarring increases the probability of more favorable appraisals by others and more opportunities in vocational and social spheres.

Interestingly and sadly, anecdotal experience indicates that individuals perceived as older are more often perceived and portrayed as "grumpy and mean." Indeed, the health problems, physical pain, and declining functional status that accompany aging can lead to a more distressed and irritable appearance. Therefore the stigmata of aging can and do often lead to both negative appraisals and negative expectations from others [9]. Cosmetic interventions can objectively and subjectively allow the aging individual to look and feel better [1]. The intervention need not be large or dramatic in nature. Interventions ranging from topical anti-aging products to plastic surgery have the potential to improve mood and activity levels while simultaneously reducing intrapsychic suffering.

Speaking with patients regarding the cosmetic intervention, it may be helpful for the clinician to refer to the fact that cosmetic interventions can be empowering. Following cosmetic intervention, patients often exude a more friendly, confident, energetic, happier, and healthier appearance [10]. While results may vary, these positive perceptions by others increase the probability of successful interactions with others. For more on the evidence behind observer reported outcomes see Chapter 10.

Outcome Studies

Cosmetic interventions have the potential to give patients both objective and subjective improvements beyond purely anatomic correction. Many studies of neurotoxins have demonstrated improved satisfaction metrics such as perception of youthfulness, self-confidence, attractiveness, and rested appearance. Improvements have even been observed in quality of life and mental health outcomes [1]. Similar quality of life outcomes have been noted with well-placed soft tissue fillers, particularly when used in multimodal treatment with botulinum toxins [11–13].

While the primary focus of cosmetic literature has traditionally been on anatomic outcomes in the Caucasian female patient, as these are the patients most likely to obtain aesthetic treatments and enter trials, psychological improvements are especially profound in populations whose appearance has been changed or altered, or deviates away from what traditional society dictates as "normal." By way of example, transgender individuals are at significantly higher risk of depression, anxiety, substance use, psychiatric hospitalizations, and suicide [14]. Surgery has been linked with better mental health outcomes with less hospitalizations and depressive episodes [14]. Facial procedures in particular can facilitate a reduction in social discrimination by creating an external appearance that is more in line with the patient's internal sense of self, resolving a major barrier faced by transgender people. As such, in this population and many others, surgery may not simply be life enhancing, it may in fact be lifesaving. (See Chapter 8 for additional information on approaches to the transgender patient.)

Likewise, well-selected cosmetic procedures can help to maintain or improve body image [15]. In addition, people living with chronic integumentary conditions can benefit from aesthetic treatments. Women with hirsutism often feel embarrassed and fear participation in social and intimate activities. Following laser treatment, multiple studies have found improvements in daily activities including work, school, and personal relationships [16, 17]. Similar improvements have been found in patients with acne vulgaris and acne scarring following treatment

with a variety of aesthetic modalities [18, 19]. Other skin conditions including rosacea have shown similar outcomes following vascular laser treatment [20], as have hyperpigmentation disorders following scar camouflage treatments [21]. Even in a poorly understood condition like photodamage-induced dysesthesia, aesthetic interventions can be of utility. It is often underappreciated that photodamaged skin frequently doesn't "feel right." Dysesthesias including extreme sensitivity, itch, and burning are common complaints that can be substantially improved with laser and light therapies [22]. Note that the degree of cosmetic "imperfection" and objective benefit from a given cosmetic intervention are not necessarily linearly correlated with the degree of psychological distress or emotional benefits after treatment. Even modest improvement of skin tone and texture, dyspigmentation, visible ectasias, dynamic wrinkling, volume loss, etc. can be emotionally or functionally liberating.

Case Study

> **Case 9.1 Aesthetics Influence on Career Performance**
>
> SG is a 47-year-old female sales representative who presents to your office seeking rejuvenation advice and services. She states that she is chronologically older than most of her professional peers who are in their mid-30s and is concerned that her "older appearance" is hindering her effectiveness as a salesperson and might potentially jeopardize her job security. SG has a fair-skinned Fitzpatrick II skin type and is a healthy vibrant person. She is an avid outdoors person with the significant photodamage that is expected with her fair skin and outdoor affinity. SG relates that the objective realities that a career in sales is a "young person's game" has been an omnipresent concern over

the past few years. She shares with you that she has become increasingly self-conscious about her obvious skin signs of sun damage and aging. She passionately believes that her readily visible stigmata of aging are fueling a growing loss of self-confidence within her. She occasionally has experienced the "humiliation" of a younger colleague asking her directly about how she feels as an older woman working among so many young and competitive others. She is married with two teenage children and states that she feels exhausted both physically and emotionally. Her husband is "a good man" who is a hard worker but emotionally distant.

Clinical Relevance and Implications

This real-life and often-repeated presentation raises several questions for ethical and compassionate aesthetic healthcare providers. These questions are as follows:

1) Is she correct in her perception that a youthful appearance matters in her professional world?
2) Is she correct in hoping and believing that the services offered by aesthetic practitioners will improve and restore her objective appearance to a sufficiently youthful state such that discrimination and potential job jeopardy can be diminished?
3) Is she correct in hoping and believing that the services offered by clinicians will sufficiently improve and restore her intrapsychic feelings and perceptions of herself to allow them forth into improvements in her functional status?

In essence, the questions become: how good are aesthetic practitioners professionally, how good are patients from an emotional standpoint, and where are patients in a reality-based pragmatic sense? These questions are important to consider as it is highly likely that her perception of a sales representative may have

been constructed through media platforms. This has ultimately led her into thinking what the "normal" would look like and subsequently altering her thought process into feeling like anything outside of that may lead to problems in her career. However, because of that media portrayal, people on the outside may become more comfortable with the "normal" representation of her job title and, as such, be more likely to engage in a business deal. This would therefore have a direct link to her potential career performance as a sales representative.

Assuming that this patient is a reasonably well-adjusted individual and that her expectations from treatment are reasonable and attainable, in all likelihood her requests for improvement and potential enhancement are valid and pragmatic from both a professional and intrapsychic perspective. Even the most modest improvements in skin appearance can provide us with the real-world evidence that we are indeed still youthful and competitive people and are embracing methods and modalities to slow our objective signs of aging. The potential functional status and career preservation/growth obtained following cosmetic interventions may be a consequence of improved physical appearance alone or, more likely, the combined physical and emotional benefits.

These improvements can also serve to answer the haunting and daunting inner voice that says "I'm not what I used to be" and, even more terrifying, "It is all downhill and deterioration from here." Stimulative therapies such as poly-L-lactic acid, topical retinoids, and growth factors all can offer the promise of gradual and gratifying benefits of subtle and ongoing rejuvenation. Treatments with hyaluronic acid fillers, botulinum toxins, laser and lights, and microdermabrasion produce more rapid improvements, allowing patients to visibly appreciate a more youthful, reflective, and healthy appearance. This can allow them to confidently answer the psychologically depressing expectation of uninterrupted deterioration and decline with more optimistic expectations.

Cosmetic interventions offer a legitimate data-proven process of ongoing rejuvenation, preservation of aging skin, and, of equal value, improved skin function [23]. Better skin function can be defined as preservation or improvements in skin sensations. Improvements in blush/flush reactions, rough texture, dyspigmentation, and skin reflectivity are often easily achieved. Each of these individually or in combination can be liberating for affected individuals. For some, one of the above may be sufficient; for others, several or all are necessary or sufficient to allow patients to readily embrace their spheres of functioning, which include but are not limited to intrapsychic, familial, vocational, recreational, and intimate.

Consequences and Ethical Concerns

Patient satisfaction with treatment outcomes is an area of great concern for all clinicians. There is a saying that "a reputation takes years to build, but seconds to destroy." Maximizing patient satisfaction and preserving our good reputations are of paramount importance. The following are several strategies to achieve patient satisfaction.

We attempt to carefully select patients whom we believe will be happy with their cosmetic intervention. We assiduously avoid those with florid psychopathology, those voicing repeated dissatisfaction with previous providers, those with evidence of extreme tissue augmentation, those that appear angry or excessively demanding, and those that make us feel uncomfortable for unknown reasons. Ideally, we utilize honest introspection, asking ourselves if this were our loved ones or ourselves, what would we suggest and what will we pursue? We listen carefully for the motivation and expectations of each patient. We try to convey warmth, empathy, and understanding. We assure patients that we are meticulous, careful, and conservative regarding quantity and intensity of treatments. We assure patients that we are passionate about maintaining a natural appearance without making them look augmented or robbing them of their unique identifying characteristics. We assure them that we will say no if ever they ask for something that is not in their best interest. In short, we ask them to trust our motivation, judgment, skill, and ethics. Do not ever deviate from an ethical and compassionate pathway. Retribution in the form of legal action and reputation destruction can be devastating.

Unfortunately, suboptimal outcomes do and will occur. Perceived clinician kindness, caring, and empathy dramatically decrease the likelihood of prolonged patient dissatisfaction and the negative associated actions on their part. The natural impulse that all of us experience when there is patient dissatisfaction is to "avoid the unpleasant." We must fight the impulse to run and hide. Make it clear to the patient that you will be available and accessible, and will stand by them until the situation is remedied.

Conclusions

There is clear supporting evidence that beyond anatomic correction or enhancement, aesthetic interventions can be associated with meaningful improvements in our patients' quality of life and satisfaction metrics. These improvements include enhancements of mood, more positive perceptions of self, increased confidence, and more positive ratings and perceptions by others. Well-chosen and carefully performed cosmetic procedures should be considered legitimate and meaningful interventions that extend from the skin to the psyche.

References

1 Wang, J. and Rieder, E. (2019). A systematic review of patient-reported outcomes for cosmetic indications of botulinum treatment. *Dermatol. Surg.* 45 (5): 668–688.

2 Kellerman, J. and Laird, J. (2006). The effect of appearance on self-perception. *J. Pers* 50 (3): 296–351.

3 Yildiz, T. and Selimen, D. (2015). The impact of facial aesthetic and reconstructive surgeries on patients' quality of life. *Indian J. Surg* 77 (3): 831–836.

4 Fried, R. (2011). Filler cheeks: a bright idea? *J. Clin. Aesthet. Dermatol.* 4 (5): 17–20.

5 Baumann, L., Weisberg, E., Mayans, M., and Arcuri, E. (2019). Open label study evaluating efficacy, safety, and effects on perception of age after injectable 20mg/mL hyaluronic acid for volumization of facial temples. *J. Drugs Dermatol.* 18 (1): 67–74.

6 Fried, R. (2008). Kindling midlife fires. *Skin Aging* 9: 68–71.

7 Slavin, B. and Beer, J. (2017). Facial identity and self-perception: an examination of psychosocial outcomes in cosmetic surgery patients. *J. Drugs Dermatol.* 16 (6): 617–620.

8 Dreno, B., Tan, J., Kang, S. et al. (2016). How people with facial acne scars are perceived in society: an online survey. *Dermatol. Ther.* 6: 207–218.

9 Rippon, I., Kneale, D., de Oliveira, C. et al. (2014). Perceived age discrimination in older adults. *Age Ageing* 43 (3): 379–386.

10 Ching, S., Thoma, A., McCabe, R., and Antony, M. (2003). Measuring outcomes in aesthetic surgery. *Plast. Reconstr. Surg.* 111: 468–480.

11 Weinkle, S.H., Werschler, P., Teller, C.F. et al. (2018). Impact of comprehensive, minimally invasive, multimodal aesthetic treatment on satisfaction with facial appearance: the HARMONY study. *Aesthet. Surg. J.* 38 (5): 540–556.

12 Molina, B., David, M., Jain, R. et al. (2015). Patient satisfaction and efficacy of full-facial rejuvenation using a combination of botulinum toxin type a and hyaluronic acid filler. *Dermatol. Surg.* 41 (1): S325–S332.

13 Rzany, B., Cartier, H., Kestemont, P. et al. (2012). Full-face rejuvenation using a range of hyaluronic acid fillers: efficacy, safety, and patient satisfaction over 6 months. *Dermatol. Surg.* 38 (7 Pt 2): 1153–1161.

14 Branstrom, R. and Pachankis, J. (2019). Reduction in mental health treatment utilization among transgender individuals after gender-affirming surgeries: a total population study. *Am. J. Psychiatry* 177: 727–734.

15 Gillen, M. (2015). Associations between positive body image and indicators of men's and women's mental and physical health. *Body Image* 13: 67–74.

16 Alizadeh, N., Ayyoubi, S., Naghipour, M. et al. (2017). Can laser treatment improve quality of life of hirsute women? *Int. J. Womens Health* 9: 777–780.

17 Maziar, A., Farsi, N., Mandegarfard, M. et al. (2010). Unwanted facial hair removal with laser treatment improves quality of life of patients. *J. Cosmet. Laser Ther.* 12 (1): 7–9.

18 Chilicka, K., Maj, J., and Panaszek, B. (2017). General qualify of life of patients with acne vulgaris before and after performing selected cosmetological treatments. *Patient Prefer. Adherence* 11: 1357–1361.

19 Porwal, S., Chahar, Y., and Singh, P. (2018). A comparative study of combined dermaroller and platelet-rich plasma versus dermaroller alone in acne scars and assessment of quality of life before and after treatment. *Indian J. Dermatol.* 63 (5): 403–408.

20 Bonsall, A. and Rajpara, S. (2015). A review of the quality of life following pulsed dye laser treatment for erythemotelangiectatic rosacea. *J. Cosmet. Laser Ther.* 18 (2): 86–90.

21 Kent, G. (2002). Testing a model of disfigurement: effects of a skin camouflage

service on well-being and appearance anxiety. *Psychol. Health* 17: 377–386.

22 Fogelman, J., Stevenson, M., and Soter, N. (2015). Idiopathic flushing with dysesthesia. *J. Clin. Aesthet. Dermatol.* 8 (8): 36–41.

23 Wollina, U. and Payne, C.R. (2010). Aging well – the role of minimally invasive aesthetic dermatological procedures in women over 65. *J. Cosmet. Dermatol.* 9: 50–58.

10

Aesthetic Interventions and the Perception of Others

Observer Reported Outcomes

Payal Shah and Evan A. Rieder

The Ronald O. Perelman Department of Dermatology, New York University Grossman School of Medicine, New York, NY, USA

Beyond the obvious desire for aesthetic correction, a consultation with a patient for a cosmetic procedure may be helpful in revealing subtle motivations for why they came into your office. While most patients will approach the aesthetic practitioner with a reality-based request to enhance or improve an anatomic deficit to improve self-esteem and well-being, not all people have such direct motivations. Some patients may allude to far-reaching effects of cosmetic procedures such as wanting to appear more beautiful to others, more attractive, or more successful. At first glance, some of these goals would seem to be naïve interpretations of what is possible with aesthetic intervention. However, emerging clinical evidence stemming from psychological research suggests otherwise. While data continue to emerge, the evidence demonstrates that individuals who undergo aesthetic enhancements by experts seem significantly different in physical appearance to others. While this may be self-evident, data also suggest that observers may view individuals' personalities before and after aesthetic intervention differently. Thus, a well-performed cosmetic procedure's success in restoring a more youthful appearance while enhancing the unique characteristics of the

individual may be a matter of "public opinion," in which the jury is made up of neutral third-party observers. To the patient, the results of these third-party observers have potential to deliver meaning to how they will be perceived by all those that surround them, including friends, family, and coworkers. This phenomenon suggests that we are now entering a time of aesthetic intervention in which the effects of cosmetic procedures may be judged not only by the practitioner and the patient, but also by the public – or more accurately, by a representative sample of the public.

Case Studies

Case 10.1   Dating Again Motivation
TK, a 56-year-old Caucasian woman with no past medical history, presents to your office requesting cosmetic consultation. She has never had a cosmetic procedure and has noticed significant change in her facial appearance over the past few years. She feels she has aged significantly and wants to feel more youthful and more attractive. As you walk through your cosmetic consultation

(Continued)

Case 10.1 (Continued)

with her, you discuss the process of facial aging and note areas where aesthetic intervention is likely to yield positive results. On review of her social history and motivations for cosmetic procedures, you learn that she divorced one year prior and has recently decided that she is open to start dating again. She has not dated in many years and recalls how difficult dating was from her early adulthood. She remembers how important a strong first impression is in the dating world because first impressions are often what lead to future encounters with a person of interest. She wants people to see her not only as attractive but also as friendly and successful.

Clinical Relevance and Implications

This case presentation brings to light how patients may begin arriving at a consultation appointment for cosmetic intervention. They may not have a particular procedure in mind at all, but rather a desire to look better or to be perceived in a more positive light by others. In addition to motivations of improving self-confidence and self-perceived beauty, many people want to improve others' perceptions of the patient's competence and youth [1–3]. Clinical evidence suggests that cosmetic intervention does in fact impact the perceptions of others [4–7]. As the evidence continues to build in this area, patient motivations to enhance how they are perceived by others may soon become a more standard question in the cosmetic consultation and even a valid indication for cosmetic intervention. Contrastingly, if a patient articulates a focused interest in a pure anatomical change, such as improving facial symmetry through cosmetic filler treatment, enhancing the perception of others may be another topic of interest that an astute clinician can raise in discussing the benefits of such a procedure.

In this particular patient case, one can begin by validating her desire to give a better first impression while dating. One can also inform the patient that recent evidence does suggest that cosmetic intervention may have a positive impact on how friendly, attractive, and successful she may appear to others. While comparative studies on which interventions specifically may enhance these particular traits are still limited, one can share which interventions have positively changed the views of others when examining a professionally aesthetically enhanced face. Face-lifts, pan-facial treatment with cosmetic fillers and neurotoxins, blepharoplasty, and rhinoplasty have all positively affected the reports of objective observers when viewing the before and after images of people who have received aesthetic procedures [7–10].

Beyond informing the initial patient consultation or informed consent discussion with the patient, quantification of how cosmetic intervention affects the perception of others can offer objective measurements for how to evaluate the success of a procedure [11–13]. While a practitioner's and patient's perspectives are important to consider, both may also be biased. The practitioner delivering the procedure may have a very particular way of viewing human faces and human anatomy based on how he or she was trained. This may bias the evaluation methodology of a patient outcome after aesthetic intervention from a more technical viewpoint. Another neutral practitioner uninvolved in the procedure who has an equivalent level of training or skill may come to an aesthetic procedure with different training in cosmetic rejuvenation and have a subtly distinct set of technical measures. Cultural and other demographic factors of the practitioner may also play roles that are more difficult to articulate. All of these factors may bias evaluation after a cosmetic procedure. Additionally, a patient's preconceived self-impressions of beauty may prevent them from viewing a cosmetic procedure through an objective lens. These issues may be complicated further by the possible presence of underlying psychological disturbance or unrealistic expectations. It could be argued that a third-party observer, unrelated to the practitioner–patient relationship or to the delivery of aesthetic intervention, may offer an interpretation of a procedure's success that is the most objective, fair, and generalizable. Importantly, appropriate outcome measures in clinical trials of interventions addressing facial aging are still in debate, demonstrating the continued challenge of defining success and who should be the one to say so in the world of cosmetic medicine [14].

Case 10.2 Workplace Promotions

BG, a 50-year-old Asian-American man with no relevant medical history, presents to your office requesting a cosmetic consultation. He says he once received laser resurfacing of acne scars in his adolescence. Prior to having the laser treatment, he endorsed being ridiculed by his peers and suffering from low self-esteem. Since the resurfacing, he has not had additional cosmetic procedures. He tells you that he has no issues with how he looks but states that he is beginning to feel like he's losing his "edge" in the workplace. In a client-facing position at work, he realizes the importance of portraying youth and strength at his job. He hesitated to say it out loud but he recently noticed how a select few younger and objectively attractive men at his work have received recent promotions and opportunities to advance their careers. He, on the other hand, feels like he's stuck at work. He hasn't received a promotion in the past five years and feels that he shares similar accomplishments in the workplace to these men. He has a theory that it has something to do with how they look. He wants others to see him as youthful, extroverted, and successful at his job. He feels these traits are important for consideration for emerging opportunities and promotions at his workplace. He asks if there is anything that can be done to give him back his youthful edge, and ultimately facilitate the pursuit of his career goals.

Clinical Relevance and Implications

Similar to the prior patient case, this patient is relatively naïve to cosmetic intervention. As BG is not familiar with all the different types of cosmetic intervention that are possible and does not have a particular facial area of concern for enhancement, he looks to you for how best to make a better impression at work through aesthetic intervention. We can again begin by validating his need to want to be perceived as more youthful, extroverted, and occupationally successful, as many other patients have similar desires. We can inform the patient that there is now clinical evidence to suggest that aesthetic intervention may offer improvement with respect to how others view him. While comparative studies on which interventions specifically may enhance these particular traits are still limited, one can share which interventions have shown positive change in these attributes. These procedures include but are not limited to perioral and nasolabial cosmetic filler, facial rejuvenation surgery, and neck-lift [4, 15–17].

While there is evidence to suggest that the impression of these personal attributes perceived by his coworkers may improve after he receives aesthetic intervention, the question of whether these newly enhanced impressions after intervention contribute to the furthering of his professional success remains unanswered. As an aesthetic practitioner, it is important to perform reality testing with the patient and emphasize that an aesthetically corrected face does not equate to future success in the workplace.

There is evidence to suggest that formulated first impressions of another's appearance may affect judicial considerations [18, 19], voting behavior [20, 21], and hiring decisions, communicating the power of the first impression. Although not yet investigated, the mere possibility of appreciable benefits to the dating success or overall life success of an individual as a result of enhanced facial appearance through aesthetic intervention is important to consider [22, 23].

As future research investigations begin to follow patient cohorts with and without cosmetic procedures, controlling for confounders such as socioeconomic status, we will hopefully one day arrive at an evolved understanding of the real-life implications of enhancing the perceptions of others.

Observer Reported Outcomes as a Novel Evaluation Tool for Cosmetic Procedures

The psychology literature suggests a biological basis for our natural tendency to judge the facial attractiveness of another individual at first glance. In this process of judging attractiveness in another's face, we have a natural tendency to form immediate impressions with respect to the degree of youth, health, and trustworthiness attributable to that individual. These impressions are ultimately linked to the evolutionary motivations of optimal mate selection and survival benefit [24–26]. In fact, studies of children passing judgment on facial images show that beautiful faces are the ones seen as more trustworthy, popular, and intelligent, suggesting that the tendency to form first impressions of others occurs early in human development [27, 28]. It may not just be the mature consciousness of the adult mind that is able to interpret a human face and evaluate how trustworthy, social, and intelligent the person is. Even children may be capable of making such decisions, meaning the process may be actually quite primal and unconscious.

In the contemporary day of skyscrapers and social media, however, the purpose of life has grown beyond the constraints of reproduction and natural selection alone. When we now aesthetically evaluate another's facial appearance and attractiveness, we may additionally unconsciously pass judgment on his or her occupational success and/or relationship success as these are traits we desire in our friends and/or life partners [29–33]. Psychological research demonstrates that particular features of the face, such as intercanthal distance, skin smoothness, mouth curvature, and eyelid openness, directly modulate how we perceive the social and character attributes of others. The specific personality traits that have been shown to associate with these facial features include one's level of submissiveness, threat, intelligence, youth, health, trustworthiness, competence, and attractiveness [34–39]. It is not a far leap of logic to think that adjusting facial beauty and particular facial features through aesthetic intervention can further modulate how the personal attributes of the individual are enhanced, diminished, or even newly introduced. These perceptions of others that are evaluated in the field of cosmetic medicine are labeled as observer reported outcomes (OROs).

What are Observer Reported Outcomes (OROs)?

In recognizing that beauty in art depends on both the physical art form itself and the interpreter, we can imagine the same can be extended to beauty of the human form. Whether a particular human being is beautiful or not beautiful depends on both the physical appearance of the individual and the eyes of the interpreter. During the process of aesthetic evaluation of any art form, a complex neurological process of evaluation is likely at play. This process involves the emotion-valuation, sensory-motor, and meaning-knowledge neural axes [40]. The concept of higher complexity judgment that takes place with aesthetic evaluation has come to be known as neuroaesthetics [40].

In the origins of cosmetic medicine, the success of aesthetic intervention was measured with objective physical markers. These included restoration of anatomic defects, improvement in symmetry, and reduction in signs of aging (e.g. wrinkling, volume loss). We have since developed standardized evaluation tools that introduce important patient reported outcomes (PROs) such as self-esteem, self-perceived beauty, and quality of life. The next

Table 10.1   Organizational schema of OROs.

Aesthetics and wellness	• Includes perception of age, attractiveness, health, sexual dimorphism, and overall first impression
Social capacities	• Includes perception of confidence, interpersonal relationships, sociability, and trustworthiness
Skills and competencies	• Includes perception of athletics, occupation and finances, and scholastics

era considers the evaluation of the interpreter. Observer reported evaluations now exist across a variety of outcomes including physical appearance and perceived personality traits of people before and after cosmetic intervention. A systematic review of OROs created an organizational schema of outcomes with three broad categories: aesthetics and wellness, social capacities, and skills and competencies (Table 10.1) [41]. In the future, as reported results on OROs after cosmetic intervention become more commonplace, our understanding of the impact of these cosmetic procedures will continue to refine itself and ultimately inform the broader risks and benefits involved in aesthetic intervention.

The diversity of physical attributes and personality traits studied to date as OROs after aesthetic intervention can be constrained to these domains; however, there may be other effects that remain unstudied which may add to this framework. Notably, negative impressions after a procedure may be possible [33], in which an undesired trait is enhanced unintentionally as a result of improper technique. More clinical research in cosmetic medicine is needed with ORO data to investigate the full range of effects on the perception of others that are possible from these interventions.

The Emerging Evidence Base for OROs in Cosmetic Procedures

How can we understand the power of first impressions and their ability to impact our perception of others? How do we create an evidence base to confirm our suspicions that

characteristics such as dating success and life success are directly connected to how attractive a person appears to be? The fields of medical and social sciences have endeavored to answer these questions from a variety of angles.

Firstly, the human brain was shown to exhibit neural activity of high-order decision-making when processing objects with varying degrees of beauty. Electrophysiological and neuroimaging studies shed light on the complexity of neurological processing that occurs when individuals interpret another person's appearance [42–44]. Specifically, human faces that are scored as more beautiful are also the ones that lead to increased levels of brain activity in the viewer. Researchers speculate that this increase in activity may indicate a need to keep these images in working memory [45]. Secondly, the relationship of brain activity during aesthetic evaluation of human facial images and during evaluation of the perceived social attributes of each of the faces has been examined. Specifically, one study demonstrated a faster neural time course for the process of pure aesthetic judgment compared to that of social judgment. This suggests that people may be primed by someone's relative attractiveness before arriving at a deeper level of judgment on their personalities [46].

Beyond brain imaging and psychological survey studies, there is a growing body of evidence in the surgical literature investigating how others perceive facial beauty and personal attributes before and after aesthetic intervention. Surgical correction of a mal-positioned chin can affect our perception of another's faithfulness, intelligence, reliability, financial status, likelihood for employment, and other personal attributes [23, 47, 48]. Similarly, alteration of oral anatomy, particularly through gingival display, can affect our perception of another's friendliness, trustworthiness, intelligence, and self-confidence [49].

In plastic and dermatologic surgery, both surgical intervention and minimally invasive interventions have demonstrated a positive impact on OROs [4, 5, 10, 15, 50]. The surgical interventions with a reported impact on observer perceptions include face-lifts, neck-lifts, hair transplants, blepharoplasty, otoplasty, rhinoplasty, lip implantation, mentoplasty, and excision of benign facial growths. Minimally invasive interventions that have a reported positive impact on observer perceptions include laser skin resurfacing, rejuvenation with botulinum toxins, soft tissue fillers (including hyaluronic acid, fat, calcium hydroxyapatite), and fat dissolving through deoxycholic acid injection [41]. Additionally, computer simulations of the changes expected by cosmetic procedures demonstrate a perceived improvement by others in the level of attractiveness or health exhibited [51].

Overall, the evidence for significant change in the perception by others is the strongest and most reproducible for the following attributes of an individual after aesthetic intervention: youth, attractiveness, health, social skills, dating success, and life success. This evidence is generated by clinical investigations before and after real patients receive cosmetic interventions, either with prospective patient cohorts undergoing procedures or with retrospective cohorts with stored photographs [41]. These results offer evidence for the complex impression that can be made at first glance of a human face and, more importantly, for the power of procedural intervention to alter this impression.

Limitations to Existing Evidence

The duration and meaning of an altered first impression remains an open question [33, 52–54]. Perhaps the perceptions of others of facial beauty, social attributes, and character attributes will fade over time, paralleling the temporary effects of cosmetic procedures themselves. Alternatively, maybe these perceptions are even more transient than the anatomical changes created by cosmetic procedures. An altered first impression may be replaced by another, perhaps more authentic, personality impression after spending more time with the individual who underwent an aesthetic intervention.

While future studies with longer follow-up are needed to answer hypotheses about OROs, the impact of cosmetic intervention on the first impression of an objective observer, while subject to change, is important to consider. It is often a first impression that may lead to a second date, a hiring decision, a judicial decision, or the confidence of an investor's belief in a startup company. However, whether transient or not, modulations in observer perception do occur. As aesthetic practitioners, we must be cognizant of the fact that we may be able to effect profound change in our patients that transcends the anatomic benefit of the placement of gel in an atrophic scar or a neurotoxin in a rhytide. The impact on the opportunities extended to and success achievable by individuals who undergo aesthetic enhancement remains an important consideration for patient care and for future research within cosmetic medicine.

Conclusions

Beyond PROs on self-perceived beauty, mood, and quality of life after aesthetic intervention, we describe an alternative metric of aesthetic interventions in the form of OROs. OROs can be conceptualized by three broad categories: aesthetics and wellness, social capacities, and skills and competencies. According to neutral third-party observers, patients of aesthetic intervention may appear younger, more attractive, healthier, more sociable, more successful at dating, and more successful at life, suggesting unexpected, far-reaching effects from these procedures. These evidence-based effects on OROs may add to the cosmetic consultation by expanding the discussion between providers and patients and offering another, arguably more objective, way of evaluating an outcome after cosmetic intervention.

As clinical evidence builds, one can imagine a not too distant future in which we may be able to say with confidence in a cosmetic consultation that aesthetic intervention can improve one's physical appearance and psychological functioning as well as one's receptivity by others.

References

1 Waldman, A., Maisel, A., Weil, A. et al. (2019). Patients believe that cosmetic procedures affect their quality of life: an interview study of patient-reported motivations. *Journal of the American Academy of Dermatology* 80 (6): 1671–1681.

2 Solish, N., Bertucci, V., Percec, I. et al. (2018). Subjective facial dynamics with the use of hyaluronic acid dermal fillers formulated for facial movement and expression. *Journal of the American Academy of Dermatology* 79 (3 Supplement 1): AB272.

3 Furnham, A. and Levitas, J. (2012). Factors that motivate people to undergo cosmetic surgery. *Canadian Journal of Plastic Surgery (Journal Canadien de Chirurgie Plastique)* 20 (4): e47–e50.

4 Dayan, S., Arkins, J.P., and Gal, T.J. (2010). Blinded evaluation of the effects of hyaluronic acid filler injections on first impression. *Dermatologic Surgery* 36: 1866–1873.

5 Parsa, K.M., Gao, W., Lally, J. et al. (2019). Evaluation of personality perception in men before and after facial cosmetic surgery. *JAMA Facial Plastic Surgery* 21 (5): 369–374.

6 Nellis, J.C., Ishii, M., Papel, I.D. et al. (2017). Association of face-lift surgery with social perception, age, attractiveness, health, and success. *JAMA Facial Plastic Surgery* 19 (4): 311–317.

7 Bater, K.L., Ishii, M., Nellis, J.C. et al. (2018). A dual approach to understanding facial perception before and after blepharoplasty. *JAMA Facial Plastic Surgery* 20 (1): 43–49.

8 Dayan, S., Rivkin, A., Sykes, J.M. et al. (2018). Aesthetic treatment positively impacts social perception: analysis of subjects from the HARMONY study. *Aesthetic Surgery Journal* 39 (12): 1380–1389.

9 Lu, S.M., Hsu, D.T., Perry, A.D. et al. (2018). The public face of rhinoplasty: impact on perceived attractiveness and personality. *Plastic and Reconstructive Surgery* 142 (4): 881–887.

10 Bater, K.L., Ishii, L.E., Papel, I.D. et al. (2017). Association between facial rejuvenation and observer ratings of youth, attractiveness, success, and health. *JAMA Facial Plastic Surgery* 19 (5): 360–367.

11 Dayan, S. and Romero, D.H. (2018). Introducing a novel model: the special theory of relativity for attractiveness to define a natural and pleasing outcome following cosmetic treatments. *Journal of Cosmetic Dermatology* 17 (5): 925–930.

12 Dey, J.K., Ishii, L.E., Nellis, J.C. et al. (2017). Comparing patient, casual observer, and expert perception of permanent unilateral facial paralysis. *JAMA Facial Plastic Surgery* 19 (6): 476–483.

13 Springer, I.N., Schulze, M., Wiltfang, J. et al. (2012). Facial self-perception, well-being, and aesthetic surgery. *Annals of Plastic Surgery* 69 (5): 503–509.

14 Schlessinger, D.I., Iyengar, S., Yanes, A.F. et al. (2017). Development of a core outcome set for clinical trials in facial aging: study protocol for a systematic review of the literature and identification of a core outcome set using a Delphi survey. *Trials* 18 (1): 359.

15 Dayan, S.H., Bacos, J.T., Gandhi, N.D. et al. (2019). Assessment of the impact of perioral

rejuvenation with hyaluronic acid filler on projected first impressions and mood perceptions. *Dermatologic Surgery: Official Publication for American Society for Dermatologic Surgery [et al.]* 45 (1): 99–107.

16 Fink, B. and Prager, M. (2014). The effect of incobotulinumtoxin a and dermal filler treatment on perception of age, health, and attractiveness of female faces. *Journal of Clinical and Aesthetic Dermatology* 7 (1): 36–40.

17 Chauhan, N., Warner, J.P., and Adamson, P.A. (2012). Perceived age change after aesthetic facial surgical procedures quantifying outcomes of aging face surgery. *Archives of Facial Plastic Surgery* 14 (4): 258–262.

18 Sigall, H. and Ostrove, N. (1975). Beautiful but dangerous: effects of offender attractiveness and nature of the crime on juridic judgment. *Journal of Personality and Social Psychology* 31 (3): 410–414.

19 Efran, M.G. (1974). The effect of physical appearance on the judgment of guilt, interpersonal attraction, and severity of recommended punishment in a simulated jury task. *Journal of Research in Personality* 8 (1): 45–54.

20 Efrain, M.G. and Patterson, E.W.J. (1974). Voters vote beautiful: the effect of physical appearance on a national election. *Canadian Journal of Behavioural Science/Revue canadienne des sciences du comportement* 6 (4): 352–356.

21 Ballew, C.C. 2nd and Todorov, A. (2007). Predicting political elections from rapid and unreflective face judgments. *Proceedings of the National Academy of Sciences of the United States of America* 104 (46): 17948–17953.

22 Olson, I.R. and Marshuetz, C. (2005). Facial attractiveness is appraised in a glance. *Emotion* 5 (4): 498–502.

23 Sena, L.M.F., Damasceno, E.A.L.A.L., Farias, A.C.R., and Pereira, H.S.G. (2017). The influence of sagittal position of the mandible in facial attractiveness and social perception.

Dental Press Journal of Orthodontics 22 (2): 77–86.

24 Nedelec, J.L. and Beaver, K.M. (2014). Physical attractiveness as a phenotypic marker of health: an assessment using a nationally representative sample of American adults. *Evolution and Human Behavior* 35 (6): 456–463.

25 Samson, N., Fink, B., and Matts, P. (2011). Interaction of skin color distribution and skin surface topography cues in the perception of female facial age and health. *Journal of Cosmetic Dermatology* 10 (1): 78–84.

26 Y.D.B. (2019). Perception and deception: human beauty and the brain. *Behavioral Science* 9 (4).

27 Ma, F., Xu, F., and Luo, X. (2015). Children's and adults' judgments of facial trustworthiness: the relationship to facial attractiveness. *Perceptual and Motor Skills* 121 (1): 179–198.

28 Rossini, G., Parrini, S., Castroflorio, T. et al. (2016). Children's perceptions of smile esthetics and their influence on social judgment. *The Angle Orthodontist* 86 (6): 1050–1055.

29 Little, A.C. and Craig Roberts, S. (2012). Evolution, appearance, and occupational success. *Evolutionary Psychology* 10 (5): 782–801.

30 Etcoff, N.L., Stock, S., Haley, L.E. et al. (2011). Cosmetics as a feature of the extended human phenotype: modulation of the perception of biologically important facial signals. *PLoS One* 6 (10): e25656.

31 Moore, F.R., Filippou, D., and Perrett, D.I. (2011). Intelligence and attractiveness in the face: beyond the attractiveness halo effect. *Journal of Evolutionary Psychology* 9 (3): 205–217.

32 Eagly, A.H., Ashmore, R.D., Makhijani, M.G., and Longo, L.C. (1991). What is beautiful is good, but . . .: a meta-analytic review of research on the physical attractiveness stereotype. *Psychological Bulletin* 110 (1): 109–128.

33 Talamas, S.N., Mavor, K.I., and Perrett, D.I. (2016). Blinded by beauty: attractiveness bias and accurate perceptions of academic performance. *PLoS One* 11 (2): e0148284.

34 Naran, S., Wes, A.M., Mazzaferro, D.M. et al. (2018). More than meets the eye: the effect of intercanthal distance on perception of beauty and personality. *Journal of Craniofacial Surgery* 29 (1): 40–44.

35 Matts, P.J., Fink, B., Grammer, K., and Burquest, M. (2007). Color homogeneity and visual perception of age, health, and attractiveness of female facial skin. *Journal of the American Academy of Dermatology* 57 (6): 977–984.

36 Tsankova, E. and Kappas, A. (2016). Facial skin smoothness as an indicator of perceived trustworthiness and related traits. *Perception* 45 (4): 400–408.

37 Talamas, S.N., Mavor, K.I., Axelsson, J. et al. (2016). Eyelid-openness and mouth curvature influence perceived intelligence beyond attractiveness. *Journal of Experimental Psychology: General* 145 (5): 603–620.

38 Oosterhof, N.N. and Todorov, A. (2008). The functional basis of face evaluation. *Proceedings of the National Academy of Sciences of the United States of America* 105 (32): 11087–11092.

39 Rojas, M., Masip, D., Todorov, A., and Vitria, J. (2011). Automatic prediction of facial trait judgments: appearance vs. structural models. *PLoS One* 6 (8): e23323.

40 Chatterjee, A. and Vartanian, O. (2016). Neuroscience of aesthetics. *Annals of the New York Academy of Sciences* 1369 (1): 172–194.

41 Shah, P.C. and Rieder, E.A. (2020). Observer reported outcomes and cosmetic procedure: a systematic review. *Journal of Dermatologic Surgery* (Online ahead of print). doi:https://doi.org/10.1097/DSS.0000000000002496.

42 Zhang, Y., Zheng, M., and Wang, X. (2016). Effects of facial attractiveness on personality stimuli in an implicit priming task: an ERP study. *Neurological Research* 38 (8): 685–691.

43 Iaria, G., Fox, C.J., Waite, C.T. et al. (2008). The contribution of the fusiform gyrus and superior temporal sulcus in processing facial attractiveness: neuropsychological and neuroimaging evidence. *Neuroscience* 155 (2): 409–422.

44 Martin-Loeches, M., Hernandez-Tamames, J.A., Martin, A., and Urrutia, M. (2014). Beauty and ugliness in the bodies and faces of others: an fMRI study of person esthetic judgement. *Neuroscience* 277: 486–497.

45 Munoz, F. and Martin-Loeches, M. (2015). Electrophysiological brain dynamics during the esthetic judgment of human bodies and faces. *Brain Research* 1594: 154–164.

46 Calvo, M.G., Gutierrez-Garcia, A., and Beltran, D. (2018). Neural time course and brain sources of facial attractiveness vs. trustworthiness judgment. *Cognitive, Affective, & Behavioral Neuroscience* 18 (6): 1233–1247.

47 Sinko, K., Jagsch, R., Drog, C. et al. (2018). Facial esthetics and the assignment of personality traits before and after orthognathic surgery rated on video clips. *PLoS One* 13 (2): e0191718.

48 Allon, D.M. and Shmuly, T. (2015). Perceived attractiveness and other characteristics of different male facial types before and after orthognathic surgery. *Refu'at ha-peh veha-shinayim (1993)* 32 (3): 19–29, 67.

49 Malkinson, S., Waldrop, T.C., Gunsolley, J.C. et al. (2013). The effect of esthetic crown lengthening on perceptions of a patient's attractiveness, friendliness, trustworthiness, intelligence, and self-confidence. *Journal of Periodontology* 84 (8): 1126–1133.

50 Nellis, J.C., Ishii, M., Bater, K.L. et al. (2018). Association of rhinoplasty with perceived attractiveness, success, and overall health. *JAMA Facial Plastic Surgery* 20 (2): 97–102.

51 Kandathil, C.K., Saltychev, M., Moubayed, S.P., and Most, S.P. (2018). Association of dorsal reduction and tip rotation with social perception. *JAMA Facial Plastic Surgery* 20 (5): 362–366.

52 Khaw, M.W., Nichols, P., and Freedberg, D. (2019). Speed of person perception affects immediate and ongoing aesthetic evaluation. *Acta Psychologica* 197: 166–176.

53 Kleisner, K., Chvatalova, V., and Flegr, J. (2014). Perceived intelligence is associated with measured intelligence in men but not women. *PLoS One* 9 (3): e81237.

54 Rantala, M.J., Coetzee, V., Moore, F.R. et al. (2013). Facial attractiveness is related to women's cortisol and body fat, but not with immune responsiveness. *Biology Letters* 9 (4): 20130255.

11

Botulinum Toxins

Beauty, Psychology, and Mood in the Cosmetic Patient

Catherine Pisano[1], Jason Reichenberg[1], and Michelle Magid[2,3]

[1] *Department of Dermatology, University of Texas Dell Medical School, Austin, TX, USA*
[2] *Department of Psychiatry, University of Texas Dell Medical School, Austin, TX, USA*
[3] *Texas A&M Health Science Center, Round Rock, TX, USA*

Introduction

Botulinum toxin is the most common cosmetic procedure performed in the United States [1]. In a cosmetic setting, botulinum toxin is used to temporarily weaken or paralyze specific muscles that contract during facial expression and lead to the development of wrinkles in the skin. It is most often used in the glabella, forehead, and periorbital regions [2], where wrinkles are often socially associated with aging. There are less well-known uses of botulinum toxin approved by the Food and Drug Administration, including the treatment of axillary hyperhidrosis, bladder dysfunction, chronic migraines, limb spasticity, cervical dystonia, blepharospasm, and strabismus [3]. In this chapter, we discuss the novel role of botulinum toxin injections in the treatment of depression.

Case Study

Case 11.1   Psychiatric Care in the Cosmetic Patient

LT, a 56-year-old Caucasian woman, presents to her psychiatrist's office for her regularly scheduled monthly appointments. LT was diagnosed with major depressive disorder over eight years ago. She has tried three different oral antidepressants and several other adjunctive psychopharmacologic medications, and has been taking a selective serotonin reuptake inhibitor for the past five years with some benefit. She has been regularly visiting her psychiatrist for psychotherapy and feels as if this modality has also been helpful. However, LT still feels depressed. She states that her friends and coworkers constantly ask her if everything is ok as they say that she "always looks stressed or sad." LT is wondering if there are any additional treatments she could try. When you opened your aesthetic practice, you introduced yourself to local primary care providers and mental health professionals. One of the local psychiatrists contacted you and asked about botulinum treatments for LT.

Psychosocial Relevance

Depression is not only a disease of the psyche, but also one of biophysical and social feedback. While depression as a disease entity is becoming less stigmatizing in our society, a physical appearance projecting anger, sadness, or depression remains less welcoming and may be socially distancing [4]. In addition, the act of frowning may trigger a feedback loop in the brain to propagate depression further.

Pathogenesis

The intricate musculature of the face provides the ability for necessary functions such as eating, drinking, and blinking, but also allows for the social function of communication through facial expressions. The repetitive contraction of the frontalis muscle, procerus muscle, corrugator supercilii muscle, and orbicularis oculi muscle initially leads to dynamic wrinkles, which resolve once the face returns to a resting position. Chronic and repeated movements of these muscles ultimately lead to static wrinkles and furrows which remain present even when the face is at rest [5]. It is posited that feeling depressed can lead to frowning, but it may be that frowning can lead to depression as well. This theory is supported by two hypothesizes: the behavioral hypothesis and the facial feedback hypothesis [6].

The *behavioral hypothesis* of how facial wrinkles and furrows play a role in depression is centered in social feedback mechanisms. People who appear more angry or sad are often received and subsequently treated in a more negative manner than people who are viewed as happy. Over time, the continued negative perception of others leads to a negative view of oneself, with increased feelings of sadness, worthlessness, and ultimately depression [7]. This increase in negative emotion is then portrayed on the patient's face, which only serves to increase the negative perception by society and continue the cycle.

The *facial feedback hypothesis* highlights the principle of biomechanical feedback of the body. This hypothesis was first described by Charles Darwin in 1872 and expanded upon by William James in the nineteenth century [8, 9]. They theorized that physical movement of facial muscles influences emotional perception via a biomechanical feedback loop. For example, when one is frowning or has a furrowed brow, the brain receives signals indicating this and assigns a negative emotion to this facial expression. Once the brain has perceived a negative emotion, one frowns more, then the brain senses more negative emotions, thus continuing the cycle [10–12]. Even if a patient is unaware that they are frowning, they respond more negatively to stimuli than a person who is inadvertently smiling [11].

To expand on the facial feedback hypothesis, studies have shown that depressed patients frequently show a relative overactivity of glabellar frown muscles, which has been confirmed via electrophysiology. When this overactivity is corrected by botulinum toxin treatment, there is a correspondent softening of negative emotions such as depression, anger, and fear [13, 14]. Studies have also shown that botulinum toxin injections in the glabellar region can lead to indirect neurochemical changes in the brain, which can help regulate mood. For instance, after glabellar botulinum toxin injections, functional magnetic resonance imaging (MRI) studies have shown that the amygdala – the brain's epicenter for processing emotional stimuli – is less reactive to negative stimuli, such as photos of angry people [7, 15]. In diseases such as depression and post-traumatic stress disorder, where the amygdala has been primed to be hypervigilant to negative stimuli, reducing distorted or misperceived responses to "harmful" stimuli via botulinum injections can lead to overall improvement in mood and social engagement.

Treatment

Botulinum toxin is a potent neurotoxin derived from the bacterium *Clostridium botulinum*. This toxin was discovered as the cause of botulism, a life-threatening systemic disease in which the toxin inhibits muscle contraction, ultimately resulting in respiratory failure and death. Botulinum toxin blocks release of acetylcholine from neurons, which eliminates the signal from nerves to the muscles to contract [2, 16]. Understanding the inhibition of muscle contraction as the pathophysiologic mechanism has allowed botulinum toxin to be developed into a treatment option used in medical settings for a variety of disorders. Botulinum toxin was initially approved by the FDA in 1989 for the treatment of strabismus and blepharospasm, but is now approved for numerous indications [3]. In 2002, botulinum toxin A, which is commercially known as Botox© (onabotulinumtoxin A), was approved by the FDA for use in cosmetic practice to reduce the appearance of facial wrinkles in the glabella [3]. There are several similar agents used worldwide, including Dysport© (abobotulinumtoxin A), Xeomin© (incobotulinumtoxin A), and Jeuveau˚ (prabotulinumtoxin A).

With the widespread use of botulinum toxin to treat facial wrinkles, a case series was published by Finzi describing 10 female patients with major depression who received botulinum toxin into the glabella. Nine patients were no longer depressed after the treatment [17]. Several randomized control trials have since been performed to determine if injection of

botulinum toxin into the glabellar region of patients with a diagnosis of major depressive disorder improves symptoms [6, 18–22]. The majority of patients in these studies had had a diagnosis of major depressive disorder for at least six months and were still experiencing depressive symptoms despite treatment with antidepressants and/or psychotherapy for at least four weeks. The patients received five injections into the glabella area with either an inert sterile saline mixture or onabotulinum toxin A at a dose of 29 units in women and 39–40 units for men (Figure 11.1). These studies showed that the patients in the treatment arm had reduced depressive symptoms by at least 50% and about one-third of patients attained remission of depression within six weeks [6, 23]. There seemed to be no difference when the dose was increased from 30 to 50 units, indicating that a higher dose may not necessarily mean a better response [22, 23]. A meta-analysis of these studies (n = 134 patients) showed that depressed patients receiving botulinum toxin into the glabellar region had a 54.2% response rate vs. a 10.7% response rate in the placebo controlled arm, according to standardized depression rating scales [24].

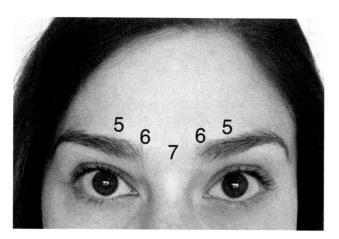

Figure 11.1 Configuration of botulinum toxin A injection for a female patient. In all discussed trials, women received a total of 29 units of botulinum toxin A, with a distribution of 7 units into the procerus, 6 units bilaterally into the medial corrugator supercilii muscles, and 5 units bilaterally into the center of the corrugator supercilii muscles. Male patients require an increased dose of botulinum toxin A, with a total of 39–40 units, in order to account for the increased average muscle density seen in male facial muscles.

Patients showed improvement in symptoms as early as two weeks after injection, which aligns with the physiologic onset of muscle paralysis over this time course [16]. This is an important clinical discovery, as antidepressant medications often require three to six weeks to take effect. Botulinum toxin A may therefore have a quicker onset of action than antidepressants, creating a treatment advantage for patients who need a faster response. Patients' depressive symptoms may reoccur several months after a single treatment, but some studies have shown that the antidepressant effect lasts even after the patient's wrinkles have reappeared [6].

While use of botulinum toxin A to treat treatment-resistant depression is an off-label use at this time, the potential benefit and time-tested safety profile offer few drawbacks. The use of botulinum toxin A injections into the glabella by a trained professional offers an extremely low risk of serious side effects. Side effects may include bleeding, infection, or bruising at the site of injection, temporary eyelid droop, and temporary asymmetry [3]. The treatment can be very cost effective as well, when compared to multiple visits to a psychiatrist or the use of brand-name prescriptions [25].

Clinical Relevance and Implications

The behavioral theory and the facial feedback hypothesis highlight the intricate pathophysiology of depression as well as the social influence on the course of this disease. As highlighted by the behavioral theory, a chain of events may be enacted when a patient feels sad. They then begin to look sad, which can cause them to be perceived negatively in society, leading to decreased interpersonal connections and communications; people are less inclined to socialize and interact with a person who looks sad than one who looks happy. This inadvertent social isolation can make the patient feel more sad, thus perpetuating the cycle. The use of

botulinum toxin A may be used to decrease the sad or negative facial expression unintentionally portrayed by the patient and evoke a more positive reception by members of society, hence improving the mood and decreasing the depressive feelings of the patient [23, 26].

With respect to the alternative hypothesis of facial feedback, botulinum toxin prevents furrowing of the brow. Because the proprioceptive feedback of a frown will be inhibited by the action of the neurotoxin, there is reduced signaling to the brain, particularly the amygdala, preventing further depressive thoughts and feelings [7, 15, 23, 26, 27].

Lewis has published two studies that may help shed light on whether the behavioral theory or facial feedback hypothesis is the "correct" explanation of the beneficial effects of botulinum toxin used in patients with major depressive disorder. In one study, he compares patients who received botulinum toxin of the forehead with those who received other cosmetic procedures including glycolic acid peels, laser treatments, and hyaluronic acid fillers to the forehead or other areas of the face. While all of the patients noted an improved perception of their appearance, only the patients who were treated with botulinum toxin of the forehead noted an improved depression score on post-treatment surveys. The results of this study contradict the behavioral theory; if the behavioral theory were to hold true, then in addition to increased self-perceived attractiveness, all patients in the study would also have an improved depression score [28].

In his second study, Lewis noted that patients who were treated with botulinum toxin in the glabella, which decreased the ability to frown, had an improved mood, whereas patients treated with botulinum toxin in the crow's feet area, which decreased smile lines, had a reduced mood. The results of this study indicate that it is not the act of injection, per se, nor the systemic absorption of botulinum toxin that results in improvement in depression. However, both the behavioral theory and facial feedback hypotheses can potentially explain these results. Botulinum toxin in the crow's feet area resulted in a decreased ability to emote a genuine smile around the eyes. According to the behavioral theory, this diminished ability to smile could have resulted in a person being perceived by others as less happy, thus making subsequent social interactions less positive. The facial feedback hypothesis dictates that the reduction of the act of smiling could have worsened a patient's mood as the brain did not perceive as much positive emotion [29].

A retrospective study performed by Reichenberg et al. in 2016 showed that the presence of glabellar frown lines at baseline was not predictive of which patients would have the most improvement in their depression following botulinum toxin injections into the glabella. These findings argue against the behavioral theory, as even patients without perceivable frown lines had improved mood following botulinum toxin injections. Furthermore, the facial feedback hypothesis can be supported by MRI studies showing that botulinum toxin A treatment of corrugator muscles decreases afferent signals from facial muscles and impacts brain areas involved in emotional processing [7, 15, 30].

Conclusions

Botulinum toxin A is well known for its use in the cosmetic world to reduce wrinkles, but its new and emerging use in the treatment of depression offers a novel adjuvant to improve the mood of patients with major depressive disorder. Though the exact mechanisms of botulinum's effects on mood are uncertain, the behavioral and facial feedback hypotheses offer compelling views on how botulinum toxin may yield its antidepressant effects. Phase II trials are currently underway to determine if botulinum toxin A will become a standard treatment for depression [22]. For now, botulinum toxin A treatment should be considered off-label for patients who are still having depressive symptoms despite standard treatment with psychotherapy and/or antidepressant medications, or patients who cannot tolerate these treatments. The aesthetic practitioner should be familiar with this emerging modality to both observe their own patients' responses to neurotoxins and potentially to offer consultation to their colleagues in the mental health professions.

References

1 (2019). The American Society for Aesthetic Plastic Surgery's Cosmetic Surgery National Data Bank: Statistics 2018. *Aesthet. Surg. J.* 39 (4): 1–27.

2 Erbguth, F.J. and Naumann, M. (1999). Historical aspects of botulinum toxin: Justinus Kerner (1786–1862) and the "sausage poison". *Neurology* 53 (8): 1850–1853.

3 Allergan (2020). Botox Cosmetic. Available from: https://www.botoxcosmetic.com/what-is-botox-cosmetic/about-botox-cosmetic-treatment?cid=sem_goo_43700047465576422&gclid=cj0kcqjwopl2brdxarisaemm9y8wwck42cficn7xgflohvkhc2grc3ilovyrsonacs888xlbk8_6uauaasgnealw_wcb&gclsrc=aw.ds.

4 Nestler, E.J. et al. (2002). Neurobiology of depression. *Neuron* 34 (1): 13–25.

5 Al Abdulmohsen, T. and Kruger, T.H. (2011). The contribution of muscular and auditory pathologies to the symptomatology of autism. *Med. Hypotheses* 77 (6): 1038–1047.

6 Magid, M. et al. (2014). Treatment of major depressive disorder using botulinum toxin A: a 24-week randomized, double-blind, placebo-controlled study. *J. Clin. Psychiatry* 75 (8): 837–844.

7 Hennenlotter, A. et al. (2009). The link between facial feedback and neural activity within central circuitries of emotion – new insights from botulinum toxin-induced denervation of frown muscles. *Cereb. Cortex* 19 (3): 537–542.

8 James, W. (1894). The physical basis of emotion. *Psychol. Rev.* 1: 516–529.

9 Darwin, C. (1872). *The Expression of the Emotions in Man and Animals*. New York: D. Appleton.

10 Larsen, R.J., Kasimatis, M., and Frey, K. (1992). Facilitating the furrowed brow: an unobtrusive test of the facial feedback hypothesis applied to unpleasant affect. *Cognit. Emot.* 6 (5): 321–338.

11 Strack, F., Martin, L.L., and Stepper, S. (1988). Inhibiting and facilitating conditions of the human smile: a nonobtrusive test of the facial feedback hypothesis. *J. Pers. Soc. Psychol.* 54 (5): 768–777.

12 Alam, M. et al. (2008). Botulinum toxin and the facial feedback hypothesis: can looking better make you feel happier? *J. Am. Acad. Dermatol.* 58 (6): 1061–1072.

13 Schwartz, G.E. et al. (1976). Facial muscle patterning to affective imagery in depressed and nondepressed subjects. *Science* 192 (4238): 489–491.

14 Greden, J.F., Genero, N., and Price, H.L. (1985). Agitation-increased electromyogram activity in the corrugator muscle region: a possible explanation of the "Omega sign"? *Am. J. Psychiatry* 142 (3): 348–351.

15 Kim, M.J. et al. (2014). Botulinum toxin-induced facial muscle paralysis affects amygdala responses to the perception of emotional expressions: preliminary findings from an A-B-A design. *Biol. Mood Anxiety Disord.* 4: 11.

16 Burgen, A.S., Dickens, F., and Zatman, L.J. (1949). The action of botulinum toxin on the neuro-muscular junction. *J. Physiol.* 109 (1–2): 10–24.

17 Finzi, E. and Wasserman, E. (2006). Treatment of depression with botulinum toxin A: a case series. *Dermatol. Surg.* 32 (5): 645–649; discussion 649–50.

18 Finzi, E. and Rosenthal, N.E. (2014). Treatment of depression with onabotulinumtoxinA: a randomized, double-blind, placebo controlled trial. *J. Psychiatr. Res.* 52: 1–6.

19 Wollmer, M.A. et al. (2012). Facing depression with botulinum toxin: a randomized controlled trial. *J. Psychiatr. Res.* 46 (5): 574–581.

20 Hexsel, D. et al. (2013). Evaluation of self-esteem and depression symptoms in depressed and nondepressed subjects treated with onabotulinumtoxinA for glabellar lines. *Dermatol. Surg.* 39 (7): 1088–1096.

21 Zamanian, A. et al. (2017). Efficacy of Botox versus placebo for treatment of patients with major depression. *Iran. J. Public Health* 46 (7): 982–984.

22 Brin, M.F. et al. (2020). OnabotulinumtoxinA for the treatment of major depressive disorder: a phase 2 randomized, double-blind, placebo-controlled trial in adult females. *Int. Clin. Psychopharmacol.* 35 (1): 19–28.

23 Kim, J., Khoury, R., and Grossberg, G.T. (2018). Botulinum toxin: emerging psychiatric indications: botulinum toxin has shown promising antidepressant effects, and might be helpful for several other indications. *Curr. Psychiatry*: 8–18.

24 Magid, M. et al. (2015). Treating depression with botulinum toxin: a pooled analysis of randomized controlled trials. *Pharmacopsychiatry* 48 (6): 205–210.

25 Beer, K. (2010). Cost effectiveness of botulinum toxins for the treatment of depression: preliminary observations. *J. Drugs Dermatol.* 9 (1): 27–30.

26 Baumeister, J.C., Papa, G., and Foroni, F. (2016). Deeper than skin deep – the effect of botulinum toxin-A on emotion processing. *Toxicon* 118: 86–90.

27 Finzi, E. (2003). *The Face of Emotion: How Botox Affects our Moods and Relationships*. New York: Palgrave Macmillan.

28 Lewis, M.B. and Bowler, P.J. (2009). Botulinum toxin cosmetic therapy correlates with a more positive mood. *J. Cosmet. Dermatol.* 8 (1): 24–26.

29 Lewis, M.B. (2018). The interactions between botulinum-toxin-based facial treatments and embodied emotions. *Sci. Rep.* 8 (1): 14720.

30 Reichenberg, J.S. et al. (2016). Botulinum toxin for depression: does patient appearance matter? *J. Am. Acad. Dermatol.* 74 (1): 171–173.e1.

Part IV

Psychological Challenges in Aesthetics

12

Boundaries

Evan A. Rieder[1] and Jacob Sacks[2,3]

[1] The Ronald O. Perelman Department of Dermatology, New York University Grossman School of Medicine, New York, NY, USA
[2] Private practice, San Francisco, CA, USA
[3] Department of Psychiatry, University of California San Francisco, San Francisco, CA, USA

Introduction

When our patients make an appointment with a mental health practitioner and walk through the door to seek treatment for a problem that they recognize, they cross both a figurative and literal threshold. Mental health clinicians are well equipped to help those patients with the insight to know that something might be psychologically wrong. The aesthetic practitioner often does not have the same opportunity to start the assessment from a place of shared understanding. Often as dermatologists, plastic surgeons, and aesthetic professionals we are faced with and put in the position of treating psychiatric disorders that come in the disguise of aesthetic concerns. In other instances, we offer consultation to people living with psychiatric disorders that they deny. Without the knowledge of psychiatric and psychological tools and tricks, we are often challenged emotionally and occupationally in our dealings with such patients. A lack of personal boundaries, disrespect for time restrictions, unreasonable expectations, inadequate reimbursement, and, sometimes, behavioral difficulties all may affect our practices and daily functioning. In some ways and at some points, especially in circumstances when a patient is highly invested in denying that mental or emotional problems underpin their complaints, our jobs can be more challenging than that of the psychiatrist, psychologist, or mental health social worker. While we attempt to provide comprehensive aesthetic services to our patients, we are forced to deal with the psychopathology of people who are unaware of or minimize their conditions. The goals of this chapter are to enforce the concept of boundary setting, offer insights to help identify problematic scenarios when they arise, and take action. By utilizing simple psychological tips, you can easily make your practice run more efficiently.

Case Studies

Case 12.1   Time Pressure
A 32-year-old woman presents to your office as a new patient for cosmetic consultation. You have scheduled her for your normal initial patient encounter, which is 30 minutes. The patient comes in on time. As you sit down to begin the consultation,

(Continued)

Essential Psychiatry for the Aesthetic Practitioner, First Edition. Edited by Evan A. Rieder and Richard G. Fried.
© 2021 John Wiley & Sons Ltd. Published 2021 by John Wiley & Sons Ltd.

Case 12.1   (Continued)

the patient begins talking about her aesthetic concerns. She continues for a few minutes then meanders into several different areas, including some concerns that seem to be tangentially relevant and others that are totally unrelated to the cosmetic consultation. You feel your heart start to race and begin to worry that this patient will begin to monopolize much more time than has been allotted for her consultation. When she finally stops talking, 15 minutes have passed and you are forced to curtail the most important parts of your examination: the discussion of potential interventions and procedures. You breeze quickly through your examination and discussion, making up the precious time that was spent listening to her talk. You then breathe a sigh of relief as you say goodbye, asking the patient to follow-up with your front desk to schedule an appointment for aesthetic intervention. As you reach for the doorknob the patient then says, "But wait, what about my hair? It has been thinning and that's the main reason why I'm here."

Clinical Relevance and Implications

One of the reasons that aesthetic practitioners enter their respective fields is to help people look and feel better about themselves. Like most medical professionals, we like our patients to feel at ease, comfortable, and heard. When patients respect our time and schedules, our jobs are often pleasant and rewarding. However, when patients violate time boundaries we often find ourselves in quandaries. Psychiatrists and psychologists, on the other hand, have both the luxury of time and wherewithal to construct treatment parameters for each patient. Mental health professionals have specific training in establishing and communicating a treatment frame. The frame is a way of referring to what happens inside the treatment and what happens outside the treatment. This includes the clear definition of clinician–patient roles and relationships and more practical boundaries – what happens during the sessions, how the time is used, what happens at the beginning and end of the appointments, and establishing expectations around personal interactions and communication [1].

When dermatologists, plastic surgeons, and aesthetic clinicians are faced with patients who routinely break time boundaries, they often do not know what to do or how to redirect patients. Some find themselves running late or going overtime. Through the maintenance of a structural treatment framework, psychiatrists are much more regimented with patients. For example, if a patient has a 45-minute appointment that begins every Monday, they have booked the therapist's time but are free to do whatever they wish with this time. If they choose to get coffee and arrive 15 minutes late, their appointment is reduced to 30 minutes in duration so as not to infringe upon the next patient. The same rules can be introduced into aesthetic practices, particularly for patients who are repeatedly late and inconvenience staff and other patients of the practice. In a similar vein, patients who routinely push the boundaries of the appointment (e.g. by being difficult to interrupt) can be redirected and reminded of the treatment parameters proactively.

When a new patient presents to the office and will not stop talking, the clinician is presented with a difficult scenario. To avoid finding yourself in the uncomfortable scenario of losing control over an office visit, the authors find two distinct approaches to be helpful in structuring the initial consultation.

Approach 1: Reactive, Less Structured

The first important element is to sit down and listen. Allowing for a few minutes of uninterrupted listening will allow most patients to feel "heard." At that point, if the patient continues to talk, ask if it is OK to interrupt the patient. This is a key step that helps to **set**

expectations for the patient going forward. You might say something like:

> Ms. Smith, is it OK if I cut you off and ask a few important questions?

Almost all patients will respond affirmatively to this simple request, and most people are understanding about the constraints on the aesthetic practitioner's schedule. There is interesting information to be gleaned about the potential future clinician–patient relationship from the patients who respond negatively. After this point, feel free to cut the patient off repeatedly as needed to be able to regain control of the conversation:

> OK Ms. Smith, I'm going to interrupt you again as I need to ask some important questions.

If the conversation continues to go in a tangential direction, pose binary ("yes"/"no") or close-ended questions to direct conversation:

> Ms. Smith, let's switch directions for a few moments. Have you ever had a soft tissue filler injection? What was the location of the procedure? Were you happy with the outcome?

Typically these simple but firm interventions will allow you to glean essential information while moving the consultation at a speed that suits you.

If you still have difficulties reining in a talkative patient, explain the realities of a busy clinic and emphasize the need for follow-up to fully address their concerns:

> Ms. Smith, hair issues are incredibly important concerns and often require substantial time to discuss. It's essential that we dedicate sufficient time to each one of your concerns or I'd be doing you a disservice. Why don't we have you schedule a follow-up at my next available appointment and we can get all of your questions answered in a time that would be satisfactory for you and sufficient for me not to give your concerns short shrift.

In cases where this intervention fails, it can be helpful to place blame for your time constraints on a third party (e.g. an employer, institution, or group) for not providing you sufficient time to work together. Such an approach can help build an alliance between you and your patient.

Approach 2: Proactive, More Structured

Another option is to be very explicit with new patients on initial consultation. Direct guidance from the aesthetic practitioner can be very effective in containing patients who may be nervous about meeting a new doctor. Those patients who have difficulty containing themselves also become apparent earlier in the encounter before things go off the rails and the doctor is in the uncomfortable position of having to interrupt and make the patient feel rejected.

> Hi Ms. Smith, it's nice to meet you. I have us scheduled for 30 minutes today. I like to start by giving you a few minutes to tell me in your own words what you think I should know and how I can help you today. At some point I might jump in if there are specific questions that would be helpful for me to know. I would like to ensure that we have 5–10 minutes to discuss the changes I am seeing on your skin (and body) and a treatment plan. We should save a few minutes at the end to review the next steps. If there is time, we may also have the opportunity to begin nonsurgical treatments today.

Once the expectations are made explicit, it becomes easier to relax and just let the patient talk. As importantly, there is a higher chance of the patient "feeling heard."

Follow-Up

Patients who come for follow-up may be easier to deal with as you can anticipate, prepare for issues, and set expectations from the onset.

> Ms. Smith we have 15 minutes today. What are the most important things that we address today?

A simple intervention such as the aforementioned opening line will allow containment from the onset of the appointment. You set the expectations and rules and can assert control over the appointment structure. For more talkative or fragile patients, it can be helpful to have regular brief visits. If you have the structure, it may be worth considering longer appointments for patients who require more time. We have found the following phrase to be particularly helpful in setting expectations and building long-term relationships:

> Remember, whatever we don't finish today we will get to at your next appointment. The aesthetic rejuvenation process is a journey that we are embarking on together.

Case 12.2 Personal Boundaries

A 22-year-old man presents to your clinic as a new patient for aesthetic consultation. You have an easy discussion about his concerns of skin quality and facial aging and make recommendations for a skin care regimen and nonsurgical injectable medications. Although the technical part of the interaction flowed smoothly, you feel somewhat uneasy about this patient. He seems overly familiar with you and sometimes even calls you by your first name. As you complete the consultation, your heart sinks as he begins asking personal questions and reveals that he knows some intimate details about your personal life. While you question if this patient is simply trying to be friendly or desiring of a more intimate relationship – whether romantic or platonic – you instinctively sense that he is attempting to move this relationship away from the professional clinician–patient encounter. He reveals that he has been following your posts on social media for months and is "a big fan."

Clinical Relevance and Implications

By explicitly defining the nature of the treatment relationship, mental health providers are much more adept at setting boundaries with their patients. The psychiatrist–patient relationship is inherently intimate, but inherently asymmetrical. While a patient will divulge intimate details of their life – including information about family, platonic and romantic relationships, occupational and social concerns – they often do not have the same level of access to the personal details of the treating clinician. With the advent of social media and patients who feel comfortable discovering information about their clinicians online and contacting them (sometimes frequently) via electronic media, aesthetic practitioners have quickly moved to promote their services through social platforms. And with large institutions including private conglomerates and academic centers allowing greater access to their clinicians through email and electronic medical records, the aesthetic practitioner may now have the sense that they may never truly have "time off."

Social media platforms may pose challenging situations for the aesthetic practitioner. While these applications are undeniably an efficient modality for wide dissemination of information about cosmetic services, they are potential pitfalls which might lead certain patients to misinterpret the depth of their connection to their clinicians. This becomes particularly thorny when the clinician shares detailed nontraditional personal information in the public sphere – including information about their families, personal relationships, social life, or even revealing photography. While people should feel free to share whatever they feel is appropriate in the public sphere, it should not be surprising that inadequate boundary setting by clinicians could lead to patients feeling more free with boundaries in their interactions with you. While sometimes these interactions are harmless in nature, in others, particularly when a patient develops a fantasy about their clinician, there is a potential for misinterpretation and a blurring of the patient and doctor roles.

The aesthetic clinician should thoughtfully consider which type of content is disseminated in the public sphere. Likewise in the office setting, it is worth considering the use of chaperones for examinations and consultations, particularly when intimate body parts are being exposed. In rare occurrences, the physical examination may be misinterpreted in patients with a history of abuse or disordered attachment to family members. And at times when patients desire more than a professional relationship with a clinician, it is advisable to refer healthy patients to colleagues. While it is ethically questionable for mental health practitioners to enter into nonprofessional relationships with their patients, aesthetic professionals may be able to refer patients to other practitioners for treatment if they wish to pursue a nonprofessional relationship.

In extreme examples of time or personal boundary violations, one might wish to consider providing patients with a copy of your practice policy or if necessary using a behavioral contract.

Approach 1: Be Proactive: A Practice Policies Document

A practice policies document establishes expectations explicitly with all patients up front rather than waiting for problematic behavior to emerge. This document should be available on your practice website and in hard copy in your office. In it, there should be clear instructions about the ways patients can contact you, including electronically and after hours, a disclaimer that you may not always be available after hours, information on reaching a covering clinician, and emergency procedures. There should also be a clause about payment and fees, unpaid bills, and privacy.

Approach 2: Be Reactive: A Behavioral Contract

Behavioral contracts are commonly utilized by teachers in interactions with students, child psychiatrists with patients, and addiction specialists with people living with substance use disorders. They are seldom used outside of the mental health professions but may be helpful to provide structure to patients who are repeatedly pushing limits in your clinic. As opposed to the proactively provided practice policies document, the behavioral contract is reactive and only introduced if repeatedly problematic behavior arises. The essential elements of a behavioral contract include:

1) A clear definition of the behavior to be exhibited both from the patient and staff
2) The positive consequences of performing the desired behavior
3) The negative consequences of not performing the desired behavior
4) Signatures of those entering into the contract [2]

Behavioral contracts can be useful in situations including repeated inappropriate behavior (e.g. verbal, physical interactions in the office), manipulative behavior, and failure to meet financial obligations. Before proposing a behavioral contract, consider whether or not the clinician–patient relationship is worth preserving, whether the behavior is an isolated incident or a pattern, if the behavior can be changed, if the behavior has been clearly documented in the patient's chart, if you are willing to follow-through on the consequences of the contract (e.g. termination of the provider–patient relationship), and if there is an immediate threat to you or your staff. In the event of immediate threat, termination of the relationship is a more prudent option. If the decision is made to use a behavioral contract, we recommend preparing your words carefully and

Heading:
Ms. Smith's Skin Care Contract
Goal:
To meet Ms. Smith's needs for skin care and rejuvenation while balancing staff's need to maintain efficiency and help other patients
Patient Agreements:
I will come to my appointment on time. I understand that my clinician needs to end our appointment on time to assist other patients. I will limit my phone calls to once per week. I will treat staff with respect and not use a demeaning tone.
Staff Agreements:
We will promptly room Ms. Smith and address all of her concerns for the duration of her visit. We will return Ms. Smith's phone calls and emails within 24 h of receipt. We will treat Ms. Smith with respect and not using a demeaning tone.
Positive Consequences:
Continued care of your skin and aesthetic concerns
Negative Consequences:
Termination of the clinician–patient relationship
Signatures: (all parties sign here)
Patient _____ Clinician_____ Ancillary Staff_____

Figure 12.1 Sample behavioral contract.

rehearsing/role-playing before presenting the contract to the patient. With respect to patient receptivity, multiple outcomes are possible. Behavioral contracts can be helpful in many scenarios but we find them particularly useful for boundary violations, such as repeated violations of your time or private life, personality issues that cause challenges for your staff, and failure to pay bills. A sample behavioral contract for an aesthetic practice is shown in Figure 12.1.

Case 12.3 Getting Patients to Mental Health
A 55-year-old woman who is a regular aesthetic patient of yours presents to your clinic for consultation for rhinoplasty. She has been a reliable patient for years, paying her bills on time and showing up for regular scheduled neurotoxin and soft tissue filler injections. However, over the past few years she has become somewhat difficult, unsatisfied with the results of many cosmetic procedures and regularly speaking to you about preoccupations with minor defects in skin quality that do not seem obvious to you. Because you are a psychologically minded clinician you screen her for body dysmorphic disorder and she does not meet the criteria. Although you do not want to lose her as a regular injectable patient, you have the sense that she is not someone who will do well with a surgical procedure without the help of a co-treating mental health practitioner. You want to refer her to see a psychologist but do not know who to refer to, when is the right time, or what to say. How do you proceed?

Clinical Relevance and Implications

One of the most common questions we face as aesthetic providers is how do I get my patient to see a psychiatrist? Unfortunately this is also one of the hardest things to do, and one for which there is no formula or easy answer. We hope the following tips will make the process of referral easier.

- **Tip 1**: *Have personal relationships with mental health providers.*
  Just like you might canvas local primary care practices for aesthetic referrals, make sure to connect with and learn who the psychologists, psychiatrists, and social work therapists are in your area. If you work in a large group or in an academic setting, make use of consultation-liaison psychiatry services. Have the contact information for these colleagues easily available in your cellphone and on business cards to give to your patients and clients.
- **Tip 2**: *Go slow and attempt to destigmatize mental healthcare.*
  It is nearly certain that a referral to a mental health provider will be rejected if offered to a patient on initial consultation. Thus it is of utmost importance to establish trust and a working relationship before introducing the concept of psychological referral. Once rapport is established, your patients will be more likely to accept a referral, particularly if it is framed as an adjunct to the primary aesthetic practitioner–patient relationship. Ideally with time, the nature of the relationships will change as will the roles, making the aesthetic practitioner–patient relationship an adjunct to a developing primary mental health practitioner–patient relationship. Having personal relationships with mental health providers will help you to pair your patients with the best-fitting mental health practitioner.

When you are ready to introduce the concept of mental health treatment, we find it helpful to remind our patients that having a person who can tend to our mental health is, in many ways, a gift to give to ourselves. Over time, a healthy relationship with a mental health provider can help your patients and clients achieve a sense of emotional well-being, including freedom from longstanding personal conflicts, expansion of interpersonal and occupational functioning, and increased self-actualization.

- **Tip 3**: *Know your limits.*
  One of the most important teachings that medical practitioners must remember is that you must find and recognize something that you like about each of your patients. If you are not able to connect with your patients on any level, consider whether this is a relationship worth pursuing. Likewise, if you feel that you are being asked to perform a procedure or take care of a patient issue that is outside of your field of knowledge or comfort zone, it is sometimes preferable to refer a patient to a trusted colleague or a known expert in the area of concern. Finally, if there is an interpersonal conflict or irreparable personal boundary violation between your patient and yourself (or your staff), it is well within your right to resign from your patient's care [3]. In instances where you have entered into a treatment relationship with a patient, it is essential to know the rules governing medical practice and patient abandonment by state. Specific areas of psychopathology and psychiatric diagnosis are discussed in Chapters 13 and 15 of this text, but we find the "SAFE" acronym to be a helpful initial screening tool for those practitioners who are not well versed in the assessment of psychiatric disease (Figure 12.2) [4].

Self-evaluation of attractiveness (Is the patient seeking a cosmetic procedure to treat a compromised self-image?)
Anxiety (Does the patient exhibit distress?)
Fear (Does the patient exhibit a preoccupation with detail that is masking underlying fears?)
Expectation (Does the patient have unrealistic expectations about social/occupational changes from a given procedure?)

Figure 12.2 SAFE acronym for psychological screening. *Source:* From ref. [4].

Conclusions

Aesthetic practitioners may be forced to reckon with multiple personal challenges in their practices. Time pressure, personal boundary violations, and even unmet financial obligations can present thorny issues for even the most experienced clinicians to navigate. Placing firm boundaries on time and interpersonal interactions can help increase practice efficiency and allow business to function smoothly. In rare instances, behavioral contracts can help redirect difficult patients or resolve thorny issues. Knowing when you are out of your comfort zone can help you know when to say no to a patient, when to refer a patient or ask for help, and if and when it's time to resign. And finally, having a network of mental health professionals and a facility with referrals can help provide your patients with comprehensive interdisciplinary care.

References

1 Gray, A. (2013). *An Introduction to the Therapeutic Frame*. New York: Routledge.

2 Medical Protective (2013). Behaviour contracts. Medical Protective Clinical Risk Management Department. Fort Wayne, IN: The Medical Protective Company. https://www.server5.medpro.com/documents/11006/16738/behavior+contracts+guideline_10-2013.pdf (accessed 7 June 2020).

3 Magid, M. and Reichenberg, J.S. (2019). Treating the difficult patient: ten pearls to reduce resentment and regain control of the doctor–patient visit. *Skinmed* 17 (1): 11–14.

4 Lavell, S. and Lewis, C. (1984). SAFE: a practical guide to psychological factors in selecting patients for facial cosmetic surgery. *Ann. Plast. Surg.* 12: 256–259.

13

Difficult Personalities and Personality Disorders in the Cosmetic Clinic

Mio Nakamura[1] and John Koo[2]

[1] Department of Dermatology, University of Michigan, Ann Arbor, MI, USA
[2] Department of Dermatology, University of California San Francisco, San Francisco, CA, USA

Introduction

Patient satisfaction is crucial to a successful aesthetic practice and an important marker of quality care [1]. Practical techniques to enhance patient satisfaction include maximizing communication, spending sufficient time in clinical interactions, providing appropriate patient education, and involving patients in therapeutic discussions [2]. Such techniques are often adequate for the average patient. However, in a minority of cases, providers may encounter a difficult patient in which even extended time, effort, and consideration are not enough to satisfy the patient. One such group of patients includes those with difficult personalities and those with personality disorders [3]. This chapter focuses on the specific types of personality disorders that are most relevant in the aesthetic practice and how to skillfully recognize and manage patients with personality disorders.

Difficult Personalities vs. Personality Disorders

Personality style is defined as enduring personal characteristics that affect how a person thinks, feels, behaves, and interacts in relationships with others and the environment [4]. Personality is an important determinant of how people react to life stress. In the aesthetic practice, personality affects how patients recognize and present their cosmetic concerns, relate to a provider, respond to treatments and procedures, and deal with discomfort [5].

Personalities can be perceived by the provider as "difficult" if they do not align with the provider's personality style. However, if a provider is able to understand the patient's unique personality style and adjust behaviors to accommodate the patient's personality traits, it is possible to establish and maintain a quality patient–provider relationship. In fact, patients who feel that they share the same personality style as their provider have been shown to be more satisfied with the care they receive [6].

Personality style is different from diagnosable personality disorders in that personality disorders are characterized by enduring patterns of maladaptive thinking and behavior that deviate from the cultural norm and are extremely rigid. Such characteristics can be harmful, not only to patients but also to others around them. No matter how much effort is put forth, the encounter may end in frustration for both the patient and the provider. Patient

Table 13.1 Diagnostic criteria for a personality disorder according to the *Diagnostic and Statistical Manual of Mental Disorders, Fifth Edition (DSM-5)*.

The essential features of a personality disorder are impairments in personality (self and interpersonal) functioning and the presence of pathological personality traits. To diagnose a personality disorder, the following criteria must be met:

A. Significant impairments in self (identity or self-direction) and interpersonal (empathy or intimacy) functioning.

B. One or more pathological personality trait domains or trait facets.

C. The impairments in personality functioning and the individual's personality trait expression are relatively stable across time and consistent across situations.

D. The impairments in personality functioning and the individual's personality trait expression are not better understood as normative for the individual's developmental stage or sociocultural environment.

E. The impairments in personality functioning and the individual's personality trait expression are not solely due to the direct physiological effects of a substance (e.g. a drug of abuse, medication) or a general medical condition (e.g. severe head trauma).

Source: Adapted from American Psychiatric Association [4].

satisfaction is largely a subjective experience reported by the individual [7]; a uniform approach that is effective for the average patient is often inadequate for patients with personality disorders.

Personality Disorders

Personality disorders are defined as stable and enduring patterns of thought, feeling, and behavior that deviate from the norms of one's culture and are pervasive and inflexible across many aspects of one's life [4]. These personality traits are generally stable over time and across situations and can affect cognition, affect, interpersonal functioning, and impulse control. Rigid personality traits cause significant distress and impairment in activities of daily living and social and occupational

functioning. The full diagnostic criteria for a personality disorder according to the *Diagnostic & Statistical Manual of Mental Disorders, Fifth Edition* (*DSM-5*) are shown in Table 13.1 [4]. To diagnose a specific type of personality disorder, the patient must meet specific criteria pertaining to that type of personality disorder. The diagnostic criteria for the types of personality disorders most relevant to the aesthetic provider will be reviewed in detail below and are summarized in Table 13.2.

Personality disorders affect approximately 15% of the general population, although the prevalence is likely higher in the medical setting [9] and even higher in the aesthetic practice [10–14]. Personality disorders often manifest in late childhood to early adulthood. Certain personality disorders including dependent, histrionic, and borderline occur more often in women, while antisocial, narcissistic, and obsessive compulsive personality disorders occur more often in men [15].

The etiology of personality disorders is thought to involve various combinations of biologic, developmental, environmental, social, and genetic triggers. Structural and morphologic differences may exist in the brains of patients with specific personality disorders, supporting a biologic etiology [16, 17]. Personality disorders, especially borderline personality disorder, are also frequently associated with disruptive childhood experiences including neglect and childhood sexual, physical, or emotional abuse [18]. Familial and twin studies estimate heritability of approximately 40% for borderline personality disorder [19].

Diagnosing personality disorders is challenging. First, to make an accurate diagnosis, it is typically necessary for the provider to get to know the patient over time to learn how the patient reacts and relates to various people and situations. Second, a true personality disorder must be differentiated from personality traits that become exaggerated under stressful situations such as a medical illness. Third, it is important to distinguish personality disorders from personality changes caused by general medical

Table 13.2 Summary of personality disorders most relevant to the aesthetic provider and practical tips for how to approach patients with each personality disorder.

Personality disorder	Clinical presentation	Clinical relevance and implications	Approach
Borderline	• Instability in interpersonal relationships, self-image, and affect • Marked impulsivity • Intense fear of rejection and abandonment • Splitting • Self-destructive behaviors	• Presenting complaint is usually due to "need to fill emptiness" • Rejection of requested services or perceived undertreatment is taken as abandonment, causing strong negative emotions	• Do not give in to patient's strong emotionality • Avoid unnecessary treatments/procedures • Provide other options rather than complete rejection • Regular follow-up appointments • Be aware of splitting and potential self-harming behavior
Histrionic	• Dramatic and excessive emotionality • Attention-seeking, provocative, seductive behavior • Perceives relationships to be more intimate than they are • Easily influenced by others	• Difficulty in medical decision-making due to impulsivity • Repeated visits due to minor defects causing anxiety • Dissatisfaction when not receiving enough attention	• Assistant or chaperone should be present at all times • Involve patient in decision-making but provide guidance, reassurance, and support • Avoid unnecessary treatment/procedures • Do not let patient's seductive behavior cloud judgment • Give appropriate attention and compliments focusing on patient as a person • Respond firmly to inappropriate seduction
Obsessive compulsive	• Preoccupation with orderliness, perfectionism, and control • Fear of losing control • Excessive attention to detail • Focus on facts and knowledge to replace or subdue emotions	• Anxiety due to fear of losing control • Knowledge and information gives sense of control over illness • Feeling of loss of control leads to anxiety, depression, and anger	• Professional, structured encounters • Set realistic expectations, be explicit about unattainable outcomes, and document discussion • Detailed explanations and plans (written information and guide to appropriate resources) • Regular follow-up appointments
Narcissistic	• Grandiosity • Uncomfortable in vulnerable or inferior position • Need for admiration • Lack of empathy • Demanding and entitled	• Underlying emptiness, low self-esteem, or insecurities • Need for admiration and power	• Do not take patient's behaviors personally • Focus on an attitude of respect • Engage patient at a medical level (discuss in medical terminology, discuss journal article, etc.) • Allow patient to have a sense of power by engaging in medical decision-making • Discuss details and risks of procedure and document discussion in medical records

Source: Adapted from Nakamura and Koo [8].

conditions such as traumatic brain injury, stroke, epilepsy, or endocrine disorders [20]. Lastly, personality disorders should not be confused with the diagnosis of other primary psychiatric conditions such as mood, anxiety, and substance abuse disorders. Like personality disorders, these primary psychiatric conditions also show unstable mood and inability to control emotions. It is important to note that a patient with a personality disorder may suffer from other psychiatric illnesses at the same time. Lastly, the provider should keep in mind that it is possible for a patient to meet diagnostic criteria for multiple types of personality disorders [21]. In fact, DSM-5 has a new diagnosis called Personality Disorder – Trait Specified (PD-TS), in which a personality disorder is considered present but the criteria for a specific personality disorder are not fully met.

Treatment of personality disorders is extremely difficult. Patients with personality disorder typically do not seek treatment because it often does not cause personal distress to the patient and there is none to minimal insight into the disorder [22]. Specific psychotherapy techniques may be effective and improvement can occur over time. Behavioral, cognitive, or interpersonal therapies in individual or group settings may be helpful [22]. In a nonpsychiatric setting, it is simply unrealistic to attempt to treat a personality disorder [23] and the best way to approach such a patient is to focus on building and maintaining a better working relationship with them.

In the following sections, the four most commonly encountered personality disorders in the aesthetic practice, borderline, histrionic, obsessive compulsive, and narcissistic personality disorders, will be reviewed. For each personality disorder, a case scenario will be followed by clinically relevant tips such as accurate recognition of the personality disorder and how to approach the patient to achieve the best outcome for both the patient and the provider. The high-yield summaries pertaining to the approach to personality disorders in the aesthetic practice are shown in Table 13.2. It is important to note that identifying the presence of a personality disorder can be helpful to understand how to better approach a "difficult" patient. However, labeling a patient with a personality disorder may serve to stigmatize the patient. This may lead to undertreatment and poorer quality of care, reduced empathy and sympathy, and negative feelings. Therefore providers should consider documenting the diagnosis of a personality disorder in the medical records and correspondence only when it is likely to be helpful in enhancing patient care. In general, it is typically advisable for the aesthetic practitioner to refer patients for whom there is concern over personality pathology to a trusted colleague in the behavioral health profession. Psychologists, psychiatrists, and social workers with behavioral health specialization can help with both the correct diagnosis and management of such challenging patients and clients.

Case Studies

Case 13.1   Borderline Personality Disorder

A 26-year-old woman comes to your office for evaluation of acne scars on the face. When you enter the room, she is visibly upset and states that all of the nursing staff are incompetent and that you are the only doctor who has ever understood her, even though you just met. On examination, she has minimal skin findings. She asks for laser resurfacing, but you do not feel that she would benefit from such a procedure. When you tell her this, she becomes very angry and begins to yell. She states that you are incompetent just like everyone else in the clinic and other doctors she has seen. How should you proceed?

Clinical Relevance and Implications

Patients with borderline personality disorder exhibit instability in their self-image, affect, and relationships with others [9], and there is a tendency toward an all-or-nothing behavior. They exhibit extreme impulsivity, presenting with self-damaging acts including suicide attempts, self-mutilating behaviors, substance abuse, and risky sexual behaviors. They often harbor a deep sense of emptiness and an intense fear of abandonment. Patients with borderline personality disorder often show a pattern of unstable and intense interpersonal relationships and exhibit splitting, characterized by extremes of idealization and devaluation where people are either all good or all bad (also known as "black and white" thinking). There is often a rapid shift in moods manifesting as inappropriate and intense anger or an inability to control anger. Self-destructive behavior is often observed during times of emotional instability. Patients with borderline personality disorder may also have difficulty differentiating reality from fantasy, and may have transient, stress-related paranoid ideation or severe dissociative clinical manifestations [9, 24]. In rare, extreme cases, there may be "micropsychotic episodes" in which the patient can briefly lose touch with reality.

In the aesthetic practice, borderline personality disorder is associated with body dysmorphic disorder [24] and various factitious disorders, such as dermatitis artefacta [25], trichotillomania [26], and psychogenic excoriation [27]. When a patient with borderline personality disorder presents to an aesthetic practice, their presenting complaint is often a "screen" to hide a real, inner, psychologic problem related to emptiness and the need to fill this emptiness. The presenting aesthetic concern may also be a result of somatization of a primary psychological problem. They are at a higher risk for postoperative depression, and therefore it is best to identify these patients quickly and approach them skillfully, including avoiding performing certain procedures, particularly those that are permanent [28]. However, rejection is often met with anger and self-destructive behavior. For example, Morioka et al. reports a patient with borderline personality disorder who cut off her own eyelids after they rejected her request for revision blepharoplasty [29].

When approaching patients with borderline personality disorder, it is important to avoid minimizing the presenting complaint, which may appear minor or purely psychologic in nature to the provider. Patients tend to have an exaggerated fear of abandonment, and rejection of any kind, including denial of requested services or perceived inadequate services, can be taken as a sign of abandonment. It is also common for patients to make the provider feel very good when the provider is idealized; however, this idealization is situational and can quickly change to the opposite extreme. The response to perceived abandonment is typically intense anger, leading to demonization of the provider. Once there is negative splitting, it can be difficult to re-establish a positive relationship, especially for physicians and other healthcare providers who are often mistrusted from the onset of the relationship [9].

In the aesthetic practice, it is crucial that the provider does not acquiesce to satisfy the patient or allow the patient's strong emotions to cloud judgment; unnecessary procedures should be avoided. Some recommend avoiding offering services to patients with borderline personality disorder altogether [28]. However, this can lead to intense anger and impulsive behavior, including self-harm and lawsuits. Instead of rejecting the patient completely, the provider may offer alternative services that are potentially less invasive and establish regular follow-up appointments to reassure that the patient does not feel abandoned because the exact requested procedure is not being offered. Trying to reason with the patient (explaining why you are not providing the requested service) is often ineffective. Furthermore, use of overly technical language may exaggerate the fear associated with the presenting complaint.

Case 13.2   Histrionic Personality Disorder

A 48-year-old woman presents for cosmetic consultation for blepharoplasty. She is dressed in a short red dress and high heels. She seductively crosses her legs and leans toward you to tell you that she had a previous blepharoplasty with a different provider a few months ago but is not satisfied with the outcome but believes that you can help her. When you lean away and begin to discuss the indications and risks of a blepharoplasty, she quickly changes her attitude, looks away, and states that maybe she will go back to her old surgeon. How should you proceed?

Clinical Relevance and Implications

Histrionic personality disorder is characterized by a pervasive pattern of emotionality and excessive attention seeking [9]. Patients are often dramatic and theatrical and express exaggerated emotions, which rapidly shift. They are often uncomfortable when they are not the center of attention. They may dress or behave in a sexually seductive or provocative fashion in an unconscious effort to engage others and draw attention to themselves. Patients often consider relationships to be more intimate than they actually are and are easily influenced by others or circumstances [22].

Histrionic personality disorder is often seen in patients with body dysmorphic disorder who seek cosmetic consultations [30] and has been found to be present in 9.7% of cosmetic surgery patients [31]. These patients tend to have unrealistic expectations for results of cosmetic procedures [32, 33]. They exhibit impulsivity and have a tendency to lack sound reasoning, which makes decision-making difficult when providing cosmetic services. Minor perceived bodily defects create ongoing anxiety, leading them to seek repeated cosmetic services that may be unnecessary. Patients with histrionic personality disorder can become angry if they feel that they are not getting enough attention, which may lead them to leave abruptly for another provider.

To manage patients with histrionic personality disorder it is essential to have an assistant or chaperone present during all clinical interactions [28]. Providers should respond calmly and firmly when patients behave seductively. To satisfy patients with histrionic personality disorder, it may be necessary to provide brief compliments on the patient's appearance made in a nonsuggestive way, while focusing on the patient as a person rather than just as an object of attention. Excessive familiarity should be avoided and effort should be made to maintain a professional relationship at all times. Providers should encourage the patient to participate in decision-making, while providing guidance, advice, and support [5]. Allowing patients to ventilate their fears and concerns while providing appropriate reassurance works better than intellectual explanations [5]. The provider's judgment should not be clouded by the patient's seductive and provocative personality; unnecessary cosmetic treatments and procedures should be avoided, as patients are likely to return dissatisfied with a minor defect, which can be a direct result of the treatment.

Case 13.3   Obsessive Compulsive Personality Disorder

A 37-year-old man presents for consultation for rhinoplasty. He is bothered by the contour of his nasal bridge and brings a picture of a celebrity whose nose he would like to have. When you discuss that it would be difficult to attain this particular celebrity's nose, he states that he has done detailed research on the matter and he knows that it is possible. As you attempt to review the risks of the procedure, he quickly interrupts and asks you for the specific percentages of people who suffer postoperative complications and the immediate and long-term consequences of each complication. You eventually agree to performing a rhinoplasty. At the postoperative follow-up visit, the patient states that his nose is not like the celebrity's nose that he had hoped for and asks you for a revision. How should you proceed?

Clinical Relevance and Implications

Obsessive compulsive personality disorder is characterized by preoccupation with orderliness, perfectionism, and mental and interpersonal control; the result is lack of flexibility, openness, and efficiency. Patients with obsessive compulsive personality disorder tend to be stubborn and controlling [22]. They are unreasonably concerned with details, rules, and organization, which interferes with efficient completion of the task. Some are overly conscientious with excessive concern for morality and ethics [9]. They find it difficult to adapt to other people and situations and instead need others to follow their plans. Thinking is often used as a way to subjugate feeling and emotion. The feeling of loss of control can lead to anxiety, tension, depression, or anger.

A study found that approximately 15% of patients in an outpatient dermatology office suffered from a personality disorder, most commonly obsessive compulsive personality disorder [34]. Specifically in the aesthetic practice, patients with obsessive compulsive personality disorder may have concurrent body dysmorphic disorder [35] and show unrealistic and excessively optimistic expectations of the procedure and its subsequent effect on their lives [28]. They fixate on minor deformities both preoperatively and postoperatively and are resistant to hearing about unattainable outcomes. They may present with a detailed plan of the corrective procedure they feel is best. Postoperatively, they tend to focus on minor imperfections rather than the overall improvement attained by the procedure [28]. Patients often focus on knowledge as a tool for controlling their fears and may ask excessive and repetitive questions about their presenting concern and various cosmetic procedures.

Encounters with patients with obsessive compulsive personality disorder should be structured and professional. A very scientific or detailed explanation may be helpful [9]. It may also be helpful to provide specific resources such as organized websites or journal papers for accurate information about the patient's presenting concern and possible treatments. Patients often become more anxious when doing their own research, especially when using unreliable sources such as social media. It is important to be explicit regarding realistic and attainable outcomes as well as possible risks of the procedure. It is critically important to document this discussion. Providers should avoid performing these procedures if the patient is not able to exhibit adequate comprehension.

When interacting with patients with obsessive compulsive personality disorder, expression of emotion should be limited because excessive emotions can create discomfort. When possible, the patient's sense of independence and control should be maximized. Lastly, periodic, close follow-up appointments may be considered in advance to avoid unexpected or unscheduled visits as a result of the patient's anxiety related to their cosmetic concerns.

Case 13.4   Narcissistic Personality Disorder

A 52-year-old man presents for consultation for botulinum toxin. He was urgently scheduled when he called yesterday saying to the receptionist, "I need to see the doctor right away. Don't you know who I am?" He brings a photograph of himself 30 years ago and states that he would like to look like this again, as the result of aging on his appearance has prohibited him from achieving the maximum position in his current job, which is "very important to growth of the economy." He looks around your office and sees your diploma on the wall and scoffs. He states that he would have tried to see a friend of a friend who is a graduate of Harvard, but the wait was too long so he came to you instead. When you bring up that fillers may be better suited for some of his concerns, the patient quickly interrupts and states that obviously he wants filler there and not botulinum toxin as he originally requested. How should you proceed?

Clinical Relevance and Implications

Narcissistic personality disorder is characterized by a long-standing, pervasive pattern of grandiosity with a need for excessive praise and admiration. Patients may have an exaggerated sense of self-importance and believe that they are unique or special. They often come off as entitled, arrogant, and haughty. They may be driven toward attaining an idealized position in terms of social, personal, romantic, or career accomplishments, while they may be envious and potentially devaluing of others whose accomplishments they perceive as exceeding their own. Patients often lack empathy and can also be manipulative or interpersonally exploitative [9, 22].

Patients with narcissistic personality disorder often present for cosmetic consultation [33] and comprise 25% of patients seeking cosmetic surgery consultations [32]. It is not uncommon for these patients to have body dysmorphic disorder [5]. Patients tend to feel that they were most attractive when they were younger and are likely to undergo cosmetic procedures in an attempt to restore a youthful appearance [33]. They tend to return for repeated consultations despite voicing dissatisfaction with previous treatment results. Some are uncomfortable presenting to a doctor's office as it may make them feel inferior, and they may attempt to compensate for this feeling of inferiority by dictating their demands. During the consultation, they interrupt frequently, demonstrating extreme resistance to active listening with a preconceived notion of what the right procedure is for them [28].

The traits of narcissistic personality disorder can be frustrating and can make the provider feel devalued and disrespected. However, it is crucial for the provider not to take this personally. It is important to remember that the personality traits are often a "screen" to hide a sense of low self-esteem and deep insecurity. The provider should remember that there is a need for praise, sense of power, and admiration, and overall, patients respond better to an attitude of respect. The best approach is to exhibit generous validation of the patient's concerns with attentive but factual response to questions [9]. Providers can give the patient a sense of uniqueness and respect by engaging the patient at a medical level as one might with a colleague, such as discussing a recent medical journal paper [5]. Most importantly, to provide appropriate medical care, it is important not to let the patient dictate the entire encounter. Instead, allowing the patient to have a sense of power by engaging in medical decision-making can be helpful, especially minor decisions that may not directly affect the outcome of the aesthetic treatment or procedure.

In the aesthetic practice, some patients with narcissistic personality disorder may be reasonable surgical candidates as long as extra precautions are taken. A witness should be present during visits, extensive written materials should be provided, and the provider should ensure that the patient exhibits understanding of the procedure, potential risks, and realistic outcomes [28], which should all be documented. However, despite these efforts, the patient may exhibit extreme hostility and anger postoperatively when their expectations are not met. It may be tempting for the provider to dismiss or discharge the patient from the practice; however, this may cause "narcissistic injury" in which the patient will do anything to "get back at you," which may include lawsuits.

Conclusions

Personality disorders are commonly encountered in the aesthetic practice. Given that personality disorders are characterized by rigid and maladaptive behavior and thinking, it is important for providers to be skillful in the approach to such patients, especially in the aesthetic practice where patient satisfaction is key. Once a personality disorder is identified, the underlying primary psychological issues should be kept in mind throughout the patient encounter. These include emptiness, neediness, and fear of abandonment in borderline personality disorder; need for attention in histrionic personality disorder; anxiety and need for control in obsessive compulsive personality disorder; and insecurity and need for admiration in narcissistic personality disorder. The behavior of the provider should then be adapted to the patient's underlying psychologic reality, keeping in mind that the presenting skin complaint is often a secondary problem, and the primary matter of importance is how the provider interacts and manages such patients. Patient satisfaction in patients with personality disorders can be maximized when the provider can understand the underlying psychodynamics of the patient. Being aware of the personality disorder and being skillful with subsequent interactions allows patients to feel that the provider is on their side, which is fundamental to providing satisfactory aesthetic care to patients with personality disorders.

References

1 Manary, M.P., Boulding, W., Staelin, R. et al. (2013). The patient experience and health outcomes. *N. Engl. J. Med.* 368: 201–203.

2 Sorenson, E., Malakouti, M., Brown, G. et al. (2015). Enhancing patient satisfaction in dermatology. *Am. J. Clin. Dermatol.* 16: 1–4.

3 Hahn, S.R., Thompson, K.S., Wills, T.A. et al. (1994). The difficult doctor–patient relationship: somatization, personality and psychopathology. *J. Clin. Epidemiol.* 47: 647–657.

4 American Psychiatric Association (2003). *Diagnostic and Statistical Manual of Mental Disorders*, 5e. Arlington, VA: American Psychiatric Association.

5 Fortin, A.H., Dwamena, F.C., Frankel, R.M., and Smith, R.C. (eds.) (2019). The clinician–patient relationship. In: *Smith's Patient-Centered Interviewing: An Evidence-Based Method*, 4e. New York: McGraw Hill.

6 Krupat, E., Bell, R.A., Kravitz, R.L. et al. (2001). When physicians and patients think alike: patient-centered beliefs and their impact on satisfaction and trust. *J. Fam. Pract.* 50: 1057–1062.

7 Williams, B. (1994). Patient satisfaction: a valid concept? *Soc. Sci. Med.* 38: 509–516.

8 Nakamura, M. and Koo, J. (2017). Personality disorders and the "difficult" dermatology patient: maximizing patient satisfaction. *Clin. Dermatol.* 35: 312–318.

9 Young, J.Q. (2020). Personality disorders. In: *Behavioral Medicine: A Guide for Clinical Practice*, 5e (eds. M.D. Feldman, J.F. Christensen and J.M. Satterfield). New York: McGraw Hill.

10 Edgerton, M.T., Jacobson, W.E., and Meyer, E. (1960). Surgical-psychiatric study of patients seeking plastic (cosmetic) surgery: ninety-eight consecutive patients with minimal deformity. *Br. J. Plast. Surg.* 13: 136–145.

11 Webb, W.L., Slaughter, R., Meyer, E., and Edgerton, M. (1965). Mechanisms of psychosocial adjustment in patients seeking "face-lift" operation. *Psychosom. Med.* 27 (2): 183–192.

12 Marcus, P. (1984). Psychological aspects of cosmetic rhinoplasty. *Br. J. Plast. Surg* 37 (3): 313–318.

13 Edgerton, M.T., Langman, M.W., and Pruzinsky, T. (1991). Plastic surgery and psychotherapy in the treatment of 100 psychologically disturbed patients. *Plast. Reconstr. Surg.* 88 (4): 594–608.

14 Hay, G.G. (1970 Jan). Psychiatric aspects of cosmetic nasal operations. *Br. J. Psychiatry* 116 (530): 85–97.

15 Anderson, K.G., Sankis, L.M., and Widiger, T.A. (2001). Pathology versus statistical infrequency: potential sources of gender bias in personality disorder criteria. *J. Nerv. Ment. Dis.* 189: 661–668.

16 Nunes, P.M., Wenzel, A., Borges, K.T. et al. (2009). Volumes of the hippocampus and amygdala in patients with borderline

personality disorder: a meta-analysis. *J. Personal. Disord.* 23: 333–345.

17 Schulze, L., Dziobek, I., Vater, A. et al. (2013). Gray matter abnormalities in patients with narcissistic personality disorder. *J. Psychiatr. Res.* 47: 1363–1369.

18 Zanarini, M.C., Frankenburg, F.R., Reich, D.B. et al. (2000). Biparental failure in the childhood experiences of borderline patients. *J. Personal. Disord.* 14: 264–273.

19 Amad, A., Ramoz, N., Thomas, P. et al. (2014). Genetics of borderline personality disorder: systematic review and proposal of an integrative model. *Neurosci. Biobehav. Rev.* 40: 6–19.

20 Ferrando, S.J. and Okoli, U. (2009). Personality disorders: understanding and managing the difficult patient in neurology practice. *Semin. Neurol.* 29: 266–272.

21 Bornstein, R.F. (1998). Reconceptualizing personality disorder diagnosis in the DSM-V: the discriminant validity challenge. *Clin. Psychol. Sci. Pract.* 5: 333–343.

22 Janowsky, D. (2008). Personality disorders. In: *Current Diagnosis & Treatment: Psychiatry*, 2e (eds. B. Nurcombe, J. Leckman and L.P. EbertM). New York: McGraw Hill https://accessmedicine-mhmedical-com. proxy.lib.umich.edu/content.aspx?bookid=3 36&sectionid=39717902 (accessed 15 October 2020).

23 Combs, G. and Oshman, L. (2016). Pearls for working with people who have personality disorder diagnoses. *Prim. Care* 43: 263–268.

24 Semiz, U., Basoglu, C., Cetin, M. et al. (2008). Body dysmorphic disorder in patients with borderline personality disorder: prevalence, clinical characteristics, and role of childhood trauma. *Acta Neuropsychiatr.* 20: 33–40.

25 Gattu, S., Rashid, R.M., and Khachemoune, A. (2009). Self-induced skin lesions: a review of dermatitis artefacta. *Cutis* 84: 247–251.

26 Christenson, G.A., Chernoff-Clementz, E., and Clementz, B.A. (1992). Personality and clinical characteristics in patients with trichotillomania. *J. Clin. Psychiatry* 53: 407–413.

27 Arnold, L.M., Auchenbach, M.B., and McElroy, S.L. (2001). Psychogenic excoriation. Clinical features, proposed diagnostic criteria, epidemiology and approaches to treatment. *CNS Drugs* 15: 351–359.

28 Davis, R.E. and Bublik, M. (2012). Psychological considerations in the revision rhinoplasty patient. *Facial Plast. Surg.* 28 (4): 374–379.

29 Morioka, D., Ohkubo, F., and Amikura, Y. (2014). Self-mutilation by a patient with borderline personality disorder. *Aesthet. Plast. Surg.* 38: 812–814.

30 Belli, H., Belli, S., and Ural, C. (2012). Psychopathological evaluation of patients requesting cosmetic rhinoplasty: a review. *West Indian Med. J.* 61 (2): 149–153.

31 Napoleon, A. (1993). The presentation of personalities in plastic surgery. *Ann. Plast. Surg.* 31: 193–208.

32 Ritvo, E.C., Melnick, I., Marcus, G.R. et al. (2006). Psychiatric conditions in cosmetic surgery patients. *Facial Plast. Surg.* 22: 194–197.

33 Malick, F., Howard, J., and Koo, J. (2008). Understanding the psychology of the cosmetic patients. *Dermatol. Ther.* 21: 47–53.

34 Rasoulian, M., Ebrahimi, A.A., Zare, M. et al. (2010). Psychiatric morbidity in dermatological conditions. *Int. J. Psychiatry Clin. Pract.* 14: 18–22.

35 Tükel, R., Tihan, A.K., and Oztürk, N. (2013). A comparison of comorbidity in body dysmorphic disorder and obsessive-compulsive disorder. *Ann. Clin. Psychiatry* 25: 210–216.

14

Normative Discontent and Social Dysmorphia in the Cosmetic Patient

Susruthi Rajanala and Neelam A. Vashi

Department of Dermatology, Boston University School of Medicine, Boston, MA, USA

Introduction

Body image dissatisfaction (BID) is a common and longstanding phenomenon in society. Originally introduced in 1985 by Rodin et al., the term "normative discontent" summarizes that this dissatisfaction is widespread and often present in women of all age groups [1]. More recent studies have shown that this sentiment is echoed across gender and cultural barriers as well [2, 3]. Although it is accepted that media platforms including social media hold a degree of responsibility for creating and evolving the accepted ideal body image over time, the extent of this influence is unknown [4]. With increasing exposure to mass media and social media usage, we are seeing a new phenomenon dubbed "social dysmorphia" – an excessive preoccupation with the body and beauty ideals present on media platforms, which may act as a trigger for body dysmorphic disorder (BDD) [5].

Body Image and Body Image Dissatisfaction

Body image has been described by psychologist David Slaade as the "mental representation of the body's shape, form, and size" which can be influenced by biological, cultural, and social factors. He notes that in addition to this perceptual component, body image comprises an attitudinal component – in other words, how an individual feels about their body [6]. BID, therefore, should be thought of as including these components – an individual's discontent with their true form when compared to the form idealized by society [2]. Overall, while rates of BID are higher among females, this phenomenon presents in both genders, although differently. Women tend to idealize a thinner body and lower weight, while men consider muscularity as well and may want to lose or gain weight to achieve a certain figure [7]. Though this phenomenon was once referred to as a "golden girl problem," suggesting that only white women were affected, a meta-analysis by Grabe et al. showed similar levels of body dissatisfaction among white, Asian, Hispanic, and black American women [8]. BID appears to be a cross-cultural phenomenon as well. A study among Nigerian young adults found that 62% of the study population was dissatisfied with their body, and these individuals tended to report a negative impact on quality of life [3].

The ideal body image that yields this comparison and discontent is not a static form.

Essential Psychiatry for the Aesthetic Practitioner, First Edition. Edited by Evan A. Rieder and Richard G. Fried.

Rather, it evolves with time and is shaped by various sociocultural factors, while being publicized and propagated by media, especially visual forms of media [9]. For instance, while a more curvaceous figure was popularized by actress Marilyn Monroe in the 1950s, most celebrities and models of today's era tend to be very thin and toned [10]. Furthermore, the body image presented as the ideal does not necessarily reflect the size of the average person, and this discrepancy has become more pronounced over time. A study assessing the anthropometric measurements of models for American retailer Victoria's Secret found that since the late 1990s, the average dress size and waist-to-hip ratio have decreased. During this same time period, the average American body mass index (BMI) has continued to steadily rise, with the average woman's size being a 16–18 [11]. An analysis of winners of the beauty pageant Miss America also reflects this trend, with the average winner in the 1920s having a BMI of 22 (considered to be in the healthy range) while several winners in the 1990s and 2000s had BMIs below 18.5, the World Health Organization's cutoff for being underweight [10]. A Canadian study assessed similar trends for men and found that the media depicted male bodies with greater muscle mass over time, while the increase in the male population BMI over the same time period was more likely due to increased body fat percentage [12].

Beyond size and figure alone, the cultural implications associated with the ideal body image may contribute to dissatisfaction. The media often depicts thinner people as being happier, more successful, and more attractive to potential partners [9]. On the other hand, overweight people are stereotyped as being lazy, less intelligent, or lacking self-control [13]. One study showed women photographs of thin subjects and gave them a social context associating the image with life success or lack thereof. The results showed that women who were exposed to thinness associated with success reported more dissatisfaction with their own bodies than those who were presented with the alternative [14].

Internalization of ideal body image begins at a young age, even if children are not yet exposed to traditional media. The most popular dolls on the market, Barbie dolls, have historically been designed to be disproportionately much taller and thinner than the average American woman [10]. Only recently have these dolls been redesigned to reflect the changing body types and diversity of the population – including dolls with conditions such as vitiligo and alopecia [15]. In a survey conducted by the Girl Scouts Research Institute, a majority of adolescent girls thought the body ideal presented in the fashion industry was "too skinny" and "unrealistic." At the same time, 60% of respondents said they compare their bodies to fashion models and 48% wished they were skinnier [16]. An earlier study by the Dove "Real Beauty" campaign showed that 81% of 10-year old-girls were afraid of becoming fat, while 42% of elementary school girls wished they were thinner [10].

Social Dysmorphia

While television, film, and print media have been the most popular propagators of body and beauty standards to date, the rise of social media has created another impactful cultural force. Uniquely, social media mainly features images of oneself and peers, as opposed to predominantly focusing on celebrities or models [17]. A recent Australian study showed that body comparison with peers in particular (compared to strangers) played a significant role in shaping body image concerns among adolescents [18]. Another phenomenon coupled with the rise of social media – and image-based platforms such as Instagram and Snapchat in particular – is the advent of filters and photo-editing apps. Both Instagram and Snapchat have built-in filters, ranging from dramatic effects like animal ears and glasses to subtler, more life-like changes such as smooth skin or long eyelashes. Beyond these built-in features, many smartphone applications exist to alter one's appearance in posted photos – from skin discoloration, to waist size and body shape. It has been shown that certain behaviors on social media, such as comparing one's appearance to others, are more likely to lead to body image concerns [19]. This finding reflects that of traditional print media, i.e. the act of comparison is what affects body image. However, an important distinction regarding social media is that users tend to share an idealized version of themselves, choosing images – possibly enhanced or filtered – that present them in the best form of appearance. While many acknowledge the editing that goes into traditional media images, the alterations that go into pictures of oneself and of those shared by peers may be more easily forgotten. One study showed that adolescent girls had trouble detecting body reshaping when shown digitally altered photos, and in fact found these altered photos to be realistic [20]. Taking into account the amount of time spent on social media platforms daily – a 2017 survey showed that a quarter of teens are spending three or more hours online per day – that yields significant exposure to these idealized, filtered images [21].

Social dysmorphia – a more generalized version of the phenomenon of Snapchat dysmorphia, introduced by cosmetic surgeon Dr. Tijion Esho [22] – can be thought of as an obsession with the ideals presented in social media and a desire to meet these standards. Social dysmorphia has been described as a potential trigger for BDD [5]. Classified on the obsessive compulsive spectrum, BDD is a preoccupation with a perceived or insignificant flaw or defect in appearance. As a result, individuals perform repetitive behavior to cope with or cover up these flaws – such as excessive grooming, skin picking, constantly seeking reassurance, or comparing oneself to others. These behaviors must be significant enough to cause impairment in functioning [23]. Those with BDD may seek cosmetic treatments as a means to fix their perceived flaw. It is important to note, however, that

the treatment for BDD involves psychiatry referral, cognitive-behavioral therapy, and antidepressants – usually in combination. Performing cosmetic procedures on these patients will not alter their self-perception and may in fact worsen BDD [24]. For more on BDD see Chapter 15.

Keeping the diagnostic criteria of BDD in mind, we can consider how social dysmorphia may serve as a trigger for it. Visual social media platforms have increased exposure to the unrealistic and unattainable beauty and body standards as individuals spend more and more time online per day [21]. Furthermore, with the ubiquity of photo-editing technology and apps, the bodies and faces we see on social media may be digitally altered to the point of being unattainable in real life [25]. Constantly seeing these filtered and seemingly perfect images of celebrities, models, and especially peers has been shown to increase body image concerns and internalizing symptoms among adolescents [26]. One study showed that increased exposure to selfies was associated with low self-esteem and decreased life satisfaction [27]. It is known that the angle and short distance at which selfies are taken can distort facial features and dimensions and may worsen a patient's self-perception [28]. In particular, higher engagement within social media platforms – such as liking, commenting, or editing one's pictures – has been associated with higher body dissatisfaction, eating concerns, and internalization of the thin ideal [29]. External pressure to filter and retouch social media posts appears to exist as well. British photographer Rankin started a project called "Selfie Harm," in which he asked adolescent girls to edit portraits of themselves until they were "social media ready." Interestingly, the subjects preferred the original images of themselves, but admitted that the edited versions would garner more attention on social media [30]. The repetitive behaviors outlined in BDD diagnostic criteria include reassurance seeking and comparison, both of which can be accomplished digitally on photosharing platforms [31].

Those experiencing social dysmorphia may seek aesthetic treatments in order to achieve the level of perfection present on social media. Dermatologists and plastic surgeons have seen a rising trend of patients seeking cosmetic procedures to emulate their filtered or digitally manipulated features [5]. Data from the 2019 Annual American Academy of Facial Plastic and Reconstructive Surgery survey show that 72% of surgeons report seeing patients who request cosmetic surgery in order to look better in selfies [32]. Another study looked into attitudes regarding cosmetic surgery in social media users and reported higher consideration of cosmetic surgery in those that used Instagram photo filters and the photo-editing app VSCO. The study also found that users of photo-editing software reported lower self-esteem scores [33]. An earlier study by Yin et al. reported that low self-esteem was a key factor in seeking cosmetic procedures [34].

Case Study

Case 14.1   The Cosmetics Consultation
A 27-year-old Caucasian woman presents to the cosmetic clinic for an initial consultation. She has never had any cosmetic treatments or procedures before, but recently has been feeling more self-conscious about her appearance. She is starting to notice a few wrinkles around the forehead and eye area, and feels like these are prominent in photos and selfies. While scrolling through her social media feeds, she notices that most women her age seem to have quite smooth and wrinkle-free skin and wonders if she is behind in starting cosmetic treatments. She wants to look and feel her best in both photos and real life.

Clinical Relevance and Implications

The rise of image-based social media has created a new avenue of comparison and feelings of inadequacy for those seeking cosmetic treatment. For the patient above, her self-consciousness about her wrinkles and feelings of being "behind" in cosmetic treatments were likely spurred by her exposure to images in her social media feed, images that may be edited or filtered, creating an unrealistic standard. While it is important to validate the patient's concerns, we should also ensure she understands that the images she is seeing and comparing herself to may be altered. In addition, we should be explicit about risks involved with cosmetic procedures, that they are not instantaneous and often require multiple treatments, and that results may not be in line with a look produced by photo-editing software.

Conclusions

Though the accepted beauty and body standards have always been influenced by social and cultural factors, the growing popularity of social media and photo-editing is reshaping how people view themselves. Images people are exposed to and idolize as being perfect may be altered to the point of being unrealistic and unattainable. Certain practices on social media may also be linked to or serve as a trigger for BDD. It is important for those who practice aesthetic medicine to be aware of the phenomenon of social dysmorphia and understand patients' motivation for seeking cosmetic procedures. Providers should be explicit about the feasibility and practicality of achieving aesthetic results that emulate edited photos. Though more research on the effect of social media on BDD is needed, clinicians need to understand its implications to better counsel patients and assess whether cosmetic procedures are warranted.

References

1 Rodin, J., Silberstein, L., and Striegel-Moore, R.H. (1984). Women and weight: a normative discontent. In: *Psychology and Gender*. Nebr. Symp. Motiv., vol. 32(2) (ed. T.B. Sondregger), 267–307.

2 Matthiasdottir, E., Jonsson, S.H., and Kristjansson, A.L. (2012 Feb). Body weight dissatisfaction in the Icelandic adult population: a normative discontent? *Eur. J. Pub. Health* 22 (1): 116–121.

3 Ejike, C.E. (2015 Dec). Body shape dissatisfaction is a "normative discontent" in a young-adult Nigerian population: a study of prevalence and effects on health-related quality of life. *J. Epidemiol. Glob. Health* 5: S19–S26.

4 Grabe, S., Ward, L.M., and Jyde, J.S. (2008 May). The role of the media in body image concerns among women: a meta-analysis of experimental and correlational studies. *Psychol. Bull.* 134 (3): 460–476.

5 Rajanala, S., Maymone, M.B.C., and Vashi, N.A. (2018 Dec). Selfies – living in the era of filtered photographs. *JAMA Facial Plast. Surg.* 20 (6): 443–444.

6 Slaade, P.D. (1994 Jun). What is body image? *Behav. Res. Ther.* 32 (5): 497–502.

7 Stanford, J.N. and McCabe, M.P. (2002 Nov). Body image ideal among males and females: sociocultural influences and focus on different body parts. *J. Health Psychol.* 7 (6): 675–684.

8 Grabe, S. and Hyde, J.S. (2006 Jul). Ethnicity and body dissatisfaction among women in the United States. A meta-analysis. *Psychol. Bull.* 132: 622–640.

9 Dakanalis, A. and Riva, G. (2013). Mass media, body image, and eating disturbances: the underlying mechanism through the lens of objectification theory. In: *Handbook on Body Image: Gender Differences, Sociocultural Influences and Health Implications* (eds. L.B. Sams and J.A. Keels), 217–236. Hauppage: Nova Science Publishers.

10 Martin, J.B. (2010 May–Jun). The development of ideal body image perceptions in the United States. *Nutr. Today* 45 (3): 98–110.

11 Maymone, M.B.C., Laughter, M., Anderson, J.B. et al. (2020 Jan). Unattainable standards of beauty: temporal trends of Victoria's secret models from 1995 to 2018. *Aesthet. Surg. J.* 40 (2): NP72–NP76.

12 Spitzer, A.L., Henderson, K.A., and Zivian, M.T. (1999 Apr). Gender differences in population versus media body sizes: a comparison over four decades. *Sex Roles* 40: 545–565.

13 ten Have, M., de Beaufort, I.D., Teixeira, J.P., and van der Heide, A. (2011 Sep). Ethics and prevention of overweight and obesity: an inventory. *Obes. Rev.* 12: 669–676.

14 Evans, P.C. (2003 Sep). "If only I were thin like her, maybe I could be happy like her": the self-implications of associating a thin female ideal with life success. *Psychol. Women Q* 27: 209–214.

15 Dockterman, E. (2016 Jan). Barbie's got a new body. Time. Available from: https://time.com/barbie-new-body-cover-story.

16 Girl Scout Research Institute (2010). Beauty Redefined. Girls and Body Image. Girl Scouts of the USA. Available from: https://www.girlscouts.org/content/dam/girlscouts-gsusa/forms-and-documents/about-girl-scouts/research/beauty_redefined_factsheet.pdf (accessed 2 March 2020).

17 Fardouly, J. and Vartanian, L.R. (2016 Sep). Social media and body image concerns: current research and future directions. *Curr. Opin. Psychol* 9: 1–5.

18 Carey, R.N., Donaghue, N., and Broderick, P. (2014 Jan). Body image concern among Australian adolescent girls: the role of body comparisons with models and peers. *Body Image* 11 (1): 81–84.

19 Fardouly, J., Diedrichs, P.C., Vartanian, L.R., and Halliwell, E. (2015 Dec). The mediating

role of appearance comparisons in the relationship between media usage and self-objectification in young women. *Psychol. Women Q.* 39: 447–457.

20 Kleemans, M., Daalmans, S., Carbaat, I., and Anschütz, D. (2018). Picture perfect: the direct effect of manipulated Instagram photos on body image in adolescent girls. *Media Psychol.* 21 (1): 93–110.

21 Cohen, R., Newton-John, T., and Slater, A. (2017 Dec). The relationship between Facebook and Instagram appearance-focused activities and body image concerns in young women. *Body Image* 23: 183–187.

22 Hosie, R. (2018 Feb 6). More people want surgery to look like a filtered version of themselves rather than a celebrity, cosmetic doctor says. Independent. Available from: www.independent.co.uk/life-style/cosmetic-surgery-snapchat-instagram-filters-demand-celebrities-doctor-dr-esho-london-a8197001.html (accessed 2 March 2020).

23 American Psychiatric Association (2013). Diagnostic and Statistical Manual of Mental Disorders, 5e. Obsessive-compulsive and related disorders;, 235–264. Philadelphia: American Psychiatric Association Publishers.

24 Vashi, N.A. (2016 Nov–Dec). Obsession with perfection: body dysmorphia. *Clin. Dermatol.* 34 (6): 788–791.

25 Coy-Dibley, I. (2016). "Digitized Dysmorphia" of the female body: the re/disfigurement of the image. *Palgrave Commun.* 2 (16040) Jul [accessed 2 March 2020]. Available from: https://doi-org.eres.qnl.qa/10.1057/palcomms.2016.40.

26 Marengo, D., Longobardi, C., Fabris, M.A., and Settanni, M. (2018 May). Highly-visual social media and internalizing symptoms in adolescence: the mediating role of body image concerns. *Comput. Hum. Behav.* 82: 63–69.

27 Wang, R., Yang, F., and Haigh, M.H. (2017 Jul). Let me take a selfie: exploring the psychological effects of posting and viewing selfies and groupies on social media. *Telematics Inform.* 34 (4): 274–283.

28 Ward, B., Ward, M., Fried, O., and Paskhover, B. (2018 Jul). Nasal distortion in short-distance photographs: the selfie effect. *JAMA Facial Plast. Surg.* 20 (4): 333–335.

29 McLean, S.A., Paxton, S.A., Wertheim, E.H., and Masters, J. (2015 Dec). Photoshopping the selfie: self photo editing and photo investment are associated with body dissatisfaction in adolescent girls. *Int. J. Eat. Disord.* 48 (8): 1132–1140.

30 Brucculieri, K. (2019 Mar.). Teenage girls in this photo series show the scary effects of editing apps. The Huffington Post. Available from: https://www.huffpost.com/entry/rankin-selfie-harm-photo-series_l_5c7d35e0 e4b0e5e313cd4a70.

31 Maymone, M.B.C., Rajanala, S., and Vashi, N.A. (2019 May). Social networks and the rhinoplasty patient – reply. *JAMA Facial Plast. Surg.* 21 (3): 265.

32 American Academy of Facial Plastic and Reconstructive Surgery (2019). Annual Survey Statistics; 2020. Available from: https://www.aafprs.org/media/press_releases/new%20stats%20aafprs%20annual%20survey.aspx?websitekey=760f3515-2fb0-441b-a8b4-28f94313fffc (accessed 2 March 2020).

33 Chen, J., Ishii, M., Bater, K.L. et al. (2019 Sep). Association between the use of social media and photograph editing applications, self-esteem, and cosmetic surgery acceptance. *JAMA Facial Plast. Surg.* 21 (5): 361–367.

34 Yin, Z., Ma, Y., Hao, S. et al. (2016 Jan–Feb). Self-esteem, self-efficacy, and appearance assessment of young female patients undergoing facial cosmetic surgery: a comparative study of the Chinese population. *JAMA Facial Plast. Surg.* 18 (1): 20–26.

15

Obsessive Compulsive Disorder and Body Dysmorphic Disorder in the Cosmetic Patient

Mary D. Sun[1] and Evan A. Rieder[2]

[1] Icahn School of Medicine at Mount Sinai, New York, NY, USA
[2] The Ronald O. Perelman Department of Dermatology, New York University Grossman School of Medicine, New York, NY, USA

Introduction

Obsessive compulsive disorder (OCD) and body dysmorphic disorder (BDD) are psychiatric conditions that disproportionately present to dermatologists, plastic surgeons, and other aesthetic providers. According to a meta-analysis, BDD occurs in 15% of plastic surgery patients and 13% of dermatology patients; its prevalence in the general population is 1–2% [1, 2]. Though fewer studies have investigated OCD in patients with skin disease, this disorder similarly presents to dermatologists at higher rates, estimated from 9 to 35% (as compared to its 2.3% global prevalence) [3]. BDD is thought to be underdiagnosed, and both disorders are considered relatively common, with overlapping symptomatology and etiologies [4]. Patients who present in the cosmetic setting are more likely to have symptoms of OCD and meet criteria for a diagnosis of BDD [5], and patients with OCD are more likely to have co-occurring BDD [6]. Often, patients with psychiatric causes of cosmetic symptoms seek out nonpsychiatric ("somatic") providers because they fear stigmatization and may not accept their underlying disease [7].

OCD is defined by the presence of obsessions, compulsions, or both, while BDD is defined as a preoccupation with perceived flaws in physical appearance that are not observable or appear slight to others [8]. If left untreated, these chronic mental illnesses can lead to clinical, social, and emotional issues that significantly decrease quality of life [9–11]. Appearance-related concerns in particular have a powerful negative effect that can extend beyond the severity of psychiatric symptoms [9]. For example, patients can become so concerned with hiding multiple aspects of their bodies that they refuse to be seen in public or engage with others [11]. In severe cases, patients can become functionally disabled and therefore unable to pursue work and other life goals.

Patients with both of these OCD-spectrum disorders suffer comorbidity with other psychiatric disorders. OCD tends to occur with multiple psychological symptoms and has been strongly associated with anxiety and depression in large multicenter studies [12, 13]. Patients who have BDD are more likely to suffer from general anxiety disorder, social phobia, major depressive disorder, OCD, attention deficit hyperactivity disorder (ADHD), and substance abuse [6, 9, 14]. Perhaps most importantly, patients with BDD have much higher rates of suicidal ideation (46%) and

Essential Psychiatry for the Aesthetic Practitioner, First Edition. Edited by Evan A. Rieder and Richard G. Fried.
© 2021 John Wiley & Sons Ltd. Published 2021 by John Wiley & Sons Ltd.

suicide attempt (18%) when compared to the general population [9–11, 15]. Patients with both OCD and BDD are similarly at higher risk of exhibiting suicidal behaviors and symptoms of eating disorders [6, 16].

Though over three-quarters of people affected by BDD pursue surgical and noninvasive cosmetic procedures [17, 18], their diagnoses are not always recognized prior to medical interventions. A survey of the American Society for Dermatologic Surgery (ASDS) found that 61% of practicing dermatologists recognized BDD in a treated patient only after a procedure was performed, though 94% were generally aware of the condition and 62% believed BDD to be a contraindication to treatment [19]. Similarly, a survey of the American Society for Aesthetic Plastic Surgery (ASPS) found that 85% of practicing surgeons recognized BDD only postoperatively; 82% of these surgeons reported poor outcomes in such patients [20]. Given the severe impacts that OCD and BDD can have on clients' and patients' lives, aesthetic providers should be able to identify these disorders early on in the clinical relationship and help arrange for appropriate mental healthcare.

Patients and clients with OCD who present in a cosmetic setting commonly have symptoms of dry skin, alopecia, and face and body excoriations due to hand washing compulsions, trichotillomania, and skin-picking disorder, respectively [21]. Patients with BDD tend to be preoccupied with facial features, skin, and hair, and most commonly seek out dermatologists for help correcting their perceived deformities [4, 10, 11]. By the time they present to a healthcare provider, they may have picked at, pulled at, or otherwise manipulated their skin, hair, or nails to the point of scarring, ulcerations, and/or bald spots [22, 23]. BDD patients concerned about looking too pale can also have undergone excessive tanning and present with burned skin and increased risk of skin cancer [17]. In a recent study, seeking aesthetic rhinoplasty was significantly associated with moderate-to-severe appearance-related symptoms of OCD and a high prevalence of fully diagnosed BDD [5].

Gender and age also play an important role in BDD symptoms, which can be helpful when identifying suspected cases. Younger, primarily female patients tend to focus on facial hair, weight, and body areas such as the arms, chest, stomach, buttocks, thighs, and legs, and may instead seek out plastic surgeons for treatment [1, 22]. The average age of women with BDD who seek out dermatologists and plastic surgeons is 27–35 [24, 25], and women display more repetitive behaviors, referred to as "camouflaging," to hide their areas of concern. Examples of camouflaging include wearing excessive amounts of makeup, purposefully loose clothing, and accessories such as hats, scarves, and gloves to physically cover areas of concern. Other examples of repetitive, appearance-focused behaviors include mirror checking, changing clothes, skin-picking, hair-pulling, and restrictive eating analogous to and sometimes indicative of an eating disorder [24]. In contrast, men with BDD tend to be preoccupied with their hair, body build, and genitalia, and are at higher risk for excessive weightlifting and substance use [24]. Symptoms appear earlier and more severely in women, but men experience greater life impairment and are more likely to receive disability and be unable to work due to their BDD [24]. In both OCD and BDD, gender incidence is roughly equal and symptoms begin during childhood and adolescence. Unless treatment is received early on, these conditions continue chronically into adulthood [7, 13, 26]. In both disorders, patients are often embarrassed about their symptoms and delay seeking treatment until early to late adulthood [5, 27]. In the case of BDD, men are less likely than women to seek medical help [28].

Developing a familiarity with the typical presentation of patients living with OCD is important to identify at-risk patients and make appropriate referrals. More importantly, developing a compassionate and structured approach is essential to treating BDD patients and protecting healthcare providers. Patients suffering from this disorder are often seeking reassurance for their beliefs from medical professionals and are unlikely to have insight into their disorder. They display high levels of delusional thinking (fixed false beliefs) and unfortunately are likely to respond negatively to psychiatric referrals [29–31]. Indeed, patients may leave and seek additional opinions with multiple providers, despite the inability of any medical procedure to truly "fix" their areas of concern [17, 32–34]. One-third of individuals with BDD display aggressive behavior related to their disorder [26, 28], and 40% of respondents in a survey of the American Society of Plastic Surgeons have been threatened with legal action, physical harm, or both by a BDD patient [20]. Accurately identifying such patients and assessing their capacity to consent, communicate a choice, understand relevant information and consequences, and reason through treatment options are critical in clinical interactions [35, 36]. To uphold the principle of nonmaleficence and prevent unnecessary cosmetic procedures, any evidence of psychotic or disordered thought process should terminate the informed consent process [35, 37]. Given the risk of harm to the patient and healthcare staff, there is an urgent need for providers in aesthetic medicine to accurately screen for and effectively manage patients with BDD [30].

Case Studies

Case 15.1   Concern for OCD

A 42-year-old Caucasian man with a history of anxiety presents to your clinic for a cosmetic consultation. He expresses embarrassment over acne scarring on his face and poor skin quality. He has never had any cosmetic procedures before but does feel self-conscious about his appearance. While he has concerns about his skin, they are not interfering with his social or occupational functioning and he is able to date and maintain full-time employment. On physical examination, he has multiple hyperpigmented and erythematous macules on his face as well as several shallow rolling acne scars. When directly questioned about his thoughts, he denies having any intrusive thoughts that cause anxiety or distress. He admits to picking his skin and examining it with a magnifying mirror, but for no more than 15–30 minutes per day. Although this behavior has become an important part of his daily routine, on days when he is not able to find the time to groom and micromanage his appearance, he functions normally.

Clinical Relevance and Implications

This case raises several concerns for OCD, namely skin-picking and overgrooming behaviors. While patients with OCD do present to aesthetic providers, they do so with less frequency than those who are living with BDD. Importantly, while this patient might raise your suspicions for OCD, he does not meet diagnostic criteria for the disorder, as he does not have any obsessive or intrusive thoughts and his behaviors do not seem to be impeding his activities of daily life. While many aesthetic-seeking patients will meet one or two criteria for OCD, having a true case of OCD in the aesthetic clinic is much less common than with BDD. That being said, his care would greatly benefit from the expert opinion and diagnostic clarity of a seasoned mental health professional. And though the treatment of OCD is outside the spectrum of practice of the aesthetic provider, it behooves the astute clinician to have familiarity with the clinical presentation and diagnostic criteria for this disorder (see Table 15.1 for a full list of DSM criteria) [8]. With appropriate concern, aesthetic providers can make referrals to mental health providers for talk therapy or medication management. Importantly,

Table 15.1 DSM-5 diagnostic criteria for obsessive compulsive disorder.

DSM-5

Disorder Class: Obsessive Compulsive and Related Disorders

A. Presence of obsessions, compulsions, or both:

   Obsessions are defined by [1] and [2]:

   1) Recurrent and persistent thoughts, urges, or impulses that are experienced, at some time during the disturbance, as intrusive and unwanted, and that in most individuals cause marked anxiety or distress.

   2) The individual attempts to ignore or suppress such thoughts, urges, or images, or to neutralize them with some other thought or action (i.e. by performing a compulsion).

   Compulsions are defined by [1] and [2]:

   1) Repetitive behaviors (e.g. hand washing, ordering, checking) or mental acts (e.g. praying, counting, repeating words silently) that the individual feels driven to perform in response to an obsession or according to rules that must be applied rigidly.

   2) The behaviors or mental acts are aimed at preventing or reducing anxiety or distress, or preventing some dreaded event or situation; however, these behaviors or mental acts are not connected in a realistic way with what they are designed to neutralize or prevent, or are clearly excessive.

   Note: Young children may not be able to articulate the aims of these behaviors or mental acts.

B. The obsessions or compulsions are time-consuming (e.g. take more than 1 hour/day) or cause clinically significant distress or impairment in social, occupational, or other important areas of functioning.

C. The obsessive compulsive symptoms are not attributable to the physiological effects of a substance (e.g. a drug of abuse, a medication) or another medical condition.

D. The disturbance is not better explained by the symptoms of another mental disorder (e.g. excessive worries, as in generalized anxiety disorder; preoccupation with appearance, as in body dysmorphic disorder; difficulty discarding or parting with possessions, as in hoarding disorder; hair pulling, as in trichotillomania [hair-pulling disorder]; skin picking, as in excoriation [skin-picking] disorder; stereotypies, as in stereotypic movement disorder; ritualized eating behavior, as in eating disorders; preoccupation with substances or gambling, as in substance-related and addictive disorders; preoccupation with having an illness, as in illness anxiety disorder; sexual urges or fantasies, as in paraphilic disorders; impulses, as in disruptive, impulse-control, and conduct disorders; guilty ruminations, as in major depressive disorder; thought insertion or delusional preoccupations, as in schizophrenia spectrum and other psychotic disorders; or repetitive patterns of behavior, as in autism spectrum disorder).

Specify if:

• With good or fair insight: The individual recognizes that obsessive compulsive disorder beliefs are definitely or probably not true or that they may or may not be true.

• With poor insight: The individual thinks that obsessive compulsive disorder beliefs are probably true.

• With absent insight/delusional beliefs: The individual is completely convinced that obsessive compulsive disorder beliefs are true.

Specify if:

• Tic-related: The individual has a current or past history of a tic disorder.

Source: Based on DSM-5 Changes: Implications for Child Serious Emotional Disturbance, Substance Abuse and Mental Health Services Administration, Center for Behavioral Health Statistics and Quality, June 2016.

patients and clients living with OCD or OCD-like symptoms are likely to have insight (a recognition and understanding of their illness) and accept referrals for mental health providers. A high degree of insight allows for a smoother provider–patient relationship, which may be less fraught with the multitude of challenges that characterize relationships with patients living with BDD. Once the patient is networked with a mental health professional, a collaborative effort between aesthetic provider and mental health professional can ensure that such patients receive comprehensive care.

Case 15.2   Concern for BDD

A 29-year-old Hispanic woman with a history of anxiety and depression presents to your clinic for a cosmetic consultation. She expresses a long-term concern about the shape of her "disgustingly bumpy" nose and has had two rhinoplasties in the past three years. She is also concerned about the condition of her skin and expresses interest in a surgical facelift, as she has been disappointed with the results of previous laser therapy and chemical peels. When you review her social history, she describes difficulty with keeping a steady job and frequent episodes of shame regarding her physical appearance in public. She prefers to stay at home and declines most social invitations.

When she does go out, she spends three to four hours putting on makeup and focuses heavily on "contouring" her features. She has not dated before and thinks that it would be "extremely difficult" for her to find a partner due to her appearance. You are the fourth aesthetic provider that she has been to in the past few months, and she expresses anger and disappointment with the results of previous procedures. She is hoping that you have the "proper skills" to "finally understand" what she sees and fix her "ugliness." Upon physical examination, her facial features appear normal and her previous rhinoplasty appears well healed.

Clinical Relevance and Implications

This case illustrates several key aspects of BDD as defined in the DSM-5 under the Obsessive–Compulsive and Related Disorders classification. There are four diagnostic criteria for BDD, with additional specifications for the presence of muscle dysmorphia and degree of patient insight (see Table 15.2 for a full list of DSM criteria, contrasting changes from the DSM-IV to DSM-5) [8]. Note that BDD is also referred to as "dysmorphophobia" and "dermatologic hypochondriasis" in the medical literature [25, 37].

When evaluating a potential case of BDD, providers should pay particular attention to criteria B listed in the DSM-5. Repetitive behaviors can usually be observed within a clinical interaction and mental acts can be reported by the patient when taking a social history.

Screening for BDD in Aesthetic Medicine

Two tools for BDD screening have been validated in a dermatology setting [18, 38]. The Dysmorphic Concern Questionnaire (DCQ) is a seven-item questionnaire that can be self-administered by the patient. While the DCQ should not be used to formally diagnose BDD, it is a valuable tool for quickly identifying individuals with excessive dysmorphic concerns who are at high risk for this condition [38]. The Body Dysmorphic Disorder Questionnaire – Dermatology Version (BDDQ-DV) is another, publicly available option that can be used for formal diagnosis. The BDDQ-DV consists of nine self-administered items, which are followed by seven clinician-administered questions; this tool demonstrates an excellent sensitivity of 100% and high specificity ranging from 90.3 to 93% in cosmetic patients [18, 39]. These question-based tools are simple to use during clinical visits and have outperformed physicians in previous studies. In a cohort of 597 patients, the BDDQ accurately identified positive screens in 9.7% of patients as compared to 4% identified by oculoplastic and facial plastic surgeons [40]. Regular use of these screening protocols can help providers recognize and provide appropriate treatment in cases of potential BDD.

Table 15.2 Comparison of DSM-IV to DSM-5 diagnostic criteria for body dysmorphic disorder.

DSM-IV	DSM-5
Disorder class: somatoform disorders	Disorder class: obsessive compulsive and related disorders
A. Preoccupation with an imagined defect in appearance. If a slight physical anomaly is present, the person's concern is markedly excessive.	A. Preoccupation with one or more perceived defects or flaws in physical appearance that are not observable or appear slight to others.
	B. At some point during the course of the disorder, the individual has performed repetitive behaviors (e.g. mirror checking, excessive grooming, skin picking, reassurance seeking) or mental acts (e.g. comparing his or her appearance with that of others) in response to the appearance concerns.
B. The preoccupation causes clinically significant distress or impairment in social, occupational, or other important areas of functioning.	C. The preoccupation causes clinically significant distress or impairment in social, occupational or other areas of functioning.
C. The preoccupation is not better accounted for by another mental disorder (e.g. dissatisfaction with body shape and size in anorexia nervosa).	D. The appearance preoccupation is not better explained by concerns with body fat or weight in an individual whose symptoms meet diagnostic criteria for an eating disorder.
	Specify if:
	With muscle dysmorphia: The individual is preoccupied with the idea that his or her body build is too small or insufficiently muscular. This specifier is used even if the individual is preoccupied with other body areas, which is often the case.
	Specify:
	Degree of insight regarding body dysmorphic disorder beliefs (e.g. "I look ugly" or "I look deformed").
	● Good or fair insight: The individual recognizes that the body dysmorphic disorder beliefs are definitely or probably not true or that they may or may not be true.
	● Poor insight: The individual thinks that the body dysmorphic beliefs are probably true.
	● Absent insight/delusional beliefs: The individual is completely convinced that the body dysmorphic beliefs are true.

Source: Based on DSM-5 Changes: Implications for Child Serious Emotional Disturbance, Substance Abuse and Mental Health Services Administration, Center for Behavioral Health Statistics and Quality, June 2016.

Guide to the Clinical Interview for BDD

In the event of a positive patient screen for BDD, providers should conduct a structured clinical interview to gain additional information that informs the treatment strategy. The guide below assumes that the patient has responded "yes" to the first question of the BDDQ-DV (Item I): "*Are you very concerned about the appearance of some part of your body, which you consider especially unattractive?*" [41].

1) Begin the interview by asking the patient if they have experienced excessive worry caused by a perceived defect in their appearance. If the patient answers yes, continue with the interview portion of the evaluation and base your questioning on the BDDQ-DV. If the patient answers no, conclude the BDD component of the cosmetic consultation.

2) Discuss the patient's concern in the context of their history of other cosmetic procedures and inquire about their experiences with other physicians and providers. Multiple procedures and consistently negative experiences raise the possibility of BDD.

3) Examine the patient's area of concern together using a handheld mirror. Ask the patient to indicate what they see. Be suspicious if the defect can only be perceived by the patient or is extremely slight.

4) Evaluate how much time the patient spends worrying about and/or trying to fix their perceived defect and if their behavior has led to impairment of social or occupational activities. Be specific in asking about the number of daily hours they spend thinking about their appearance. Do their concerns cause them to miss work or school, or refrain from socializing?

5) Ask questions to help gauge the risk of self-harm and suicidality. Does the patient have thoughts about or a plan to harm themselves? Ask these questions without fear of planting an idea for suicidality.

6) Respond supportively, knowing that many patients with BDD will be defensive and/or resistant, and provide the patient with information about BDD. If you are concerned that a patient may have this disorder, make sure to deliver a set of key messages (Table 15.3).

7) If the patient is open to learning more, discuss the possibility of multidisciplinary care and provide a referral to a trusted mental health professional. This intervention is best presented as an adjunct to the dermatologist–patient relationship and saved for a follow-up visit once rapport has been established.

Table 15.3 Key messages for aesthetic medicine patients with a positive BDD screen.

Key message	Example phrasing
The possibility of BDD	I'm concerned that you might have a common body image condition called body dysmorphic disorder.
A discrepancy between others' perceptions and patient's view of themselves	People suffering from BDD see themselves as deformed but appear objectively normal and attractive to others.
Excessive time and money spent	People with BDD may not feel understood by their friends, family, or doctors, and may spend lots of time and money trying to hide or fix their perceived deformity.
Acknowledgment of suffering	People with BDD suffer from poor quality of life, depression, and sometimes suicidal thoughts and behaviors.
Lack of response of BDD to cosmetic procedures	BDD does not respond to cosmetic dermatologic or plastic surgery treatments.
Availability of effective treatments	BDD is a treatable condition but requires the use of cognitive-behavioral therapy and/or serotonin-reuptake inhibitor medications.

Source: Adapted from Sun and Rieder [41].

Patients who (i) display excessive worry about a perceived imperfection that is not noticeable to others or observed upon physical examination and (ii) suffer disruptions in one or more aspects of their daily lives as a result should be considered to have BDD.

Clinical Approaches to BDD in Aesthetic Medicine

If a patient is determined to have BDD, providers should inform them of their potential diagnosis in a respectful and nonjudgmental way. Simply advising patients to stop repetitive behaviors and/or dismissing their cosmetic concerns will likely be ineffective [29]. Educating patients about the nature and symptoms of their condition can be more helpful, with emphasis on the fact that BDD is treatable. Building rapport with the patient and communicating clearly and consistently is vital to providing appropriate treatment options. Table 15.3 highlights key messages that should be used in cases of a positive BDD screen.

Outside of procedures done to repair damage from BDD-related behaviors, psychiatric experts counsel that cosmetic procedures are best avoided in these patients [22, 31, 34]. Past studies show that while there may be a temporary reduction in nonsevere BDD symptoms after treatment, these improvements rarely last long term [42]. Indeed, these results may actually represent false positives that only reflect a shift of BDD-related preoccupations from one part of the body to another [43]. Furthermore, a study of cosmetic rhinoplasty in adult patients found that more severe BDD symptoms preoperatively predict worse postoperative satisfaction in the short and long term [19]. Sadly, reports of attempted and completed suicides in postoperative BDD patients persist [42]. In general, research shows that cosmetic treatments do not improve overall outcomes for patients with BDD and emphasizes the importance of accurate detection and screening.

Most patients with BDD benefit from referrals to mental health providers for cognitive-based therapy or pharmacotherapy [42], rather than to other aesthetic providers. In the case of patients who have substantially damaged their body and have a medical need for cosmetic procedures (e.g. severe cases of skin-picking, hair-pulling, or body mutilation), a combination of psychiatric and aesthetic treatment can be used. Aesthetic treatments should only occur after a stable relationship and meaningful progress has been made with a mental health professional. When discussing treatment options with such patients, aesthetic providers should emphasize that psychiatric referrals are adjuvant to the primary therapeutic relationship; patients should not feel dismissed or disbelieved. Understand that patients are likely to reject information about BDD early on in the clinical relationship, which should be met with an understanding and empathetic approach on behalf of the provider(s). Developing relationships with trusted mental health professionals to better understand the treatment pathways for BDD can also be beneficial.

Conclusions

OCD and BDD, two psychiatric disorders that are more likely to co-occur in cosmetic patients, present commonly in patients of aesthetic providers much than the general population. These conditions can have serious comorbidities and consequences for a patient's quality of life and the pursuit of their life goals. In severe cases, they may cause functional disability and are correlated with significantly high rates of suicidal ideation, behavior, and attempt. Importantly, these conditions can also adversely affect the provider–patient relationship and multiple aspects of the treating clinician's life.

BDD is currently underdiagnosed by healthcare providers, and specifically underrecognized by dermatologists and plastic surgeons. Cosmetic procedures are unlikely to help patients and can be actively harmful in the long term. Additionally, BDD patients who are refused treatment or dissatisfied with results of their procedures may harass, attempt to harm, or file legal suit against their providers. To protect patients and healthcare workers alike, there is an urgent need for regular and accurate screening in the cosmetic setting.

Dermatologists, plastic surgeons, and other aesthetic practitioners should be able to recognize both OCD and BDD and discuss appropriate treatment options and referrals. In the case of a positive BDD screen, key messages should be clearly conveyed to patients with an emphasis on psychiatric referrals, psychoeducation, and multidisciplinary care. By recognizing and referring patients with suspected OCD to mental health professionals and taking an understanding and structured approach to the treatment of potential BDD cases, cosmetic providers can better recognize and help relieve the suffering of patients living with these disorders.

References

1 Ribeiro, R.V.E. (2017). Prevalence of body dysmorphic disorder in plastic surgery and dermatology patients: a systematic review with meta-analysis. *Aesthetic Plastic Surgery* 41 (4): 964–970.

2 Veale, D., Gledhill, L.J., Christodoulou, P., and Hodsoll, J. (2016). Body dysmorphic disorder in different settings: a systematic review and estimated weighted prevalence. *Body Image* 18: 168–186.

3 Ruscio, A.M., Stein, D.J., Chiu, W.T., and Kessler, R.C. (2010). The epidemiology of obsessive-compulsive disorder in the National Comorbidity Survey Replication. *Molecular Psychiatry* 15 (1): 53–63.

4 Mufaddel, A., Osman, O.T., Almugaddam, F., and Jafferany, M. (2013). A review of body dysmorphic disorder and its presentation in different clinical settings. *Primary Care Companion for CNS Disorders* 15 (4) PCC.12r01464.

5 Ramos, T.D., de Brito, M.J.A., Suzuki, V.Y. et al. (2019). High prevalence of body dysmorphic disorder and moderate to severe appearance-related obsessive–compulsive symptoms among rhinoplasty candidates. *Aesthetic Plastic Surgery* 43 (4): 1000–1005.

6 Jafferany, M., Osuagwu, F.C., Khalid, Z. et al. (2019). Prevalence and clinical characteristics of body dysmorphic disorder in adolescent inpatient psychiatric patients – a pilot study. *Nordic Journal of Psychiatry* 73 (4–5): 244–247.

7 Sheikhmoonesi, F., Hajheidari, Z., Masoudzadeh, A., and Mozaffari, M. (2014). EPA-0054 – prevalence and severity of obsessive-compulsive disorder and its relationships with dermatological disease. *European Psychiatry* 29: 1.

8 American Psychiatric ssociation (2017). *Diagnostic and Statistical Manual of Mental Disorders (DSM-V)*. Springer-Verlag.

9 Marques, L., LeBlanc, N., Robinaugh, D. et al. (2011). Correlates of quality of life and functional disability in individuals with body dysmorphic disorder. *Psychosomatics* 52 (3): 245–254.

10 Möllmann, A., Dietel, F.A., Hunger, A., and Buhlmann, U. (2017). Prevalence of body dysmorphic disorder and associated features in German adolescents: a self-report survey. *Psychiatry Research* 254: 263–267.

11 Zakhary, L., Weingarden, H., Sullivan, A., and Wilhelm, S. (2017). *Clincal Features, Assessment, and Treatment of Body Dysmorphic Disorder. Oxford Medicine Online*. Oxford University Press.

12 Dalgard, F.J., Gieler, U., Tomas-Aragones, L. et al. (2015). The psychological burden of skin diseases: a cross-sectional multicenter study among dermatological out-patients in

13 European countries. *Journal of Investigative Dermatology* 135 (4): 984–991.

13 Horwath, E. and Weissman, M.M. (2000). The epidemiology and cross-national presentation of obsessive-compulsive disorder. *Psychiatric Clinics of North America* 23 (3): 493–507.

14 Frias, Á., Palma, C., Farriols, N., and González, L. (2015). Comorbidity between obsessive-compulsive disorder and body dysmorphic disorder: prevalence, explanatory theories, and clinical characterization. *Neuropsychiatric Disease and Treatment* 11: 2233–2244.

15 Angelakis, I., Gooding, P.A., and Panagioti, M. (2016). Suicidality in body dysmorphic disorder (BDD): a systematic review with meta-analysis. *Clinical Psychology Review* 49: 55–66.

16 Conceição Costa, D.L., Chagas Assunção, M., Arzeno Ferrão, Y. et al. (2012). Body dysmorphic disorder in patients with obsessive-compulsive disorder: prevalence and clinical correlates. *Depression and Anxiety* 29 (11): 966–975.

17 Koblenzer, C.S. (2017). Body dysmorphic disorder in the dermatology patient. *Clinics in Dermatology* 35 (3): 298–301.

18 Dey, J.K., Ishii, M., Phillis, M. et al. (2015). Body dysmorphic disorder in a facial plastic and reconstructive surgery clinic. *JAMA Facial Plastic Surgery* 17 (2): 137–143.

19 Barone, M., Cogliandro, A., and Persichetti, P. (2013). Preoperative symptoms of body dysmorphic disorder determine postoperative satisfaction and quality of life in aesthetic rhinoplasty. *Plastic and Reconstructive Surgery* 132 (6): 1078e–1079e.

20 Sarwer, D.B., Spitzer, J.C., Sobanko, J.F., and Beer, K.R. (2015). Identification and management of mental health issues by dermatologic surgeons. *Dermatologic Surgery* 41 (3): 352–357.

21 Mavrogiorgou, P., Bader, A., Stockfleth, E., and Juckel, G. (2015). Obsessive-compulsive disorder in dermatology. *Journal der Deutschen Dermatologischen Gesellschaft* 13 (10): 991–999.

22 Phillips, K.A., Didie, E.R., Menard, W. et al. (2006). Clinical features of body dysmorphic disorder in adolescents and adults. *Psychiatry Research* 141 (3): 305–314.

23 Crerand, C.E., Sarwer, D.B., and Ryan, M. (2017). *Cosmetic Medical and Surgical Treatments and Body Dysmorphic Disorder*. *Oxford Medicine Online*. Oxford University Press.

24 Phillips, K.A., Menard, W., and Fay, C. (2006). Gender similarities and differences in 200 individuals with body dysmorphic disorder. *Comprehensive Psychiatry* 47 (2): 77–87.

25 França, K., Roccia, M.G., Castillo, D. et al. (2017). Body dysmorphic disorder: history and curiosities. *Wiener Medizinische Wochenschrift* 167 (S1): 5–7.

26 Bjornsson, A.S. (2017). *Age at Onset and Clinical Course of Body Dysmorphic Disorder*. *Oxford Medicine Online*. Oxford University Press.

27 Phillips, K.A., Menard, W., Quinn, E. et al. (2012). A 4-year prospective observational follow-up study of course and predictors of course in body dysmorphic disorder. *Psychological Medicine* 43 (5): 1109–1117.

28 Reddy, K.K. and Besen, J. (2015). *Body Dysmorphic Disorder: Epidemiology and Specific Cohorts. Beauty and Body Dysmorphic Disorder*, 127–137. Springer International Publishing.

29 Phillips, K.A. and Dufresne, R.G. (2000). Body dysmorphic disorder. *American Journal of Clinical Dermatology* 1 (4): 235–243.

30 Simberlund, J. and Hollander, E. (2017). *The Relationship of Body Dysmorphic Disorder to Obsessive-Compulsive Disorder and the Concept of the Obsessive-Compulsive Spectrum*. *Oxford Medicine Online*. Oxford University Press.

31 Phillips, K.A. (2017). *Body Dysmorphic Disorder in Children and Adolescents*. Oxford Medicine Online. Oxford University Press.

32 Phillips, K.A. and Stein, D.J. (2015). *Obsessive-Compulsive and Related Disorders: Body Dysmorphic Disorder, Trichotillomania (Hair-Pulling Disorder), and Excoriation*

(Skin-Picking) Disorder, 1129–1141. Psychiatry: Wiley.

33 Bowyer, L., Krebs, G., Mataix-Cols, D. et al. (2016). A critical review of cosmetic treatment outcomes in body dysmorphic disorder. *Body Image* 19: 1–8.

34 Wang, Q., Cao, C., Guo, R. et al. (2016). Avoiding psychological pitfalls in aesthetic medical procedures. *Aesthetic Plastic Surgery* 40 (6): 954–961.

35 Rieder, E. (2015). Approaches to the cosmetic patient with potential body dysmorphia. *Journal of the American Academy of Dermatology* 73 (2): 304–307.

36 Appelbaum, P.S. (2007). Assessment of patients' competence to consent to treatment. *New England Journal of Medicine* 357 (18): 1834–1840.

37 Sun, M. and Rieder, E. (2020). Psychosocial issues and body dysmorphic disorder in aesthetics: review and debate. *Clinics in Dermatology* In press.

38 Picavet, V., Gabriëls, L., Jorissen, M., and Hellings, P.W. (2011). Screening tools for body dysmorphic disorder in a cosmetic surgery setting. *The Laryngoscope* 121 (12): 2535–2541.

39 Dufresne, R.G., Phillips, K.A., Vittorio, C.C., and Wilkel, C.S. (2001). A screening questionnaire for body dysmorphic disorder in a cosmetic dermatologic surgery practice. *Dermatologic Surgery* 27 (5): 457–462.

40 Joseph, A.W., Ishii, L., Joseph, S.S. et al. (2017). Prevalence of body dysmorphic disorder and surgeon diagnostic accuracy in facial plastic and oculoplastic surgery clinics. *JAMA Facial Plastic Surgery* 19 (4): 269–274.

41 Sun, M. and Rieder, E. (2020). How we do it: body dysmorphic disorder for the cosmetic dermatologist. *Dermatologic Surgery*. Epub ahead of print. doi:https://doi.org/10.1097/DSS.0000000000002506.

42 Crerand, C.E., Menard, W., and Phillips, K.A. (2010). Surgical and minimally invasive cosmetic procedures among persons with body dysmorphic disorder. *Annals of Plastic Surgery* 65 (1): 11–16.

43 Tignol, J., Biraben-Gotzamanis, L., Martin-Guehl, C. et al. (2007). Body dysmorphic disorder and cosmetic surgery: evolution of 24 subjects with a minimal defect in appearance 5 years after their request for cosmetic surgery. *European Psychiatry* 22 (8): 520–524.

16

Protecting Your Patients

When Enough Is Enough – Saying No and Satisfying the Dissatisfied Patient

Jacqueline Watchmaker[1], Prasanthi Kandula[2,3], and Michael S. Kaminer[2-4]

[1] Department of Dermatology, Boston University School of Medicine, Boston, MA, USA
[2] Department of Dermatology, Brown University School of Medicine, Providence, RI, USA
[3] SkinCare Physicians, Inc., Chestnut Hill, MA, USA
[4] Department of Dermatology, Yale University School of Medicine, New Haven, CT, USA

Introduction

Medical students throughout the world learn the Latin phrase "primum non nocere" [1] ("first, do no harm"). However, the phrase's applicability to modern medicine is hotly debated, and while appealing in theory, many physicians find it impractical, especially if taken to its extremes [2, 3]. For example, does one forego prescribing medication because it might have a side effect?

Because physicians must often inflict harm – by inserting a needle, prescribing immunosuppressive medication, or causing purpura from a laser treatment – the better analysis is to balance potential benefits to the patient against potential harm. Sometimes this balance is straightforward (e.g. in the case of lifesaving surgery), but sometimes, especially in the field of aesthetic medicine where procedures are elective, this balance is more difficult. Often, it is wise for aesthetic providers to err on the side of "do no harm" by telling patients no. "No," however, is not always easy to say, especially to demanding cosmetic patients with the ability to self-pay.

This chapter discusses two previously described techniques that can be utilized during patient encounters to optimize patient satisfaction. We review the LEAP (Listen, Educate and Empower, Align, Perform) technique [4] for conducting cosmetic consultations (including, where necessary, saying no) and the BLAST technique [5, 6] for satisfying the dissatisfied patient.

The LEAP Technique for a Successful Cosmetic Consult

While established practitioners develop their own methods to maneuver through difficult consultations, younger physicians and medical professionals new to aesthetic medicine may benefit from some guidance. The LEAP technique is an efficient, easy to remember mnemonic and set of steps that helps ensure a positive experience for both the patient and provider – even if the physician must say "no" to a patient's initial desires (Table 16.1).

Listen

Uninterrupted, active listening forms a good foundation for the consultation and strengthens the doctor–patient relationship [7]. Active,

Essential Psychiatry for the Aesthetic Practitioner, First Edition. Edited by Evan A. Rieder and Richard G. Fried.
© 2021 John Wiley & Sons Ltd. Published 2021 by John Wiley & Sons Ltd.

Table 16.1 The LEAP technique is a framework for a successful cosmetic consult.

L	Listen
E	Educate and empower
A	Align
P	Perform

uninterrupted listening is critical [8] and allows the patient to express their concerns, wants, and expectations, which may differ from those of the provider. While listening throughout the consultation is important, devoting time at the beginning of the consultation allows the provider, early on, to understand the patient's perspective and identify potential unrealistic expectations.

Listening is a key component of patient-centered communication. A growing body of literature demonstrates a correlation between patient satisfaction and patient-centered care and communication [9–11]. Unfortunately, despite this, a large number of patient visits remain "physician-centered," with only 20% of specialty clinicians asking patients to discuss their concerns [12]. In encounters in which physicians do directly elicit the patient's concerns, clinicians often interrupt before patients have completed speaking [12]. Clinicians must make time to listen; "being listened to" is often rated as one of the most important factors contributing to patient satisfaction [13].

The *quality* of listening is also important. Active listening not only demonstrates empathy but ultimately helps people communicate more efficiently [14]. The efficient aesthetic practitioner might also take the opportunity at this point in the consultation to observe the patient's candid facial dynamic, which can be especially valuable to an aesthetic provider who performs neurotoxin and soft tissue filler augmentation procedures.

Educate and Empower

When a practitioner thoroughly discusses the benefits, shortcomings, alternatives, downtime (if applicable), and realistic outcomes of a proposed intervention, the patient feels like an active participant in their treatment. This feeling in and of itself can be empowering. More informed patients lead to more satisfied patients [15–17].

Align

The majority of patients favor partnership over the traditional paternalistic model of the doctor–patient relationship [18, 19]. When patients feel educated, an alliance is formed with an emphasis on shared decision-making [20] as well as shared responsibility for potential negative outcomes. Although in an ideal world aesthetic practitioners and their patients would always agree on the best method of intervention, this harmony is not always the case. Even if the patient's views differ from those of the provider, suggesting alternative options rather than simply saying "no" makes the patient feel that their treatment is a collaboration with an overall common goal.

Perform

At this point in the consultation, the patient should feel that their practitioner has listened to their concerns; the patient should feel empowered and informed; and the patient should feel like an alliance was formed with their provider. Cosmetic intervention in this setting will ultimately lead to more satisfied patients. If, however, a practitioner believes a certain aesthetic intervention would be more harmful than good, the aesthetic provider has an obligation to "do no harm" and persuade the patient that this is the wrong course of action. Rather than simply saying "no," clinicians should explain the reasoning behind a decision. While some studies have showed not fulfilling a patient's request leads to reduced satisfaction [21], others do not [22, 23]. Even when an initial request is denied, patients are often satisfied when physicians express personal interest, offer reassurance, and provide some form of treatment, even if different from what the patient initially had in mind [22].

Case Study

Case 16.1   Using the LEAP Technique

A 60-year-old woman comes to you for a cosmetic consultation. She has received multiple hyaluronic acid filler treatments by local aesthetic providers, the most recent of which was one month ago. You notice that her face appears overfilled and unnatural. Despite this, she would like additional filler in her perioral region to "erase" her persistent fine lines. She does not want bruising given that she has a large social event next week. You think that injecting more filler in this patient will lead to a poor aesthetic outcome.

- **Listen:** During the listening phase, the practitioner gains insight into the patient's wants (improvement of rhytides), concerns (downtime/ecchymoses), and sometimes unrealistic expectations ("erasing" of all rhytides). The practitioner can also observe the patient's dynamic rhytides during this portion of the consultation and start to formulate a treatment plan.
- **Educate and empower:** In this case, the practitioner might say: "I understand that you would like to improve the wrinkles around your mouth. Given that you recently had filler treatment and are not completely satisfied with your results, we could try an alternative approach. Filler is one method to improve fine lines, but laser and microneedling are also effective treatments with minimal downtime, low risk of bruising, and natural-looking results. It is important to understand that no treatment will remove your wrinkles

completely. All treatment options have potential side effects, which we can discuss. What questions do you have? Which treatment do you think is best for you?"
- **Align:** Ideally, at this point the patient and aesthetic provider align and agree on the best treatment option. If their preferred method of reaching a goal differs, the practitioner should still make the patient feel as though they are working together toward a common goal. The practitioner might say: "I am here to help you achieve your goals. Let's talk further about how we can best do that."
- **Perform:** At this point a therapeutic alliance has been formed and if the provider and patient agree on a treatment, e.g. laser or microneedling, cosmetic intervention can take place. For the patient in the case example, deferring treatment until after her social event would be ideal. Performing the cosmetic treatment is sometimes the easiest and quickest part of a cosmetic consult. If, however, the patient continues to request filler, the practitioner should gently persuade the patient this is not the ideal treatment plan and explain the reasoning behind that decision. In this example, the physician might say: "In your particular case more filler will result in an unnatural look and will not accomplish your goal of erasing all wrinkles around your mouth. If you would like to pursue other options, I would be happy to move forward with those treatments."

The BLAST Technique for Dealing with Unhappy Patients

Unhappy patients are challenging – especially unhappy cosmetic patients. The BLAST technique [5, 6] is a tool to help clinicians new to

aesthetic medicine successfully manage uncomfortable encounters with displeased patients (Table 16.2).

Believe

The clinician should believe the patient's feelings – even if the clinician does not agree with

Table 16.2 The BLAST technique is a framework for dealing with unhappy patients.

B	Believe
L	Listen
A	Apologize
S	Satisfy
T	Thank

the patient's complaint. Belief and empathy are directly related [24]; it is difficult to feel empathy toward someone you do not believe. Therefore, believing the patient's feelings, even in situations where the clinician thinks the patient is incorrect, helps the provider be more empathetic. Furthermore, as physicians and aesthetic practitioners we are trained to make every effort to not only heal but also ensure patient satisfaction. When a patient is unhappy with the result or care they receive, it is natural for medical professionals to become uncomfortable and sometimes even defensive. Starting a difficult conversation while harboring negative internal feelings is a recipe for poor outcomes when communicating with patients. Taking a moment to breathe deeply and making a conscious decision to believe the patient, preferably before entering the room to begin the discussion, allows the aesthetic practitioner to control their own emotions, and lays a better foundation for a productive conversation with the unhappy patient.

Listen

Focused, active listening strengthens the clinician–patient relationship in difficult situations [25]. Listening can also help the clinician better understand exact unmet expectations. It is essential to focus efforts on active listening to communicate to the patient that one is being supportive of their concerns. Patients may be unhappy due to a number of reasons, many of which may be surprising to the provider. For example, in minimally and noninvasive aesthetic

procedures many dissatisfied patients cite an expected side effect from treatment (i.e. bruising or swelling) as the reason for their discontent [26]. In more surprising circumstances, patients may be unhappy because of uncommon side effects or unrealistic expectations. Listening can help the clinician discern the precise reason for dissatisfaction so they can more accurately address the issue.

Apologize

Ethically, when a medical error occurs, clinicians are responsible for disclosing the error and apologizing. Apologizing decreases blame and anger, promotes forgiveness, and is known to strengthen the doctor–patient relationship [27, 28]. Legally and practically, however, apologizing is less straightforward, given fear of malpractice litigation. To address the intersection between the ethical responsibility and the potential legal repercussions, apology laws were introduced in the 1990s which made apologies after a medical error inadmissible as evidence in legal trials in certain jurisdictions. Still, there is little evidence that apology laws achieve their goal of reducing litigation [29]. Despite this, we advise physicians and aesthetic professionals to prioritize their ethical responsibility over fear of litigation.

While true medical errors do occur in aesthetic medicine, more commonly, patients are unhappy due to unmet expectations rather than a true error [26]. In this situation, an apology that expresses empathy with the patient's feelings rather than an acknowledgment of wrongdoing is more appropriate. Apologies such as "I'm sorry you are unhappy," "I apologize that you had to make an extra trip to see me," and "I'm sorry you don't feel the treatment has worked as well as you expected" show sympathy for how the patient is feeling but do not directly apologize for the clinical outcome. Apologizing for the conflict the patient is feeling, rather than the result itself, can be a powerful tool to improve communication and ultimately patient satisfaction.

Satisfy

If the patient suggests a solution that is reasonable, the aesthetic practitioner may satisfy the patient by proceeding with the proposed solution. Alternatively, providing the patient with options on how to best solve the problem and then allowing the patient to choose allows the clinician to direct the conversation. This approach still allows the patient to feel in control, and ultimately satisfied. In contrast, if the patient is given the opportunity to propose a solution without direction, the provider risks potentially not being able to satisfy the request if it is either unreasonable or not within the realm of what the practitioner can provide. In some cases, there is no option but to agree to disagree if a mutually satisfactory solution cannot be reached. In these cases, it can be helpful to address an unrelated yet troublesome problem to help satisfy the patient.

Thank

Genuinely thanking the patient for expressing his or her concerns at the conclusion of a visit lets the patient know the clinician was not bothered, but rather happy to help resolve an issue. Thanking the patient for being open and recognizing that it may not have been easy for them to candidly express their discontent will further strengthen the therapeutic relationship. The physician or aesthetic practitioner should thank the patient not only for their confidence to speak their mind, but also for having confidence in you to fix their issue. In some cases, the clinician can thank the patient for coming to them, even if the situation may be difficult for both patient and clinician. This can often lead to a stronger treatment relationship than going to a colleague, competitor, or even a lawyer.

Case Study

Case 16.2   Using the BLAST Technique

A 32-year-old woman presents to your office four months after undergoing one session of cryolipolysis to her outer thighs. She is frustrated that she has not seen a more dramatic improvement in her cellulite. You examine the patient and compare before and after pictures. You realize she had about a 20% decrease in adiposity as you had discussed prior to the procedure. The appearance of her cellulite is similar in the before and after pictures.

- **Believe:** Although as the clinician you believe the treatment was a success, it is important to believe the patient's feelings. In this case, the clinician needs to believe the patient thought cryolipolysis would treat her cellulite. Instead of becoming defensive because the clinician knows that cryolipolysis does not treat cellulite, the clinician must believe that the patient had

a different understanding and did not get what she was expecting. This belief in the patient is key to getting BLAST started on the correct path. In turn, this will help the clinician control their emotions and formulate a plan, rather than allowing negative emotions to lead down a destructive path.

- **Listen:** Listening in this case allowed the practitioner to realize the patient's major concern is the persistence of her cellulite rather than ineffective decrease in adiposity.
- **Apologize:** No medical error occurred in this scenario so the practitioner should not offer an apology that acknowledges wrongdoing. Instead they should offer an apology that sympathies with the patient's feelings such as "I am sorry you feel the treatment did not achieve the results you were hoping for," "I'm sorry you were under

the impression that cryolipolysis would treat your cellulite," or "I'm sorry that this has upset you."

- **Satisfy:** Discussing and moving forward with treatment that specifically targets cellulite will potentially satisfy this patient. Alternatively, sharing the before and after photos demonstrating a decrease in adiposity could help satisfy the patient. If the patient remains unhappy, this may be an example where the clinician and patient need to agree to disagree (presuming the practitioner explained clearly at the initial consult that cellulite would be unaffected by the treatment). If this is the case, helping the patient with an unrelated but bothersome issue may be the best way to satisfy the patient.

- **Thank:** At the end of the appointment the aesthetic provider should thank the patient for returning to express their concerns despite their initial discontent.

Conclusions

A positive patient experience is important in aesthetic medicine. The LEAP and BLAST techniques may help practitioners maintain a positive experience in difficult patient encounters. While recognizing when to say "no" may be simple, elegantly conveying a difference in opinion while maintaining good patient rapport proves more difficult. Similarly, dealing with unhappy patients in a methodical, empathetic, and productive manner can be challenging. The LEAP and BLAST techniques are proven strategies to help practitioners navigate these hurdles gracefully and effectively.

References

1 Smith, C.M. (2005). Origin and uses of primum non nocere – above all, do no harm! *J. Clin. Pharmacol* 45 (4): 371–377.

2 Sokol, D.K. (2013). "First do no harm" revisited. *BMJ* 347: f6426.

3 Hughes, G. (2007). First do no harm; then try to prevent it. *Emerg. Med. J* 24 (5): 314.

4 Watchmaker, J., Kandula, P., and Kaminer, M.S. (2020). L.E.A.P.ing into the cosmetic consult. *J. Cosmet. Dermatol.* 19 (6): 1499–1500.

5 Barneto, A. Dealing with Customer Complaints – B.L.A.S.T. https://www. customerservicemanager.com/dealing-with-customers-complaints (accessed 29 September 2019). Published 2009.

6 Steinman, H.K. (2013). A method for working with displeased patients – BLAST. *J. Clin. Aesthet. Dermatol.* 6 (3): 25–28.

7 Jagosh, J., Donald Boudreau, J., Steinert, Y. et al. (2011). The importance of physician listening from the patients' perspective: enhancing diagnosis, healing, and the doctor–patient relationship. *Patient Educ. Couns* 85 (3): 369–374.

8 Davis, J., Foley, A., Crigger, N., and Brannigan, M. (2008). Healthcare and listening: a relationship for caring. *Int. J. Listening* 22: 168–175.

9 Rathert, C., Wyrwich, M.D., and Boren, S.A. (2013). Patient-centered care and outcomes: a systematic review of the literature. *Med. Care Res. Rev* 70 (4): 351–379.

10 Stewart, M., Brown, J.B., Donner, A. et al. (2000). The impact of patient-centered care on outcomes. *J. Fam. Pract* 49 (9): 796–804.

11 Wanzer, M.B., Booth-Butterfield, M., and Gruber, K. (2004). Perceptions of health care providers' communication: relationships between patient-centered communication and satisfaction. *Health Commun* 16 (3): 363–383.

12 Singh Ospina, N., Phillips, K.A., Rodriguez-Gutierrez, R. et al. (2019). Eliciting the patient's agenda – secondary analysis of recorded clinical encounters. *J. Gen. Intern. Med* 34 (1): 36–40.

13 Wolf, J.A. (2018). The consumer has spoken: patient experience is now healthcare's core differentiator. *Patient Exp. J.* 5 (1): 1–4.

14 Bavelas, J.B., Coates, L., and Johnson, T. (2000). Listeners as co-narrators. *J. Pers. Soc. Psychol.* 79 (6): 941–952.

15 Bradford, A. and Meston, C. (2007). Sexual outcomes and satisfaction with hysterectomy: influence of patient education. *J. Sex. Med.* 4 (1): 106–114.

16 Ong, L.M., de Haes, J.C., Hoos, A.M., and Lammes, F.B. (1995). Doctor–patient communication: a review of the literature. *Soc. Sci. Med.* 40 (7): 903–918.

17 Parascandola, M., Hawkins, J., and Danis, M. (2002). Patient autonomy and the challenge of clinical uncertainty. *Kennedy Inst. Ethics J.* 12 (3): 245–264.

18 Bailoor, K., Valley, T., Perumalswami, C. et al. (2018). How acceptable is paternalism? A survey-based study of clinician and nonclinician opinions on paternalistic decision making. *AJOB Empir. Bioeth.* 9 (2): 91–98.

19 deBronkart, D. (2015). From patient centred to people powered: autonomy on the rise. *BMJ Br. Med. J.* 350: h148.

20 Stiggelbout, A.M., Pieterse, A.H., and De Haes, J.C. (2015). Shared decision making: concepts, evidence, and practice. *Patient Educ. Couns.* 98 (10): 1172–1179.

21 Bell, R.A., Wilkes, M.S., and Kravitz, R.L. (1999). Advertisement-induced prescription drug requests: patients' anticipated reactions to a physician who refuses. *J. Fam. Pract.* 48 (6): 446–452.

22 Sanchez-Menegay, C., Hudes, E.S., and Cummings, S.R. (1992). Patient expectations and satisfaction with medical care for upper respiratory infections. *J. Gen. Intern. Med.* 7 (4): 432–434.

23 Peck, B.M., Ubel, P.A., Roter, D.L. et al. (2004). Do unmet expectations for specific tests, referrals, and new medications reduce patients' satisfaction? *J. Gen. Intern. Med.* 19 (11): 1080–1087.

24 Bloom, P. (2017). *Against Empathy: The Case for Rational Compassion*. Random House.

25 Hull, S.K. and Broquet, K. (2007). How to manage difficult patient encounters. *Fam. Pract. Manag.* 14 (6): 30–34.

26 Watchmaker, L.E., Watchmaker, J.D., Callaghan, D. et al. (2020). The unhappy cosmetic patient: lessons from unfavorable online reviews of minimally and noninvasive cosmetic procedures. *Dermatol. Surg.* 46 (9): 1191–1194.

27 Allan, A. and McKillop, D. (2010). The health implications of apologizing after an adverse event. *Int. J. Qual. Health Care* 22 (2): 126–131.

28 Robbennolt, J.K. (2009). Apologies and medical error. *Clin. Orthop. Relat. Res.* 467 (2): 376–382.

29 McMichael, B.J., Van Horn, R.L., and Viscusi, W.K. (2019). "Sorry" is never enough: how state apology laws fail to reduce medical malpractice liability risk. *Stanford Law Rev.* 71 (2): 341–409.

17

Protecting Yourself

Legal Issues in Aesthetic Medicine – Informed Consent, Discharge, and Lawsuits

Brian P. Hibler and Mathew M. Avram

Dermatology Laser and Cosmetic Center, Massachusetts General Hospital, Harvard Medical School, Boston, MA, USA
Wellman Center for Photomedicine, Massachusetts General Hospital, Harvard Medical School, Boston, MA, USA

Introduction

In recent years, there has been a dramatic increase in the volume of patients seeking aesthetic procedures. In 2018, members of the American Society of Plastic Surgeons performed nearly 18 million cosmetic procedures in the United States, with an estimated annual spending over US$16 billion [1]. Minimally invasive cosmetic procedures are on the rise, with significant demand for injectable neuromodulators and dermal fillers, body sculpting, and laser treatments [2]. To meet this demand, increasing numbers of physicians and nonphysicians are performing these procedures. Approximately half of all medical malpractice claims result in litigation, which can be expensive, time-consuming, emotionally stressful, and harmful to professional reputation [3]. Knowledge of common causes for litigation in aesthetic medicine and how to avoid them may protect a medical provider from facing a malpractice suit and may, in turn, help strengthen the provider–patient relationship.

Key Legal Terms

Negligence

Most legal claims that arise against cosmetic providers pertain to negligence. *Negligence* is defined as a failure to behave with the level of care that someone of ordinary prudence would have exercised under the same circumstances. Negligent conduct may consist of either an act or an omission to act when there is a duty to do so. Four elements are required for a plaintiff to establish a prima facie ("true until proven otherwise") case of negligence: (i) the provider owed a professional duty to the patient; (ii) the provider breached this duty by deviating from the standard of care; (iii) the patient suffered personal injury or adverse event; and (iv) the injury inflicted was directly caused by the provider's infringement on such duty (Table 17.1) [4].

As it pertains to aesthetics, the "duty" is to perform the cosmetic procedure in accordance with the standard of care. It is generally accepted that a poor result of treatment in

Table 17.1 Informed consent doctrine.

Duty	The provider owed a professional duty to the patient
Standard of care	The provider breached this duty be deviating from the standard of care
Injury	The patient suffered personal injury or adverse event
Causation	The injury inflicted was directly caused by the provider's infringement on such duty

itself is not evidence of negligence (see *Miller v. Kennedy 1978*) [5]. As long as the treating provider can prove they acted as a reasonably prudent person, performing *lege-artis* (according to the law of the art [medicine]) is a method or technique that is acceptable within the medical community [4]. It is irrelevant whether the majority use this method or technique, so long as the technique is considered within the standard of care. Nevertheless, negligence is among the most common causes of action for litigation pertaining to aesthetic procedures, including laser treatments and body contouring procedures [6, 7].

Standard of Care

Even though cosmetic surgery is elective, a provider is still responsible for maintaining the appropriate standard of care in their specialty. *Standard of care* is generally defined as what a competent aesthetic provider would have done if they were treating a similarly situated patient undergoing the same procedure. Importantly, as it pertains to cosmetic medicine, where providers span a wide range of medical specialties and levels of training, a dermatologist, plastic surgeon, ophthalmologist, physician extender, and nurse aesthetician are all held to an equal standard based on the way in which a majority of providers in a similar medical community practice. They need not be the most talented in their specialty, but must be able to perform the procedure at hand in a manner that is considered by an objective standard as reasonable [8]. Under

normal circumstances, a provider is not held liable for a mistake in judgment unless the mistake was so gross that it made the professional conduct substandard (see *Boyanton v. Reif 1990*) [9].

There are often differences and inconsistencies between the medical profession, legal system, and public definitions of standard of care. From a medical profession standpoint, recommendations, guidelines, and policies for treatment modalities published by nationally recognized boards, societies, and commissions help establish the appropriate standard of care. Knowledge of these clinical guidelines and position statements as they pertain to the practice of cosmetic procedures developed by specialty societies including the American Academy of Dermatology, American Society for Dermatologic Surgery, American Society for Laser Medicine and Surgery, American Society of Plastic Surgeons, etc. is important, as they help define the standard of care.

In order for a successful case, a plaintiff must be able to demonstrate that they did not receive the standard of care they would have expected to receive from a reasonably competent, skilled specialist performing aesthetic treatments, and that they suffered harm as a result. Expert witnesses serve as a critical part of the litigation process in medical malpractice cases, providing insight for the judge and jurors who may be unfamiliar with both the medical and specialty-specific aspects of the case. The trial judge has discretion to determine whether the physician meets the standard for qualifying as an expert. Often, a plaintiff will use their own expert witness to establish negligence, which might be proven in multiple ways: (i) using clinical practice guidelines; (ii) cross-examining the physician defendant's expert witness; (iii) obtaining admission by the defendant that he/she was negligent; (iv) obtaining testimony by the plaintiff in the situation they are a medical expert qualified to evaluate the allegedly negligent physician's conduct; or (v) using common knowledge where a layperson could understand the negligence without the assistance of an expert [8]. Ultimately, expert testimony is required to introduce the standard of care and establish its sources and relevance.

Case Studies

Case 17.1   Informed Consent

JG, a 30 year-old man, presents to your clinic for evaluation of deep furrows on his forehead and between his eyes, which he feels give him an "angry" appearance. In a particularly busy clinic day, Dr. Vessel discusses off-label treatment with a dermal filler to fill in the deep rhytides. While he sees his next patient, his assistant briefly counsels the patient regarding risks of the procedure, including bleeding, bruising, and infection. Believing other risks, such as intravascular occlusion and blindness, to be very rare, these are not discussed. Dr. Vessel returns from his other patient, asks the patient if he has any questions, and the consent form is signed. During the procedure, JG notes intense pain with one of the injections. In the hours following the procedure, his pain increases and he notes a violaceous rash appearing on his forehead, along with diminished vision in his right eye. He returns to Dr. Vessel with retiform purpura in the distribution of the supratrochlear artery, and Dr. Vessel recognizes this as an intravascular complication. He treats the area with hyaluronidase, with improvement in the pain. Over the following weeks, the area on the forehead heals with atrophic scarring. John is now filing a lawsuit against Dr. Vessel, stating he would not have undergone this procedure if he had been informed of the risks of intravascular complications.

Clinical Relevance and Implications

In a review of litigation cases surrounding dermal fillers, deficiencies of informed consent were a commonly cited factor [10, 11]. This is also true for chemical peels, body-contouring, and laser procedures [6, 12–15]. Informed consent is a legal practice to ensure a patient has enough information about their diagnosis, proposed treatment, prognosis, and possible risks of proposed therapy (and alternatives) to allow them to make a knowledgeable decision [16]. Legal disputes over informed consent for aesthetic treatments often result from providers failing to disclose particular risks or not explaining the potential lack of benefit from a procedure [17]. Providers of aesthetic treatments have a responsibility (duty of care) to explain the procedures and potential risks to ensure a valid informed consent is obtained.

Informed consent is more than obtaining a patient's initials on a list of risks and complications. Consent should include the condition, indications for treatment, other therapeutic options, number of treatments anticipated, expected results, possible adverse events, and need to follow pre- and postprocedural instructions. Multiple studies have demonstrated patients do not recall much of the details of the informed consent process. In a study of patients' recall of risks related to carotid endarterectomy, only 1 of 71 patients, one month after surgery, could quote the risks they were told preoperatively [18]. In a study of patients undergoing elective or trauma-related orthopedic surgery, only 22% of patients could recall the potential complications and over 40% could not recall any of the possible complications [19]. Brochures and handouts containing this information may help physicians avoid malpractice claims. They should be written in simple, comprehensible sentences. Showing patients photos of actual complications that could arise from cosmetic treatments, such as burns, dyschromia, and post-treatment infections might improve patient understanding of potential risks and dissuade plaintiffs from stating they were not properly informed prior to treatment [15].

The provider who is going to perform the procedure is responsible for obtaining consent. In *Shinal v. Toms*, the Pennsylvania Supreme Court held that informed consent may not be delegated to a physician assistant, nurse, or other intermediary acting on the physician's behalf [20]. Courts in other jurisdictions, including Connecticut, Louisiana, Texas, South Dakota, and New Mexico, have similarly ruled that obtaining informed consent is the responsibility of the treating physician [21, 22]. However, other staff may serve as witnesses and are advised to sign the consent form.

Patients should also fill out a consent form each time a procedure is to take place. In the case of *Gustafson v. Baribeau*, the plaintiff sought full-face Erbium laser resurfacing and blepharoplasty [23]. The blepharoplasty was scheduled for two weeks after the laser resurfacing, and the defendant performed a second laser resurfacing of the full face, without consent, when he performed the blepharoplasty. The plaintiff sustained scattered areas of second and third degree burns, requiring scar revision surgery and further treatment to correct the dyspigmentation. Baribeau was charged with negligence and medical battery. There was a verdict for US$377 288. Providers must uniformly handle consent forms and adhere to performing only the treatments that were discussed and for which they have written informed consent.

Proper informed consent fosters a discussion between the provider and the patient, promoting communication and shared decision-making. For informed consent to be considered valid, the patient must be competent and give consent voluntarily. It is important to give the patient adequate time for reflection; they should not feel rushed or pressured. Significantly, in a study of legal cases following body-contouring surgery, cases that alleged a lack of informed consent were 50% less likely to result in favor of the plaintiff. The authors of the study believe this is because juries consider the signed consent form a legally binding document and the plaintiff's signature conveys full understanding [6].

Risks to Discuss

In the current healthcare environment, there is an increasing propensity for dissatisfied patients to consider litigation. In addition to inadequate informed consent, other major factors for litigation in cosmetic procedures include severe injury and poor cosmesis [6, 10, 11, 15]. Knowledge and discussion of reported adverse events, including those that have led to litigation, may improve the patient education process and should certainly be included in any preprocedural counseling.

When counseling patients on potential risks, one needs to examine the probability of risk and the severity of the side effect. Common complications of dermal fillers include bruising, pain, swelling, and infection. More serious complications including vascular occlusion and blindness can occur and have been raised in cases involving litigation [10]. Thus even the small chance of blindness with soft tissue filler injections warrants inclusion in the consent form. Procedure-specific consent forms are recommended, as they focus on particular adverse events associated with the procedure being performed. Providers should use plain language terminology and avoid using medical jargon on consent forms (Table 17.2).

Table 17.2 Medical consent terms.

Medical jargon	Plain language
Purpura	Bruising
Ptosis	Drooping
Bullae	Blisters
Hyperpigmentation	Skin darkening
Hypopigmentation	Skin lightening
Edema	Swelling
Necrosis	Ulceration
Crusting	Scabbing

Providers should use plain language and avoid medical jargon on their written consent forms.

In a study of litigation over informed consent in cosmetic procedures in Australia, 70% of cases alleged that the doctor failed to disclose risks and 39% said the potential lack of benefit was not explained [17]. In addition to the potential adverse outcomes that may occur, such as disfigurement, pain, or nerve injury, it is important to discuss the possibility that treatment may confer limited benefit or possible need for further treatment. Although cosmetic procedures have lower risks of catastrophic outcomes than many other types of surgery, the high expectations and low tolerance for risk on the patient side, in concert with competitive market pressures on the provider, may explain the prevalence of lawsuits regarding informed consent [17]. Complications of cosmetic procedures are usually visible and out-of-pocket payments are common, contributing to reduced patient tolerance for risk. Through a nuanced and comprehensive discussion, cosmetic providers can get to know their patients and determine and explain the risks, benefits, and possible outcomes that are relevant to the procedure at hand.

Off-Label Use of Cosmetic Treatments

With the rising demand for cosmetic procedures and the rapidly expanding field of aesthetic medicine, providers are quick to implement new innovations and techniques. Injectable neuromodulators and dermal fillers are US Food and Drug Administration (FDA)-cleared for use in designated anatomic locations for designated indications; yet they are often used in an off-label manner. For example, poly-L-lactic acid, FDA-cleared for HIV lipoatrophy, is more commonly used for off-label, non-FDA-cleared, facial volume enhancement in non-HIV patients. Most off-label use not only is legal but also represents an appropriate physician standard of care [24]. Manufacturers of cosmetic drugs and devices are not allowed to promote off-label aspects of their products. Moreover, federal law prohibits use of non-FDA-approved

cosmetic injectables obtained from foreign countries. Providers using non-FDA-approved drugs and devices risk enforcement actions by the FDA, licensing actions by state medical boards, and professional liability actions from dissatisfied patients [25].

Teaching Points

Deficiencies of informed consent are a commonly cited factor in litigation for cosmetic procedures. The informed consent process fosters communication and builds rapport between the patient and provider. Providers should discuss the diagnosis, prognosis, proposed treatment, and possible risks of proposed therapy (and alternatives) to allow patients to make an informed decision. Knowledge and discussion of reported adverse events, including those that have led to litigation, may improve the patient education process and should be included in any preprocedural counseling. For informed consent to be considered valid, the patient must be competent and the consent given voluntarily, and an informed consent should take place before every procedure, even if it has been previously performed on a patient. In addition to adverse events, providers should discuss the possibility that treatment may confer limited benefit or possible need for further treatment.

Case 17.2   Discharge

A 65-year-old female patient has been coming to your practice for the past year for various cosmetic treatments. Prior to finding your clinic, she had been seen by four other providers in the area for cosmetic treatments and recently filed a claim against one of them for dissatisfied results. She is consistently canceling her appointments, and when she shows up she is more than an hour late. She has been verbally abusive to the front desk staff and your

(Continued)

Case 17.2 (Continued)

assistant. Following her last appointment for a chemical peel, despite your counseling, she went to the beach and sustained postinflammatory hyperpigmentation, resulting in numerous angry phone calls to your clinic. Today, she presents for consultation regarding neuromodulation of dynamic wrinkles and consideration of dermal fillers.

Clinical Relevance and Implications

Patient Selection

Patient selection is among the most important elements in medical liability. The role of consultation is to connect with a patient before a patient–provider relationship has been established. A history of prior cosmetic procedures and level of satisfaction from those procedures can help assess the expectations and level of risk. Dissatisfaction with multiple prior providers can be a red flag [16]. Prior legal proceedings or threats toward former cosmetic specialists are even worrisome for the potential of future litigation. Standardized history-taking forms can be effective tools for developing patient rapport, understanding their expectations, and determining if they are a good candidate for a procedure [26].

The patient who has a personal conflict with the provider or staff, has unrealistic expectations for cosmetic results, or raises your concern for body dysmorphia should generally be avoided [27]. Staff can play a role in identifying potentially problematic patients through their interactions. It is important to resist pressure for treatment from a patient with unrealistic expectations. For elective procedures, you have discretion to refuse any services you do not feel are appropriate.

Patient compliance is also an important factor to predict a successful treatment and satisfied patient. A provider can control aspects related to the performance of the cosmetic procedure; however, it is up to the patient to make lifestyle modifications and adhere to a

postprocedural regimen to ensure optimal results. Providers should ask about social history and recreational activities that can inform whether the patient's lifestyle allows sufficient downtime for the procedure. For example, a history of smoking can impair wound healing, and over-the-counter supplements and anti-platelet drugs may result in excessive bruising or bleeding, which may increase the risk of a poor outcome or patient dissatisfaction.

While patients are under your care after having a procedure, they should be asked to report any unusual or unexpected events that occur. The treating provider must be made available for early diagnosis and management of possible complications. The need for follow-up visits and anticipated time course to see results should be discussed before the procedure, and patients should agree to the necessary postprocedural care. For example, to prevent nodule formation after poly-L-lactic acid filler for lipoatrophy, it is important to massage the area five times a day for five minutes for five days [28].

Typically, providers will not be held liable for a poor cosmetic outcome as long as they can prove they acted as a reasonably prudent person performing *lege-artis*. Important elements of a successful defense case of a malpractice claim include the following: the individual performing the procedure can prove they have been trained and certified for it; documentation that the individual acted as a prudent provider, performing a well-accepted technique in accordance with the standard of care; and the furnishing of documentation of discussion of all aspects of the procedure, including early and late complications. Pre- and postprocedure photography should be performed to allow a provider to better demonstrate results and prevent a patient from perceiving a defect that was present prior to any treatment.

Discharge and Abandonment

The law governing medical abandonment is predicated on the status of the patient–physician relationship. *Abandonment* is a form of medical malpractice that occurs when a physician terminates the doctor–patient relationship without reasonable notice and fails to provide the patient with a qualified replacement care provider. Once engaged in providing care to a patient, the physician is obligated to care for them as long as the physician–patient relationship continues. It is important to note that medical abandonment can occur between other healthcare providers and patients, not just between a physician and patient. Only proper termination of that relationship will relinquish the provider of their duty.

There are certain steps a provider can take to discharge a patient and avoid liability. First, the treating provider should provide the patient with a written notice of the termination; the reasons for termination are optional. It is recommended to have an attorney draft a standard patient discharge letter, as there may be some jurisdictional variability in the requirements for patient discharge. The letter should be sent via certified mail to confirm receipt, and a copy should be placed in the patient's medical record. Discharging physicians are required to provide care for a reasonable period of time to allow the patient to arrange for alternative care from another competent provider. Once the patient has identified another provider, the physician must provide patients access to their medical records.

Teaching Points

Patient selection is among the most important elements in medical liability. The role of consultation is to develop patient rapport, understand their expectations, and determine if they are a good candidate for a procedure before establishing a patient–provider relationship. For elective procedures, you have discretion to refuse any services you do not feel are appropriate. Once engaged in providing care to a patient, the physician is obligated to care for them as long as the physician–patient relationship continues. Taking the proper steps to discharge a patient can help avoid liability.

> **Case 17.3   Lawsuits**
>
> A 40-year-old man with fair skin presents to your clinic after suffering burns and scarring after receiving intense pulsed light (IPL) treatment at a local medical spa for facial rejuvenation. Immediately following treatment, he noted pain and erosions forming at the sites treated. You call the medical spa but are told the medical director is a podiatrist who is not on site. The patient is considering legal action against the medical director.

Clinical Relevance and Implications

Procedures utilizing laser and light-based energy devices have been dramatically increasing since the late 2000s [1, 2]. With the increased use of laser technology and procedures performed by nonphysicians has come a concomitant rise in lawsuits alleging malpractice arising out of misuse of a laser device [14]. It is important to understand the most common causes for litigation in laser procedures, the complex landscape of laser operator laws, and other medicolegal issues arising from physician delegation of cosmetic procedures.

Laser Litigation

Claims related to cutaneous laser surgery are increasing, with payments exceeding the previously reported average across all medical specialties [14]. Common allegations include permanent injury, disfigurement/scarring, inadequate informed consent, unnecessary/inappropriate procedure, and burns [12]. The most common litigated procedures were laser hair removal, rejuvenation (mostly IPL), and vascular treatments [14]. The most common causes of action were standard of care, informed consent, and fraud (exaggeration of benefits). Similarly, for ablative laser procedures, inadequate informed consent was alleged in 64% of malpractice cases, and the most common alleged injuries included scarring (57%), discoloration (14%), and infection (9.5%) [13]. Appropriate training in the physics, safety, and surgical techniques of sophisticated laser and light-based energy devices is paramount for all laser operators to select the right patient, treatment modality, and parameters and ultimately mitigate risk of these adverse events. Laser operators may consider conducting a test spot prior to performing a full treatment, although this is not a requirement. Nevertheless, patient counseling for all laser procedures should include the most common and severe adverse events.

Physician Liability for Extenders

The laws and regulations in the United States governing laser operation are highly complex and vary state-to-state. A 2018 review article demonstrated the convoluted landscape of laws and regulations of laser operation, where each state varies in which supervisory board regulates laser procedures [29]. Some states do not have any regulations in place, others have ambiguous laws, and in some states the medical and nursing boards have conflicting interpretations of the law [29, 30]. As such, it is important for physicians, especially those who delegate procedures to nonphysicians in states where it is legal, to understand the unique delegation, supervision, and operation laws in their state. Qualified assistants, including physician extenders, can be a valuable asset in the realm of cosmetic medicine; however, adequate training, appropriate supervision, and reporting of patient outcomes are warranted.

There has been an increase in lawsuits alleging misuse of a laser device, in part attributable to more nonphysicians performing these procedures, and the supervising physicians are often held accountable. Although nonphysician operators perform only about one-third of all laser hair removal procedures, upwards of 75–86% of lawsuits were brought against nonphysician operators, and almost two-thirds took place outside of a traditional medical practice without any direct physician supervision [31]. In a study of litigation in laser surgery, physicians were named as a defendant in 138 cases, even though only 100 procedures were physically performed by physicians [14]. These studies highlight that if a nonphysician is legally performing laser treatments and is performing within the scope of his or her duty, both the physician extender and the supervising physician may be found liable for negligence for any complication that arises, regardless of whether or not the physician saw the patient at the time of the visit [8, 32]. Similarly, physicians have been held liable for facial dermabrasion and chemical peels performed by nonphysician ancillary staff [15]. These studies reinforce the fact that nonmedical personnel failing to perform procedures commensurate with the standard of care will be held liable for any adverse outcome.

A physician's vicarious liability is rooted in the doctrine of *respondeat superior* – Latin for "let the master answer." This law doctrine is often used to hold the employer responsible for the actions of their employees if and when the employee is acting within the scope of his or her employment. In a medical setting, a physician may be held vicariously liable for the negligence of their subordinates, including nurses, physician extenders, and other staff. Specific allegations against the physician might include failure to properly supervise, failure to train and hire appropriate staff, or negligent entrustment. Negligent entrustment means the physician provided another individual with a potentially dangerous instrument and is responsible if this instrument is used for a procedure that results in injury to a patient. The physician liability is predicated on the fact that a reasonable person in similar circumstances would not have entrusted someone without proper training, licensing, or supervision with the equipment. Numerous complications can arise when individuals without proper experience or supervision perform laser procedures. These complications may be due to insufficient training, unsuitable patient selection, or inappropriate treatment parameters [33]. As a result, almost all malpractice cases arising from the negligence of nonphysicians performing laser procedures are coupled with vicarious liability claims against the employer, either the medical spa or supervising physician [31].

In a similar vein, a study of litigation involving soft-tissue fillers found that 50% of legal actions were related to a nonphysician performing the procedure, and a majority of disciplinary actions were reprimanding physicians (often serving as director of a medical spa) for not being present while a nonphysician employee injected patients [34]. In some states, medical spas operate with physicians off-site and nonphysicians can perform most, if not all, services [35]. A 2012 survey showed wide variation across state medical boards regarding the delegation and supervision of minimally invasive cosmetic procedures [36]. Variations included on-site versus off-site supervision, the type and numbers of nonphysician providers who can be supervised, and the requirements for reporting adverse events. In a more recent survey of medical spas, only 52% stated the medical director is on site at least 50% of the time, and almost one-third (29.3%) stated most or all procedures are not performed by a physician [35]. Some medical spas reported nonphysician medical directors, including nurse practitioners, nurses, and naturopaths. Medical specialty position statements can provide guidance regarding medical spa supervision [37]. Until there is more standardization, knowledge of local state laws and regulation of cosmetic procedures is paramount.

In the end, it is the physician's responsibility to ensure that any nonphysicians providing cosmetic treatments, whether it be administering injectables or performing laser procedures, possess the proper education and training. The individual physician of record is ultimately responsible for both understanding and abiding by applicable local and state professional practice regulations. Along those lines, there are a number of physicians who are offering laser procedures outside the scope of their specialty [14]; physicians who are not specifically trained in the use of medical laser devices should keep in mind that they will be held to the same standard of care expected of physicians trained in delivering these treatments.

Teaching Points

Physicians must know the laws and regulations in their state regarding delegation of cosmetic procedures. Even if supervision is not required, physicians may still be liable for the misconduct of their employees under the legal doctrine of *respondeat superior*. Nonphysicians and physicians who are not specifically trained in the use of medical laser devices (or performing other cosmetic procedures) will be held to the same standard of care expected of physicians trained in delivering these treatments. To minimize liability, individuals performing laser procedures should seek out the requisite training and/or licensing.

Case 17.4 Body Dysmorphic Disorder and the Law

A 34-year-old woman presents to your clinic for a cosmetic consultation stating "I dislike everything about my face." She is bothered by her "wide" nose, "asymmetrical" smile, "flat" cheeks, "terrible" complexion, and multiple other perceived abnormalities. She has had prior rhinoplasties, dermal fillers, and laser procedures, some of which were repeated due to dissatisfied results. She states she spends hours each day obsessing over these imperfections. Prior to leaving the house, she excessively checks herself in the mirror, tries numerous different hairstyles, and finds herself comparing her appearance to that of others. She has become more socially isolated over the past two years and notes her obsession with her appearance has negatively impacted her performance at work. She believes, with your aesthetic eye, you can help "fix" her appearance with only a few more treatments.

Clinical Relevance and Implications

This patient clearly raises suspicion for the diagnosis of body dysmorphic disorder (BDD). BDD may be more prevalent in patients seeking cosmetic treatments than previously believed. A recent review found the prevalence of BDD in patients seeking cosmetic surgery to be 13.2%, and as high as 20.2% for patients seeking surgical rhinoplasty [38]. With rising trends in cosmetic procedures, fueled in part by greater visibility through social media platforms alongside reality television shows and perhaps embellished advertising claims, many individuals may believe anything is possible with the right procedure. Moreover, varied age groups, ethnicities, and gender identities are pursuing cosmetic treatments; thus the aesthetic provider must be wary for signs to look out for when patients have unrealistic expectations or a perception that their appearance is flawed despite successful treatment – key signs of BDD.

Patients with BDD often have a poor outcome following aesthetic surgery, and it is well accepted that BDD is probably a contraindication to cosmetic procedures [39, 40]. In order to avoid unknowingly performing cosmetic procedures on a patient with BDD, it is important to understand the psychopathology of BDD and develop strategies to accurately screen patients.

The key indicator of BDD is an obsessive fixation on a perceived defect in one's appearance not readily apparent to others. During the initial consultation, several behaviors or warning signs may become apparent, which can signal to the provider the patient might have BDD. Detailed information on the clinical presentation, diagnostic criteria, and screening for BDD can be found in Chapter 15.

Though the long-term treatment of BDD is often best managed by mental health professionals, it is important for providers of cosmetic procedures to identify and appropriately manage individuals with BDD initially. Oftentimes, these patients will present for an elective cosmetic procedure prior to being given a formal diagnosis of BDD; thus the cosmetic provider is the one responsible for eliciting the diagnosis. Though aesthetic practitioners should be encouraged to and commended for suggesting the diagnosis of BDD to patients who raise their suspicion, they should also recognize that the treatment of BDD is often best managed with assistance from mental health professionals. Particularly in instances in which patients exhibit demanding behavior, it can be extremely helpful to obtain additional outside records or request a psychological consultation prior to considering treatment.

Legal Issues Related to BDD

Performing cosmetic procedures in patients with BDD is usually the wrong course of action, as the rate of satisfaction is typically very low and procedures in one area can shift patients' focus to other parts of the body [41]. Many patients will continue to perceive the defect as present or even exacerbated. As such, patients may attempt retaliation toward the physician. In a study of aesthetic surgery providers, 40% stated they had been threatened legally or physically by a patient with BDD [42].

Some argue that patients with BDD are unable to reliably provide informed consent due to mental impairment associated with their perceived physical flaw. In the case of *Lynn G v. Hugo*, plastic surgeon Dr. Hugo was sued for dissatisfied postoperative results, medical malpractice, and lack of informed consent [43]. Plaintiff Lynn G visited defendant Dr. Hugo more than 50 times over a six-year period for various elective treatments which produced satisfied results. However, she had an abdominoplasty and was dissatisfied with the residual scar. Prior to the procedure she had acknowledged in writing that the defendant had discussed the risks of scarring. Her attorneys claimed that her history of multiple "unnecessary" procedures together with her history of antidepressant medication should have alerted the plastic surgeon to her condition and she should have been referred to a psychiatrist; the defendant stated that she was adequately informed of risks and alternatives, and that he did not deviate from acceptable medical practice by not referring to a psychiatrist. Ultimately, since Lynn G had no documented history of BDD the case was dismissed. This case suggests providers of aesthetic treatments may be entering into uncertain medicolegal territory when performing procedures on patients with behaviors concerning for BDD. To date, no other cases with this cause of action have been published, so the legal risk at this time appears minimal. However, if Lynn G had a prior documented diagnosis of BDD, it is uncertain if the case would have been dismissed, as BDD may be considered prima facie evidence of inability to provide informed consent as a result of their mental impairment associated with their perceived physical defect [44].

Capacity and Competence

Capacity and competency are not considered synonymous. *Capacity*, assessed by a physician, is the ability of an individual to understand, appreciate, and manipulate information and form rational decisions. In contrast, *competence* is a legal state, not a medical one, assessed by a court. It refers to the mental ability and cognitive capabilities required to execute a legally recognized act rationally [45]. Incompetence is defined by one's functional deficits (e.g. due to mental illness, intellectual disability, or other mental condition), which are judged to be sufficiently great that the person cannot meet the demands of a specific decision-making situation, weighed in light of its potential consequences. In some jurisdictions, providers may meet their responsibility when they make a "reasonable effort to convey sufficient information, [even] though the patient, without fault of the physician, may not fully grasp it" [40]. However, BDD may become so severe that it impacts their ability to make rational decisions concerning the risks of associated cosmetic procedures, and these associated cognitive deficits would preclude them from competency, invalidating their consent [46].

Experts have suggested including an additional checklist to the preprocedure consent paperwork for patients where there is a suspicion of BDD [40]. The checklist contains a description of BDD and includes five statements the patient has to agree to: (i) I have never been diagnosed with or treated for BDD; (ii) I have undergone plastic surgery procedures in the past and I have not been unhappy with these procedures; (iii) I consent to contacting my previous plastic surgeon(s); (iv) I recognize that there is a significant emotional component in choosing an elective plastic surgery procedure; and (v) I understand that the procedure I am seeking may not have the exact outcome that I desire [40, 47].

If patients present without a visible deformity or have excessive preoccupation regarding a minor imperfection, screening questionnaires such as the Body Dysmorphic Disorder Questionnaire, Body Dysmorphic Questionnaire – Dermatology Version, or Modified Pisa Body Dysmorphic Symptom Scale (among others) may be used to screen patients [39]. If a mild deformity exists and the questionnaires diagnose possible BDD, further psychological workup is advised prior to treatment [48].

Teaching Points

Patients with a documented diagnosis of BDD are poor candidates for elective cosmetic procedures, not only because they are unlikely to yield patient satisfaction but also because of the patients' potential inability to provide informed consent for cosmetic procedures. A key indicator of BDD is an obsessive fixation on a perceived defect in one's appearance not readily apparent to others. A preprocedure checklist may provide additional legal protection for aesthetic providers [40] and several BDD questionnaires exist which can help screen patients [48]. Suspicion of BDD may warrant referral to a mental health professional for full evaluation prior to treatment to improve patient satisfaction and prevent cosmetic providers from poor outcomes.

Conclusions

Knowledge of legal issues that may arise within the practice of aesthetic medicine is important to mitigate risk of litigation. Careful patient selection, good counseling, fully informed consent, proper training and oversight of procedures, and ensuring patient compliance with postprocedure care and follow-up are critical to minimize risks. Knowledge of malpractice claims for cosmetic procedures may serve as a safeguard against the most common allegations. Moreover, physicians must know the laws and regulations in their state regarding delegation of cosmetic procedures and that they may be liable for misconduct of their employees. Any individual performing cosmetic procedures should seek appropriate training and/or licensing to maintain the appropriate standard of care and minimize liability. Ultimately, the patient's perception of their relationship with the provider is one of the most important factors in deciding whether or not the patient will file a lawsuit [16].

References

1 American Society of Plastic Surgeons (2018). Plastic Surgery Statistics Report. https://www.plasticsurgery.org/documents/ News/Statistics/2018/plastic-surgery-statistics-full-report-2018.pdf (accessed 6 May 2020).

2 American Society for Dermatology Surgery. ASDS Survey on Dermatologic Procedures. https://www.asds.net/portals/0/images/ body-procedures-survey-results-infographic-2018.jpg (accessed 6 May 2020).

3 Jena, A.B., Chandra, A., Lakdawalla, D. et al. (2012). Outcomes of medical malpractice litigation against US physicians. *Archives of Internal Medicine* 172: 892–894.

4 Mavroforou, A., Giannoukas, A., and Michalodimitrakis, E. (2004). Medical litigation in cosmetic plastic surgery. *Medicine and Law* 23: 479–488.

5 Miller v. Kennedy, 11 Wn. App. 272 (Wash. Ct. App. 1974).

6 Paik, A.M., Mady, L.J., Sood, A. et al. (2014). Beyond the operating room: a look at legal liability in body contouring procedures. *Aesthetic Surgery Journal* 34: 106–113.

7 Halepas, S., Lee, K.C., Higham, Z.L. et al. (2020). A 20-year analysis of adverse events and litigation with light-based skin resurfacing procedures. *Journal of Oral and Maxillofacial Surgery* 78: 619–628.

8 Goldberg, D.J. (2009). Cosmetic dermatology: legal issues. *Dermatologic Clinics* 27: 501–505, vii.

9 Boyanton v. Reif, 798 P.2d 603 (Okla. 1990).

10 Rayess, H.M., Svider, P.F., Hanba, C. et al. (2018). A cross-sectional analysis of adverse events and litigation for injectable fillers. *JAMA Facial Plastic Surgery* 20: 207–214.

11 Beauvais, D. and Ferneini, E.M. (2020). Complications and litigation associated with injectable facial fillers: a cross-sectional study. *Journal of Oral and Maxillofacial Surgery* 78: 133–140.

12 Svider, P.F., Carron, M.A., Zuliani, G.F. et al. (2014). Lasers and losers in the eyes of the law: liability for head and neck procedures. *JAMA Facial Plastic Surgery* 16: 277–283.

13 Pierce, R.R. and Martell, D.W. (2018). Ablative lasers: 24 years of medical malpractice cases in the United States. *Dermatologic Surgery* 44: 730–731.

14 Jalian, H.R., Jalian, C.A., and Avram, M.M. (2013). Common causes of injury and legal action in laser surgery. *JAMA Dermatology* 149: 188–193.

15 Svider, P.F., Jiron, J., Zuliani, G. et al. (2014). Unattractive consequences: litigation from facial dermabrasion and chemical peels. *Aesthetic Surgery Journal* 34: 1244–1249.

16 Sacchidanand, S.A. and Bhat, S. (2012). Safe practice of cosmetic dermatology: avoiding legal tangles. *Journal of Cutaneous and Aesthetic Surgery* 5: 170–175.

17 Bismark, M.M., Gogos, A.J., McCombe, D. et al. (2012). Legal disputes over informed consent for cosmetic procedures: a descriptive study of negligence claims and complaints in Australia. *Journal of Plastic, Reconstructive & Aesthetic Surgery* 65: 1506–1512.

18 Lloyd, A.J., Hayes, P.D., London, N.J. et al. (1999). Patients' ability to recall risk associated with treatment options. *Lancet* 353: 645.

19 Sahin, N., Ozturk, A., Ozkan, Y. et al. (2010). What do patients recall from informed consent given before orthopedic surgery? *Acta Orthopaedica et Traumatologica Turcica* 44: 469–475.

20 Shinal v. Toms, 162 A.3d 429 (Pa. 2017).

21 Sawicki, N. IRBs advise physician involvement in informed consent. *Harvard Law Bill of Health* 2017; https://blog. petrieflom.law.harvard.edu/2017/09/13/ irbs-advise-physician-involvement-in-informed-consent/ (accessed 17 May 2020).

22 Fernandez Lynch, H., Joffe, S., and Feldman, E.A. (2018). Informed consent and the role of the treating physician. *New England Journal of Medicine* 379: e25.

23 Baribeau v. Gustafson, Texas Court of Appeals (Bexar County). Case No. 04–01-000732-CV (2002).

24 Goldberg, D.J. (2006). Legal ramifications of off-label filler use. *Dermatologic Therapy* 19: 189–193.

25 (2006). ASPS Executive Committee and the ASAPS Executive Committee. Injectables and fillers: legal and regulatory risk management issues. *Plastic and Reconstructive Surgery* 118: 129s–132s.

26 Blackburn, V.F. and Blackburn, A.V. (2008). Taking a history in aesthetic surgery: SAGA – the surgeon's tool for patient selection. *Journal of Plastic, Reconstructive & Aesthetic Surgery* 61: 723–729.

27 Shiffman, M.A. (2005). Medical liability issues in cosmetic and plastic surgery. *Medicine and Law* 24: 211–232.

28 Burgess, C.M. and Quiroga, R.M. (2005). Assessment of the safety and efficacy of poly-l-lactic acid for the treatment of HIV-associated facial lipoatrophy. *Journal of the American Academy of Dermatology* 52: 233–239.

29 DiGiorgio, C.M. and Avram, M.M. (2018). Laws and regulations of laser operation in the United States. *Lasers in Surgery and Medicine* 50: 272–279.

30 Gillum, J.D. and Dellavalle, R.P. (2013). Contradictory state administrative regulation of minimally invasive cosmetic procedures in Kentucky and North Carolina. *JAMA Dermatology* 149: 137–138.

31 Jalian, H.R., Jalian, C.A., and Avram, M.M. (2014). Increased risk of litigation associated with laser surgery by nonphysician operators. *JAMA Dermatology* 150: 407–411.

32 Goldberg, D.J. (2005). Laser physician legal responsibility for physician extender treatments. *Lasers in Surgery and Medicine* 37: 105–107.

33 Hammes, S., Karsai, S., Metelmann, H.R. et al. (2013). Treatment errors resulting from use of lasers and IPL by medical laypersons: results of a nationwide survey. *Journal der Deutschen Dermatologischen Gesellschaft [Journal of the German Society of Dermatology: JDDG]* 11: 149–156.

34 Ezra, N., Peacock, E.A., Keele, B.J. et al. (2015). Litigation arising from the use of soft-tissue fillers in the United States. *Journal of the American Academy of Dermatology* 73: 702–704.

35 Gibson, J.F., Srivastava, D., and Nijhawan, R.I. (2019). Medical oversight and scope of

practice of medical spas (med-spas). *Dermatologic Surgery* 45: 581–587.

36 Choudhry, S., Kim, N.A., Gillum, J. et al. (2012). State medical board regulation of minimally invasive cosmetic procedures. *Journal of the American Academy of Dermatology* 66: 86–91.

37 American Society for Dermatologic Surgery Association. (October 2015). Position on Physician Oversight in Medical Spas; https://www.asds.net/portals/0/pdf/asdsa/asdsa-position-statement-physician-oversight-in-medical-spas.pdf (accessed 17 May 2020).

38 Veale, D., Gledhill, L.J., Christodoulou, P. et al. (2016). Body dysmorphic disorder in different settings: a systematic review and estimated weighted prevalence. *Body Image* 18: 168–186.

39 Higgins, S. and Wysong, A. (2018). Cosmetic surgery and body dysmorphic disorder – an update. *International Journal of Women's Dermatology* 4: 43–48.

40 Sweis, I.E., Spitz, J., Barry, D.R. Jr. et al. (2017). A review of body dysmorphic disorder in aesthetic surgery patients and the legal implications. *Aesthetic Plastic Surgery* 41: 949–954.

41 Phillips, K.A. (2006). The presentation of body dysmorphic disorder in medical settings. *Primary Psychiatry* 13: 51–59.

42 Sarwer, D.B. (2002). Awareness and identification of body dysmorphic disorder by aesthetic surgeons: results of a survey of American Society for Aesthetic Plastic Surgery members. *Aesthetic Surgery Journal* 22: 531–535.

43 Lynn G. v. Hugo, 96 N.Y.2d 306 (N.Y. 2001).

44 Rieder, E. (2015). Approaches to the cosmetic patient with potential body dysmorphia. *Journal of the American Academy of Dermatology* 73: 304–307.

45 Leo, R.J. (1999). Competency and the capacity to make treatment decisions: a primer for primary care physicians. *Primary Care Companion to the Journal of Clinical Psychiatry.* 1: 131–141.

46 Newell, B.L. (2011). Informed consent for plastic surgery. Does it cut deeply enough? *Journal of Legal Medicine* 32: 315–335.

47 Veale, D., Ellison, N., Werner, T.G. et al. (2012). Development of a cosmetic procedure screening questionnaire (COPS) for body dysmorphic disorder. *Journal of Plastic, Reconstructive & Aesthetic Surgery* 65: 530–532.

48 Nachshoni, T. and Kotler, M. (2007). Legal and medical aspects of body dysmorphic disorder. *Medicine and Law* 26: 721–735.

Part V

Psychological Tools to Assist Your Practice

18

Psychological Tools to Assist Your Practice

Progressive Muscle Relaxation, Deep Abdominal Breathing, Mindfulness, and Guided Imagery

Nicholas Brownstone[1], Bridget Myers[1], and Josie Howard[1,2]

[1] *Department of Dermatology, University of California San Francisco, San Francisco, CA, USA*
[2] *Private practice, San Francisco, CA, USA*

Introduction

Cosmetic procedures can present a particularly intense psychological experience for patients. In addition to the usual stresses and concerns regarding side effects and untoward events, aesthetic patients bring hopes and expectations regarding improved self-image [1]. High levels of anxiety have been reported among patients undergoing cosmetic procedures [2] and there may be a higher prevalence of anxiety disorders among patients who choose to undergo cosmetic procedures [3]. The anxiety–pain cycle is well documented, as is the contribution of higher levels of pain and anxiety to poorer treatment outcomes [4, 5]. By addressing patients' anxieties, treatment outcomes may be improved, pain can be minimized, and the treatment experience itself can be more therapeutic, satisfying, and enjoyable for patients.

In this chapter, we focus on nonpharmacologic therapies to assist patients undergoing elective aesthetic procedures. These treatment strategies, both structured and unstructured modalities, include progressive muscle relaxation, deep abdominal breathing, mindfulness, and guided imagery. In mitigating symptoms of anxiety or peri- or postprocedural pain, these treatment strategies may allow for decreased pain and anxiety medication use and help patients feel more empowered in their care.

The goal of all of these techniques is an overall physiologic calming preceding, during, and after the procedure. Here we outline three distinct techniques and how they could be applied in specific cases. In practice, there is often significant overlap between patient needs and techniques employed in real time. Given this overlap in symptomology, patients often benefit from a mix of multiple techniques. Much of the art of using these techniques involves establishing rapport and trust, listening to the patient's needs, and conveying a sense of sincere confidence in their efficacy.

Case Studies

Case 18.1   Needle Phobia: Applied Relaxation and Applied Tension
LS is a 31-year-old Caucasian woman with no past medical history who presents to your office requesting a cosmetic consultation for forehead rhytides. She is interested in neurotoxin injection for her forehead and glabella before an upcoming wedding

(Continued)

Essential Psychiatry for the Aesthetic Practitioner, First Edition. Edited by Evan A. Rieder and Richard G. Fried.
© 2021 John Wiley & Sons Ltd. Published 2021 by John Wiley & Sons Ltd.

Case 18.1 (Continued)

where she will be the maid of honor. She reports her best friend has received the same treatment and was happy with the results. She has never had any cosmetic or medical procedures before. She endorses a fear of needles as does her mother. She has donated blood once and during that time became lightheaded, but she did not lose consciousness. While she reports that the thought of needles causes her anxiety, she also endorses feeling a reduction in her self-confidence secondary to her forehead lines and is highly motivated to have them treated. After the risks and benefits are explained, the patient elects to have the procedure done.

Clinical Relevance and Implications

This case highlights the issue of needle phobia. Needle phobia is found to occur in about 20–30% of young adults. It is more prevalent in women and tends to decrease with age [6]. In 2018, neurotoxin and soft tissue filler (both needle-based therapies) were the top two noninvasive cosmetic procedures performed by plastic surgeons, with 7.4 million neurotoxin injections performed (a 4% increase from 2017) [7]. This patient likely meets the diagnostic criteria for specific phobia, a subset of anxiety disorders involving an intense, persistent, irrational fear of a specific object, situation, activity, or person. Patients that have specific phobias are highly distressed about having the fear and often go to great lengths to avoid the object or situation in question. This patient suffers from a form of needle phobia, formally classified as blood–injection–injury (BII)-type phobia in the *Diagnostic Statistical Manual of Mental Disorders, 5th Edition (DSM-5)* (see Table 18.1). Many different forms of behavior therapy have been used to treat BII-type phobia, including rapid desensitization [8], cognitive behavioral therapy, systematic desensitization [9], and progressive muscle relaxation.

This patient would likely benefit from the use of progressive muscle relaxation (PMR) or a similar applied relaxation (AR) method to relieve her needle anxiety. These methods are useful for their ease of delivery in an office-based setting, rapid onset of relief, and application for the patient to ease other anxieties beyond needle phobia. AR encompasses a number of different techniques which are empirically supported, long-standing, efficacious treatments and the gold standard of behavioral therapy for anxiety disorders. They have the potential to meaningfully improve patients' overall quality of life, as they are portable tools one can use when anxiety is encountered in daily life in addition to office-based settings. Because anxiety involves interacting systems of cognitive, physiological, affective, and behavioral responses, by decreasing sympathetic activation AR reduces the overall level of anxiety that a person experiences [10]. Applied relaxation has been shown to be as effective as exposure to *in vivo* therapy in the treatment of blood phobia [11]. AR was originally developed to treat phobic patients but has also been used successfully in the treatment of headaches, pain, and insomnia [12].

PMR is delivered as a behaviorally based therapy for the treatment of phobias. It is traditionally taught by and practiced with a therapist over the course of multiple sessions but can be adapted for use in an office-based and time-limited clinical setting. The large muscle groups are divided into two parts and worked through in the following way: face, neck, shoulders, arms, hands; and back, chest, stomach, hips, legs, feet. The patient closes their eyes and should be instructed to tense each muscle group for a 5-second period followed by 10–15 seconds of relaxation before proceeding to the next area, working sequentially from head to toe. The technique's goal is to help the patient achieve a relaxed state quickly, often within 20–30 seconds. It is hypothesized that AR reduces sympathetic activation, thereby decreasing the overall level of anxiety experienced by the patient [13].

Follow-up

Your patient, LS, has practiced her AR/PMR before her injections and this has greatly

Table 18.1   DSM-5 criteria for specific phobia (also known as simple phobia).

Specific phobia – diagnostic criteria

A) Marked fear of anxiety about a specific object or situation (e.g. flying, heights, animals, receiving an injection, seeing blood).

B) The phobic object or situation almost always provokes immediate fear or anxiety.

C) The fear or anxiety is out of proportion to the actual danger posed by the specific object or situation and to the sociocultural context.

D) The phobic object or situation is actively avoided or endured with intense fear or anxiety.

E) The fear, anxiety, or avoidance causes clinically significant distress or impairment in social, occupational, or other important areas of functioning.

F) The fear, anxiety, or avoidance is persistent, typically lasting for six months or more.

G) The disturbance is not better explained by the symptoms of another mental disorder, including fear, anxiety, and avoidance of situations associated with panic-like symptoms or other incapacitating symptoms (as in agoraphobia); objects or situations related to obsessions (as in obsessive compulsive disorder); reminders of traumatic events (as in post-traumatic stress disorder); separation from home or attachment figures (as in separation anxiety disorder); or social situations (as in social anxiety disorder).

Specify if:

Animal

Natural environment

Blood–injection–injury (e.g. needles, invasive medical procedure)

Situational

Other

Source: Adapted from Blood-Injection-Injury (BII) Type Phobia in the Diagnostic Statistical Manual of Mental Disorders, 5th Edition (DSM-5).

helped her tolerate the current procedure. She is currently sitting up in an examination chair. However, during the last set of injections to the glabella, she reports a sudden feeling of light-headedness and says that she is about to faint.

The most outstanding characteristic of BII phobic individuals is their unique physiological response when confronted with phobic stimuli. As a group, they display what Graham, Kabler, and Lunsford (1961) called a diphasic response, characterized by an initial increase in blood pressure (BP) and heart rate (HR) followed by a rapid drop that eventually leads to fainting if no adjustments have been made [14]. You describe the diphasic pattern and tell the patient that it is the rapid drop in BP and cerebral blood flow during the second diphasic response phase that causes the patient to feel dizzy and eventually faint. In order to reverse this, the patient needs to learn a coping skill that they can easily and quickly apply in almost any situation.

One coping skill that also produces an increase in BP and cerebral blood flow is applied tension. To apply it successfully a patient should first learn to tense the gross body muscles and second learn to identify the earliest signs of a drop in BP (such as light-headedness) and use them as cues to apply the tension technique. The patient is instructed in this technique as follows: tense the muscles of the arms, torso, and legs and maintain contraction for 10–15 seconds – long enough to feel warmth rising in the face. Then release the tension, but not to a relaxed state, just back to normal. After 20–30 seconds the patient should repeat the tension again and then release it. This procedure should be repeated five times. This method was studied in patients who had blood phobias, and there was demonstrated to be a mean increase in systolic BP of 13.6 mmHg (range of 3–34 mmHg) and significant improvement in clinical/behavioral measures (rating of fainting behavior, self-rating of anxiety, and time watching a phobia-inducing film) [15].

LS applied the techniques mentioned above and found that they reduced her anxiety to a much more manageable level. She was able to successfully tolerate repeated treatments by using PMR.

Case 18.2   Preprocedural Anxiety: Guided Imagery

42-year-old woman presents to your office desiring right forearm tattoo removal. She explains that she had the tattoo done when she was in her early twenties when many of her friends were doing the same. She no longer wants any visible tattoos, worrying that they are frowned upon in her current, more conservative line of work. She explains that she has wanted to remove her tattoos for many years, but feels significant anxiety regarding the procedure itself and fears the pain involved.

Clinical Relevance and Implications

Preprocedural anxiety is common among patients undergoing procedures, with some studies estimating it to be as prevalent as 47% of patients [16]. Guided imagery is a relaxation technique that has been shown in some studies to be successful in reducing perioperative anxiety [17]. It has also been shown to decrease pain and anxiety in intensive care unit (ICU) patients [18]. Stress and anxiety can interfere with the results of surgical procedures in part by inducing physiological changes, such as elevated BP or syncope, as well as producing considerable discomfort. Guided imagery encompasses relaxation and visualization techniques in which the individual imagines desirable physical responses in order to reduce psychological stress and attain a calm state of mind [19]. Guided imagery may be performed by the patient independently or with an instructor (either individually or in a group setting) using audio or scripts [20].

A blinded-randomized controlled study on guided imagery relaxation therapy demonstrates its ability to significantly reduce preoperative anxiety scores and cortisol levels. Participants listened to an audio tape with soft background music, nature sounds, and an audio track that led participants through a guided imagery exercise. These patients experienced, compared to a control group, reduced anxiety and cortisol levels in the immediate preoperative period, possibly through mind–body-induced neurochemical changes that led to an anxiolytic effect [21].

Guided imagery can be easily taught and can help calm and rebalance the autonomic nervous system, reducing sympathetic overactivation that could contribute to anxiety [22]. In a prospective randomized controlled trial, Shenefelt observed reduced anxiety in patients undergoing dermatologic procedures when they used guided imagery (combined with hypnotic induction) [23]. When using guided imagery as a technique, the use of prerecorded tapes or provider-directed imagery is often likely to be less effective than self-directed imagery [24]. With self-directed imagery, topics chosen by patients are highly individualistic and can include imagined scenes such as a beach, a walk, travel, or floating down a river or through the air. Interestingly, recorded guided imagery tapes have been shown to reduce surgeon anxiety during procedures as well [25].

Muscle relaxation has been shown to be an effective technique in reducing pain and anxiety during laser removal of tattoos. In a pilot study of 56 patients undergoing laser tattoo removal, patients received approximately 30 minutes of muscle relaxation training using biofeedback orientation and verbal instruction prior to scheduled laser treatment. The muscle relaxation method significantly reduced the levels of pain and anxiety, measured using the Beck Anxiety Inventory and the visual analog pain scale, compared to previous treatment sessions [26]. Reducing preoperative anxiety has been shown to have many benefits, including improved surgical outcomes, decreased length of hospital stay, minimized postoperative disruption, and increased overall patient satisfaction [27].

Case 18.3 Postprocedural Pain: Mindfulness

A 53-year-old woman, MH, comes to your office with a chief complaint of "age spots" or facial solar lentigines. Her medical history is significant for anxiety and hypothyroidism, for which she takes levothyroxine, and she has Fitzpatrick skin type one. The patient endorses regular tanning during her twenties without sunscreen. She has been feeling self-conscious about the brown lesions over her chin, forehead, and cheeks, which she says have progressed in size over the last five years. She denies itching, bleeding, or change in color. She previously completed a seven-month trial of hydroquinone cream which was stopped because of skin irritation. She also tried three sessions of chemical peel treatments with only slight improvement. On physical examination she has $0.5-1.0\,cm^2$ hyperpigmented macules scattered over her face.

After discussing the patient's desired treatment outcomes and the therapeutic options available, you and MH decide to try fractionated carbon dioxide (CO_2) laser resurfacing. You tell her that she may require multiple treatments in order to achieve desired effects and that the healing process after the procedure may take two to four weeks. The first treatment goes well with no complications; however, postoperative day two MH calls complaining of sharp, stinging, constant facial sensitivity with 4 out of 10 severity. She has been taking ibuprofen regularly and applying ice to her face with only minimal relief in pain. She says her face is red, swollen, and "raw"-appearing, but denies fever, chills, bleeding, and discharge. She reports that her pain is most bothersome at night and that she only slept "maybe three hours" due to the pain over the past two nights. She expresses concern that the pain will continue to keep her from sleeping and wonders whether something may have gone wrong during the procedure. How should you proceed?

Clinical Relevance and Implications

This case represents the challenge of pain management in aesthetic medicine. Pain is a potential side effect of many cosmetic procedures and for the first two weeks after laser resurfacing some pain and facial sensitivity is often normal. It is important for the aesthetic provider to be able to offer patients a variety of effective resources and tools to manage postprocedural pain, as good pain control is shown to improve patient satisfaction following various procedures [28]. While pharmacologic approaches to pain management, such as nonsteroidal anti-inflammatory drugs (NSAIDs), local anesthetics, and narcotics, provide adequate pain control in many patients, these medications may have only partial efficacy for some and may be contraindicated or undesirable in others because of side effects or issues regarding tolerance.

A nonpharmacologic adjunct to pain management that has been more recently explored is mindfulness, the ability to consciously be aware of one's present experience in a deliberate and nonjudgmental manner [29]. This patient who has a history of anxiety and insomnia is likely to benefit from a mindfulness-based intervention (MBI), as MBIs have proved effective in managing anxiety [30] and insomnia [31], which both can have detrimental effects on pain perception [32, 33]. MBIs include a variety of practices such as mindfulness meditation, breathing techniques, and movement exercises such as gentle yoga [34]. MBIs may help with pain management by diverting attention away from the pain sensation and toward the present moment [35]. To date, several studies have been done suggesting that MBIs are effective in reducing postoperative pain. For example, a study by Yi et al. assessed the efficacy of mindfulness-based stress reduction as an adjuvant to standard treatment following lumbar surgery for degenerative disease, detecting significantly lower back pain scores in MBI-treated patients versus controls [36]. Mindfulness has also been shown to affect how one experiences acute pain, as researchers Zeidan et al. detected a 57% decrease in pain unpleasantness and 40% decrease in pain intensity in individuals exposed to noxious stimuli during mindfulness meditation versus rest. Using neuroimaging, they saw that these changes corresponded with more activity in brain regions involved in cognitive regulation of nociceptive and sensory processing, suggesting that MBI may recruit higher-order brain areas to suppress ascending nociceptive input [37].

You inform the patient about the studies you have read, suggesting that a mindfulness practice could help her with the pain and insomnia she has been experiencing. The patient is interested in trying mindfulness meditation. You advise the patient to increase her ibuprofen dose and begin meditating for 10 minutes at a time, one to two times per day. You direct her to a few guided meditations available online and provide instructions on how she may practice mindfulness meditation on her own. These include sitting comfortably in an area that she will be left undisturbed, with eyes closed or open maintaining a soft gaze. Her attention should be directed toward her breath moving in and out, counting her inhales and exhales if helpful. If she has a thought come up, you tell her to first acknowledge it, then return to noticing her breath.

Follow-up

At a follow-up visit two and a half weeks later, your patient reports that she has been practicing mindfulness meditation most days. In the morning and evening she has been using a mobile application offering a series of guided 10-minute meditations but says that she struggles sitting still for that long and "not doing anything." While she has some slight facial sensitivity still, she is no longer experiencing pain and has not had any trouble sleeping over the past week.

You commend the patient on meditating, even though it is difficult for her. You tell her that while meditation is one way to practice mindfulness, there are other ways as well such as breathing techniques, creative practices such as drawing or playing music, and movement exercises such as yoga. She is interested in trying yoga and thinks it may be easier for her to practice mindfulness when in motion. She asks when to schedule an appointment for her next laser resurfacing treatment and you tell her that you want to wait one to two months, after her skin has properly healed. You advise that she try to maintain a regular yoga practice up until then, as it could help with minimizing postprocedural pain from her next treatment. There are data to suggest that a preoperative mindfulness practice is efficacious in reducing postoperative pain, as Weston et al. found an inverse correlation between preoperative mindfulness and postoperative pain scores in individuals following a minimally invasive hysterectomy [38]. In another study by Dowsey et al., researchers observed that an eight-week mindfulness training program prior to receiving a total joint arthroplasty significantly improved knee pain scores at 12 months post-operation [39]. For the aesthetic provider, in a patient with a history of pain after an aesthetic procedure or symptoms of anxiety or depression, recommending a mindfulness practice prior to receiving treatment could also be beneficial.

Conclusions

Aesthetic procedures present an opportunity to enhance patients' quality of life but are often also complicated by patients' anxieties. In this

Table 18.2 Summary of techniques described in this chapter.

Technique	Brief summary	Examples used in this chapter
Progressive muscle relaxation	The large muscle groups are divided into two parts and worked through in the following way: face, neck, shoulders, arms, hands; and back, chest, stomach, hips, legs, feet. The patient closes their eyes and should be instructed to tense and relax the different muscle groups for 5 seconds. Subsequent relaxation should be held for 10–15 seconds before proceeding to the next area, working sequentially from head to toe.	Injection phobia, periprocedural anxiety
Applied tension	The patient tenses the muscles of the arms, torso, and legs and keeps the tension for 10–15 seconds, long enough to feel the warmth rising in the face. Then the patient releases the tension, but not to a relaxed state, just back to normal. After 20–30 seconds the patient repeats the tension and releases it. This procedure is usually repeated five times.	Syncope/presyncope associated with phobic stimuli (e.g. injection phobia)
Guided imagery	Guided imagery encompasses relaxation and visualization techniques. Topics chosen by patients are highly individualistic and can include imagined scenes such as a beach, a walk, travel, or floating down a river or through the air, and are practiced while the patient is in a comfortable position with their eyes closed.	Periprocedural anxiety
Mindfulness	Interventions include a variety of practices such as mindfulness meditation, breathing techniques, and movement exercises such as gentle yoga. Mindful meditation includes sitting comfortably in an area where the patient will be undisturbed, with eyes closed or open maintaining a soft gaze. Attention should be directed toward the breath moving in and out, counting the inhales and exhales if helpful. If the patient has a thought come up, you tell the patient to first acknowledge it, and then return to noticing the breath.	Postprocedural pain

chapter, we reviewed nonpharmacologic therapies to assist patients undergoing elective aesthetic procedures with the goal of decreasing pain and anxiety and helping patients feel more empowered in their care (Table 18.2). Our goal here was to present a select group of techniques which may be incorporated relatively easily into clinical practice to ease patients' anxiety, thereby improving clinical outcomes. The use of these skills will not only improve the patient experience but also offer patients and clients the opportunity to enhance their coping skills and improve their quality of life for years to come.

References

1 Rankin, M. and Borah, G.L. (1997). Anxiety disorders in plastic surgery. *Plast. Reconstr. Surg.* 100 (2): 535–542.
2 Sönmez, A., Bişkin, N., Bayramiçli, M., and Numanoğlu, A. (2005). Comparison of preoperative anxiety in reconstructive and cosmetic surgery patients. *Ann. Plast. Surg.* 54 (2): 172–175; discussion 176–7.
3 Özkur, E., Altunay, İ.K., and Aydın, Ç. (2020). Psychopathology among individuals seeking minimally invasive cosmetic procedures. *J. Cosmet. Dermatol.* 19 (4): 939–945.

4 Perković, I., Romić, M.K., Perić, M., and
Krmek, S.J. (2014). The level of anxiety and
pain perception of endodontic patients. *Acta
Stomatol. Croat.* 48 (4): 258–267.

5 Gan, T.J. (2017). Poorly controlled
postoperative pain: prevalence,
consequences, and prevention. *J. Pain Res.*
10: 2287–2298.

6 McLenon, J. and Rogers, M.A.M. (2019). The
fear of needles: a systematic review and
meta-analysis. *J. Adv. Nurs.* 75 (1): 30–42.

7 American Society of Plastic Surgeons. 2019
Plastic Surgery Statistics. Available from:
https://www.plasticsurgery.org/news/
plastic-surgery-statistics.

8 Fernandes, P.P. (2003). Rapid desensitization
for needle phobia. *Psychosomatics* 44 (3):
253–254.

9 Jenkins, K. (2014). II. Needle phobia: a
psychological perspective. *Br. J. Anaesth.* 113
(1): 4–6.

10 Hayes-Skelton, S.A. and Roemer, L. (2013). A
contemporary view of applied relaxation for
generalized anxiety disorder. *Cogn. Behav.
Ther* 42 (4) https://doi.org/10.1080/16506073
.2013.777106.

11 Öst, L.-G., Lindahl, I.-L., Sterner, U., and
Jerremalm, A. (1984). Exposure in vivo vs
applied relaxation in the treatment of blood
phobia. *Behav. Res. Ther.* 22 (3): 205–216.

12 Ost, L.G. (1987). Applied relaxation:
description of a coping technique and review
of controlled studies. *Behav. Res. Ther.* 25 (5):
397–409.

13 Ayala, E.S., Meuret, A.E., and Ritz, T. (2009).
Treatments for blood-injury-injection
phobia: a critical review of current evidence.
J. Psychiatr. Res. 43 (15): 1235–1242.

14 Graham, D.T., Kabler, J.D., and Lunsford, L.
(1961). Vasovagal fainting: a diphasic
response. *Psychosom. Med.* 23: 493–507.

15 Ost, L.G. and Sterner, U. (1987). Applied
tension. A specific behavioral method for
treatment of blood phobia. *Behav. Res. Ther.*
25 (1): 25–29.

16 Bedaso, A. and Ayalew, M. (2019).
Preoperative anxiety among adult patients

undergoing elective surgery: a prospective
survey at a general hospital in Ethiopia.
Patient Saf. Surg. 13: 18.

17 Álvarez-García, C. and Yaban, Z.Ş. (2020).
The effects of preoperative guided imagery
interventions on preoperative anxiety and
postoperative pain: a meta-analysis.
Complement. Ther. Clin. Pract. 38: 101077.

18 Hadjibalassi, M., Lambrinou, E.,
Papastavrou, E., and Papathanassoglou, E.
(2018). The effect of guided imagery on
physiological and psychological outcomes of
adult ICU patients: a systematic literature
review and methodological implications.
Australian Critical Care. 31 (2): 73–86.

19 Astin, J.A., Shapiro, S.L., Eisenberg, D.M.,
and Forys, K.L. (2003). Mind-body
medicine: state of the science, implications
for practice. *J. Am. Board Fam. Pract.* 16 (2):
131–147.

20 Daake, D.R. and Gueldner, S.H. (1989).
Imagery instruction and the control of
postsurgical pain. *Appl. Nurs. Res.* 2 (3):
114–120.

21 Felix MM dos, S., Ferreira, M.B.G., de
Oliveira, L.F. et al. (2018). Guided imagery
relaxation therapy on preoperative anxiety: a
randomized clinical trial. *Rev. Lat. Am.
Enfermagem* 26: e3101.

22 Shenefelt, P.D. (2010). Relaxation strategies
for patients during dermatologic surgery. *J.
Drugs Dermatol.* 9 (7): 795–799.

23 Shenefelt, P.D. (2013). Anxiety reduction
using hypnotic induction and self-guided
imagery for relaxation during dermatologic
procedures. *Int. J. Clin. Exp. Hypn.* 61 (3):
305–318.

24 Fick, L.J., Lang, E.V., Logan, H.L. et al.
(1999). Imagery content during
nonpharmacologic analgesia in the
procedure suite: where your patients would
rather be. *Acad. Radiol.* 6 (8): 457–463.

25 Alam, M., Roongpisuthipong, W., Kim, N.A.
et al. (2016). Utility of recorded guided
imagery and relaxing music in reducing
patient pain and anxiety, and surgeon
anxiety, during cutaneous surgical

procedures: a single-blinded randomized controlled trial. *J. Am. Acad. Dermatol.* 75 (3): 585–589.

26 Huang, F., Chou, W.-J., Chen, T.-H. et al. (2016). Muscle relaxation for individuals having tattoos removed through laser treatment: possible effects regarding anxiety and pain. *Lasers Med. Sci.* 31 (6): 1069–1074.

27 Rosiek, A., Kornatowski, T., Rosiek-Kryszewska, A. et al. (2016). Evaluation of stress intensity and anxiety level in preoperative period of cardiac patients. *Biomed. Res. Int.* 2016: 1–8.

28 Hanna, M.N., González-Fernández, M., Barrett, A.D. et al. (2012). Does patient perception of pain control affect patient satisfaction across surgical units in a tertiary teaching hospital? *Am. J. Med. Qual.* 27 (5): 411–416.

29 Anava, A.W., Ross, A.C., D'Souza, G. et al. (2019). Multidisciplinary pain management for pediatric patients with acute and chronic pain: a foundational treatment approach when prescribing opioids. *Children (Basel)* 6 (2): 33.

30 Hearn, J.H. and Cross, A. (2020). Mindfulness for pain, depression, anxiety, and quality of life in people with spinal cord injury: a systematic review. *BMC Neurol.* 20 (1): 32.

31 Ong, J. and Sholtes, D. (2010). A mindfulness-based approach to the treatment of insomnia. *J. Clin. Psychol.* 66 (11): 1175–1184.

32 Woo, A.K. (2010). Depression and anxiety in pain. *Rev. Pain.* 4 (1): 8–12.

33 Finan, P.H., Goodin, B.R., and Smith, M.T. (2013). The association of sleep and pain: an update and a path forward. *J. Pain* 14 (12): 1539–1552.

34 Baer, R.A. (2003). Mindfulness training as a clinical intervention: a conceptual and empirical review. *Clin. Psychol. Sci. Pract.* 10 https://doi.org/10.1093/clipsy.bpg015.

35 Ahmad, A.H. and Zakaria, R. (2015). Pain in times of stress. *Malays. J. Med. Sci.* 22 (Spec Issue): 52–61.

36 Yi, J.L., Porucznik, C.A., Gren, L.H. et al. (2019). The impact of preoperative mindfulness-based stress reduction on postoperative patient-reported pain, disability, quality of life, and prescription opioid use in lumbar spine degenerative disease: a pilot study. *World Neurosurg.* 121: e786–e791.

37 Zeidan, F., Martucci, K.T., Kraft, R.A. et al. (2011). Brain mechanisms supporting the modulation of pain by mindfulness meditation. *J. Neurosci.* 31 (14): 5540–5548.

38 Weston, E., Raker, C., Huang, D. et al. (2019). The association between mindfulness and postoperative pain: a prospective cohort study of gynecologic oncology patients undergoing minimally invasive hysterectomy. *J. Minim. Invasive Gynecol.* 27 (5): 1119–26.e2.

39 Dowsey, M., Castle, D., Knowles, S. et al. (2019). The effect of mindfulness training prior to total joint arthroplasty on post-operative pain and physical function: a randomised controlled trial. *Complement Ther. Med.* 46: 195–201.

19

Hypnotic Techniques for the Aesthetic Practitioner

Philip D. Shenefelt

Department of Dermatology, University of South Florida, Tampa, FL, USA

Introduction

Hypnosis may sound mysterious and inapplicable to the aesthetic practitioner. However, hypnosis is simply the Western approach to inducing and utilizing trance for the benefit of the patient. Trance is a transition or passage into an alternative state of consciousness. Most of us have experienced light trance while being absorbed in reading a book, watching a movie, daydreaming, or thinking about something while driving and then suddenly realizing that we had safely gotten somewhere without paying attention to the driving. Listening to a fascinating story also induces a light trance. Sometimes surprise will induce a trance.

Recognizing or inducing and utilizing an altered state of consciousness can prove quite helpful in many instances involving patient care. Altered states, while seemingly totally unrelated to the practice of cosmetics, may play a significant role for the aesthetic practitioner as many cosmetic patients bring with them unresolved psychological issues, worries, fears, and anxieties. The altered state of consciousness can occur spontaneously or be induced intentionally. Many patients who visit us are already in an altered state consisting of narrowed focus, increased suggestibility, and increased dissociation [1]. Part of our task during the encounter is to recognize or induce trance and utilize it to help our patients get through the office visit and procedure. This need not necessarily be a formal process.

Informal Hypnotic Techniques

Humans naturally cycle through more alert and less alert phases about every 90–120 minutes while awake, shifting between normal alertness and drifting into light trance [2]. This is similar to how we cycle between lighter dreaming sleep and deep sleep about every 90–120 minutes when asleep. A patient coming into an encounter with us often has already shifted toward trance. One can often recognize and use "hypnomoments" [3], moments of light trance during the regular encounter, to explore issues or make positive suggestions. Examples of hypnomoments might include an eyelid flutter or a sustained fixed or vacant gaze. These moments can be helpful for the aesthetic provider to insert suggestions through nonverbal means as well as to carefully choose words to help patients relax. Hypnomoments may also be induced by exercises such as slow deep breathing. Matched, paced, and gradually slowed breathing exercises done in concert between aesthetic practitioner and patient may help to calm patients and potentially induce trance. It is equally important to refrain from giving negative suggestions (nocebos) during the encounter [4] and to investigate whether the patient has been given a nocebo by someone else. In other situations a more formal trance induction may be needed.

Hypnotizability

About 15% of individuals are considered to be low hypnotizable, meaning that it is difficult for them to lose the power of voluntary action and be responsive to suggestion or direction. About 70% of people are medium hypnotizable and about 15% are high hypnotizable [1]. The hypnotizability trait remains quite stable throughout life. However, even those who are low hypnotizable can often benefit from trance when their motivation is high, as is often the case in medical situations. The power of suggestion can be particularly useful in clinical situations, especially when patients may be under stress of an unfamiliar or new procedure or meeting a new practitioner. Those who are low hypnotizable may respond better to suggestions for distraction (e.g. telling the patient a story of interest to them), those who are medium hypnotizable may respond better to suggestions for distortion of time or sensation (e.g. imagining numbing of the hand, wearing an imaginary purple glove, and then transferring numbness to the affected area), and those who are high hypnotizable may respond better to suggestions for dissociation or fantasy (e.g. asking your patient "imagine where you would rather be"). High hypnotizables will usually be very responsive to suggestions, both positive and negative, so it is important to be impeccable with words when talking to them. Listing possible adverse effects of a treatment unless very carefully done can produce nocebo results, especially in high hypnotizables.

Formal Hypnotic Techniques

Training in clinical hypnosis such as that offered by the American Society of Clinical Hypnosis (www.asch.net) facilitates recognizing trance and hypnomoments as they occur and teaches appropriate methods of trance utilization that can benefit the patient. Other approaches to the positive use of trance include the Eastern methods of mindfulness meditation or of concentrative meditation. While these meditative techniques may be generally beneficial for overall health for many individuals, they lack the kinds of specific suggestions and explorations that are available using hypnosis. The Eastern meditation approach is more about centering and balance, while the Western hypnosis approach is more about exploring and reframing specific issues.

Hypnotic techniques include establishing rapport by matching breathing and then slowing down to pace the patient to a calmer rate, matching the patient's preference of visual versus auditory versus kinesthetic mode of expression, speaking in a slower more soothing voice, having the patient focus on an object or thought, and/or one of many other methods of trance induction [5]. The Spiegel eye-roll induction [1] is a quick and fairly reliable method of trance induction that is easy to learn and use (Figure 19.1). The Spiegel induction allows the practitioner to assess the hypotizability of a patient. In short, during the induction, the practitioner has the patient roll their eyes up into the top of their head while keeping their eyelids open. The more the eyes roll up into the head (the more the bottom whites of the eyes are seen), the more susceptible to hypnotic induction the person is believed to be. The amount of eye roll is graded on a scale of 0–4, with four being the most susceptible to hypnosis. The patient is then instructed to allow the eyes to close slowly.

Deepening of trance can be used if needed. Once the person is in a light trance it is possible to explore past events, make positive

EYE-ROLL SIGN FOR HYPNOTIZABILITY

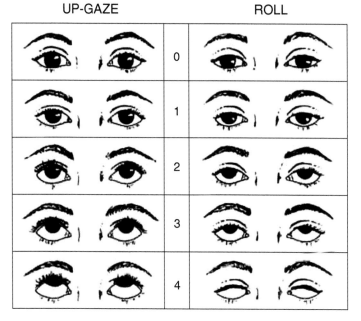

Figure 19.1 Spiegel eye-roll induction. Now look toward me. As you hold your head in that position, look up toward your eyebrows – now toward the top of your head. As you continue to look upward, close your eyelids slowly. That's right – close, close, close, close. Keep your eyelids closed and continue to hold your eyes upward. Take a deep breath, hold – now exhale, and let your eyes relax while keeping the lids closed, and let your body float. Imagine a feeling of floating, floating right down through the chair/table. There will be something pleasant and welcome about this sensation of floating.

suggestions, and/or have the person alter some aspect of their physiology that is normally not consciously possible. Examples for conditions that can be modified by hypnosis include altering blood flow, sensation, or habits such as scratching or picking. It is also possible to modulate the immune system [6] relative to the skin. We are just beginning to understand some of the neuropeptide and other molecular mediator mechanisms of communication between the nervous system and skin. The cutaneous and nervous systems develop side by side in the embryo and remain intimately connected and highly communicative throughout life. What affects the skin can affect the nerves and vice versa. Informed use of hypnotic techniques can assist the patient in ways not otherwise available.

Case Studies

Case 19.1 Study of Psychogenic Picking

A 32-year-old pregnant woman living with acne desired to stop picking excessively at her acneiform lesions. She had evidence of multiple recent excoriations on her face as well as mild acneiform lesions. Because of her pregnancy her only acne treatment was topical erythromycin. She did not want to take any psychopharmacologic medications because she was pregnant. She had had prior experience with hypnosis for pain control. A 30-second Spiegel eye-roll induction followed by suggestions that she visualize the word "scar" anytime she reached for her face, and suggestions that "natural

(Continued)

Case 19.1 (Continued)

is more beautiful than is perfection" induced her to cease picking at her acne on her face. Her improvement was dramatic with healing of the excoriations within a week. She augmented the effect with clinician-taught self-hypnosis. The avoidance of picking at her acne lesions persisted for months [7].

Clinical Relevance and Implications

This case illustrates the ease of inducing and utilizing hypnosis during a regular clinic encounter. The keys to success are knowing how to induce and/or utilize trance and providing suitable suggestions to help the patient. Learning how to do this is no more complex that learning how to perform a basic surgical or cosmetic procedure such as an excision or an injection of neurotoxin. As one becomes familiar with the signs of trance one begins to pick them up in everyday encounters and to recognize when and how to use them. Some cases may require formal trance induction, deepening, and therapeutic explorations and suggestions, while other cases may permit momentary utilization of a spontaneous or quickly induced light trance (a hypnomoment). In this case a simple quick eye-roll induction and a set of direct suggestions along with a post-hypnotic suggestion for self-hypnosis were sufficient to obtain the desired results. The suggestions were chosen to counteract the picking habit. She did not want to cause a "scar." Reframing slight imperfections as more naturally beautiful than "artificial" perfection allowed her to accept the slight imperfections and not attempt to improve them through scratching them away. The patient was asked to continue with self-hypnosis to maintain the effect and she was successful in avoiding picking using self-hypnosis for months after the initial session.

Case 19.2 Study of Relaxation for a Procedure

A 51-year-old woman was diagnosed with melanoma of her upper arm and came to a dermatologic surgeon's office for excision. As she lay on the operating table, she revealed that she had a severe needle phobia and asked that the procedure be halted after it had already begun. Attempts to reassure her with words were not successful, but given the nature of the diagnosis, the dermatologist knew that this procedure was essential to undertake without delay. She was given an option of hypnotic trance induction. Within less than a minute the Spiegel eye-roll technique had shifted her into trance and she was instructed to go in her mind to someplace that she would rather be. She quickly became calm and relaxed. The trance was reinforced every few minutes. She remained calm during the remainder of the procedure. When re-alerted after the procedure she said she had gone on an imaginary shopping trip in Italy. This trip was similar to one she had previously made. She was thoroughly enjoying herself and had not made all of the purchases she wanted to before she was re-alerted [8]. She was very relieved that the procedure was over and pleased that she had tolerated it well once in trance.

Clinical Relevance and Implications

Patients are often anxious before and during procedures and hypnotic trance is often an excellent way of relaxing them [8]. Having them go where they would rather be gives them the option of becoming deeply absorbed in some personally pleasing hobby, event, gathering, view, or other experience while shifting their thinking away from the procedure. It is most helpful to allow the patient to identify their own special location and not suggest a location based on the practitioner's own fantasies. It has been shown in a randomized control trial that hypnotic relaxation can significantly reduce anxiety during dermatologic procedures [9]. In that study, recorded suggestions were less effective at reducing anxiety than live suggestions were. This approach of shifting the person into a self-guided trance results in a much more positive and enjoyable experience for the person and may allow for more rapid completion of the procedure. Being able to provide this service for the patient can give the practitioner a competitive advantage.

The aforementioned case scenarios are fairly simple and straightforward; success can easily be accomplished by a practitioner with basic hypnosis training. While there are a myriad of more complex case scenarios that require more experience in hypnosis, these cases can be paradigmatic for the aesthetic practitioner because of their utility and ease of administration. While many aesthetic practitioners may be disinclined to obtain basic hypnosis training and rely on referrals to hypnotherapists or other modalities of psychological treatment instead, basic hypnosis training can open the practitioner's awareness and allow them to revise approaches during many patient encounters.

There is much going on beneath the surface that can be modified in constructive ways if one has the understanding and appreciation that comes from having had basic training in hypnosis. Psychologist Teresa Robles [10] referred to this as a concert for four hemispheres in psychotherapy. She utilized hypnosis in her clinical practice and it helped her to understand the complex interpersonal relationships that occur between two people, a helping professional and a patient, during the conscious and unconscious interactions of the left and right hemispheres of each with the other person. Having some comprehension of this complex set of interactions can be quite enlightening for the aesthetic practitioner as rarely are patients' motivations solely for anatomic correction without any underlying psychological undertones. About 30% of regular dermatology visits have some psychological overlay [6], and those who seek cosmetic improvement from an aesthetic practitioner of any training background may have even higher levels of psychiatric dysfunction. Beyond the screening for disorders that are discussed in other chapters of this text, if the practitioner has personal experience in utilizing hypnosis, this modality can often help sensitize the practitioner to their patients' potential underlying psychiatric or personality issues.

For Additional Information

Hypnosis training typically is done starting at the basic level with training extending over about 20 or more hours over one or several weekends. After completing the basic training, the practitioner can obtain an intermediate level of training, often tailored more specifically to the subject area where the practitioner is active. Again the training typically lasts about 20 hours. At this level the practitioner should be comfortable working with relatively simple use of hypnosis for relaxation and for direct suggestions to patients. Further mentoring can also help the neophyte to develop more assuredly. Advanced training is available at regional or national meetings or online where the practitioner can further expand their training in the areas relevant to their needs. For those at the masters level licensed in a health or mental health profession the American Society of Clinical Hypnosis offers excellent training. Practitioners at the Bachelor of Science in Nursing (BSN) nursing level and above can obtain similar training through the Society for Clinical and Experimental Hypnosis. Further mentoring is then available as the practitioner becomes more comfortable and competent in inducing and utilizing hypnosis.

Conclusions

The basics of clinical hypnosis are easy to learn and implement for clinicians of a variety of backgrounds and trainings. While seemingly unrelated to the practice of an aesthetic practitioner, these modalities can be very helpful for decreasing patient psychological dysfunction and improving the practitioner–patient relationship. Having this training can give the aesthetic practitioner a competitive advantage over others not so trained in terms of offering patients more pleasant encounter and procedure experiences. It can also make practice more interesting and pleasant.

References

1 Spiegel, H. and Spiegel, D. (2004). *Trance and Treatment: Clinical Uses of Hypnosis*, 2e. Washington DC: American Psychiatric Publishing.

2 Rossi, E.L. (1999). *The Twenty Minute Break: Reduce Stress, Maximize Performance, Improve Health and Emotional Well-Being Using the New Science of Ultradian Rhythms*. Los Angeles, CA: JP Tarcher.

3 Shenefelt, P.D. (2019). Inducing and utilizing hypnomoments in routine medical communications with patients. *J. Altern. Med. Res.* 11 (1): 45–51.

4 Shenefelt, P.D. (2017). Noxious nocebos in dermatology. *Cutis.* 100 (3): 100–101.

5 Barabasz, A. and Watkins, J.G. (2005). *Hypnotherapeutic Techniques*. New York: Brunner Routledge.

6 Shenefelt, P.D. (2000). Hypnosis in dermatology. *Arch. Dermatol.* 136 (3): 393–399.

7 Shenefelt, P.D. (2004). Using hypnosis to facilitate resolution of psychogenic excoriations in acne excoriée. *Am. J. Clin. Hypn.* 46 (3): 239–245.

8 Shenefelt, P.D. (2003). Hypnosis-facilitated relaxation using self-guided imagery during dermatologic procedures. *Am. J. Clin. Hypn.* 45 (3): 225–232.

9 Shenefelt, P.D. (2013). Anxiety reduction using hypnotic induction and self-guided imagery for relaxation during dermatologic procedures. *Int. J. Clin. Exp. Hypn.* 61 (3): 305–318.

10 Robles, T. (1995). *A Concert for Four Hemispheres in Psychotherapy*. New York: Vantage Press.

20

Acceptance and Commitment Therapy in the Aesthetic Setting

Vanessa J. Cutler

Department of Psychiatry, New York University Grossman School of Medicine, New York, NY, USA

Introduction

My life would be so much better with smoother skin ...

I would probably have an easier time dating if my smile were just a little less toothy ...

I think that my forehead is getting in the way ... of everything!

Many people have fantasized about changing a certain aspect of their appearance – weight, breast size, cheekbone definition – and it's normal to wonder how one might look and feel with a small tweak or even a more invasive surgical procedure like liposuction or rhinoplasty. In a survey, "Body Image 1996" [1], *Psychology Today*, a popular magazine targeting the general public, found that 56% of female respondents were dissatisfied with their overall appearance, while approximately 43% of men were unhappy with their overall appearance. Though few people actually seek out a cosmetic procedure [2], it seems that the overwhelming majority of patients who do undergo intervention experience an improvement in body image, including a reduction in the degree of dissatisfaction with the specific feature altered by surgery or nonsurgical intervention [3–5]. But, for the patient who remains insistent or unrealistic in their beliefs about how a cosmetic procedure may change their life, acceptance and commitment therapy may be a helpful tool in the aesthetics toolbox.

Understanding Acceptance and Commitment Therapy

Acceptance and commitment therapy (ACT) is a psychological coping practice that can be useful when a patient and a practitioner do not agree on the need for additional interventions or when the patient has unrealistic expectations of an aesthetic intervention. ACT has been used successfully as a strategy to alleviate chronic pain [6], substance use [7], diabetes [8], and eating disorders [9]. At the heart of ACT is the understanding that language has a dual purpose not only as a method of expression but also as a means to construct a worldview through both internal and external experiences [10]. Language is dual-natured, being used both to describe celebratory occasions and to provide derogatory judgments, like destructive comparisons to peers or harmful self-criticisms. It is through this conscious awareness of language as a scaffold that an individual can start to change their behaviors. ACT utilizes this awareness to facilitate acceptance and behavioral change.

Purposeful behavioral change is the intended objective of ACT. ACT (said as a word and not as the initials) [11] strives to help individuals change behaviors through mindfulness of uncomfortable or destructive thoughts, feelings, or sensations in the present moment with the intention of learning to accept these uncomfortable thoughts or feelings as simply an experience of existence [12]. ACT challenges the notion that everyone must be happy all of the time. Instead, ACT teaches the individual how to live mindfully with negative thoughts by increasing his or her psychological flexibility [13].The literature is rife with brief exercises to help patients increase psychological flexibility, and these brief exercises can be an effective strategy to aid those who persistently request unnecessary aesthetic procedures that may actually be harmful due to unrealistic beliefs about themselves. ACT techniques are flexible and workable in a variety of different settings and can also be adapted for individuals who may have unrealistic expectations of how cosmetic interventions may help them.

The underpinnings of psychological flexibility are rooted in the complex interaction between cognitive, emotional, and sensory experiences and the way in which this intricate interaction influences an individual's behavior [14]. In the simplest of terms, psychological flexibility is the ability to go comfortably outside of one's comfort zone, and the capacity to expand a rigid set of beliefs that may actually be inhibiting true personal growth. Through accommodation of new ways of conceptualizing old problems and a willingness to expand beyond one's comfort zone, growth can occur. Flexibility requires conscious and unrestricted contact with thoughts and feelings, an analytical appraisal of the weight of a given situation, and the simultaneous alignment of one's behaviors with one's goals and values. Expressive language plays a key role in psychological flexibility as does the observation that an expressed sentiment can affect or guide behavior, the degree to which depending upon other factors within the same context [14]. Conversely, psychological rigidity or inflexibility can actually block one from living a life that is, in reality, aligned with one's true values. Central to psychological rigidity is an inability to take a perspective independent of thoughts and feelings and a preoccupation with the past or the future [15].

For example, the patient who states that the bump on their nose is ruining his life and who insists that rhinoplasty is his only way to a better future is likely acting out of a psychologically inflexible and rigid place. A more psychologically flexible patient may seek out aesthetic intervention with the understanding that the bump on his nose is causing a facial asymmetry that affects their self-esteem while dating. Though both individuals are seeking out similar intervention, it is clear that the second patient has a realistic, values-aligned expectation of what cosmetic intervention may offer his – namely, facial symmetry that may increase his physical attractiveness.

Within the framework of ACT, a psychologically rigid individual can be thought to be living in FEAR [16, 17]. FEAR stands for:

- Fusion with thoughts that are incorrectly perceived as reality
- Evaluation of experiences as a subordinate to the experience
- Avoidance of a negative experience because it might lead to discomfort
- Reason-giving or justification to rationalize poor coping skills.

In ACT, FEAR comprises the barriers that allow an individual to function in alignment with negative ideas or perceptions. FEAR is what holds people back from embracing constructive attitudes and acting from a stance of psychological flexibility. FEAR enables psychological rigidity. FEAR is truly to be feared!

However, one can overcome FEAR with ACT [17]:

- Accepting negative reactions and being present and accommodating of those reactions

- Choosing a valued direction in alignment with personal goals to move past rigidity
- Taking action to meet those goals to become psychologically flexible.

By accepting that negative thoughts will be a part of life and choosing to act purposely toward valued goals, psychological flexibility can be achieved.

Incorporating ACT into an Esthetics Practice

Inherent to the framework of ACT are six overlapping tenets that enable psychological flexibility (Table 20.1) [10]. Known as *cognitive defusion, acceptance, mindfulness, sense of self, values identification*, and *commitment to values-based goals*, these can best be thought of as new attitudes to accepting and embracing the existence of negative thoughts, such as overwrought concerns about facial wrinkles or the occasional pimple. After all, blemishes, like negativity, are just a part of living. At first, these practices may not come easily to either the practitioner or the patient. And they aren't meant to – changing a linguistic and cognitive schema takes time and effort. However, with a little motivation and repetition the core concepts of ACT can easily be learned and can ultimately encourage the patient to expand their worldview beyond the mirror.

Cognitive fusion occurs when an individual becomes entangled with his thoughts, often confusing thoughts for facts or the truth. Cognitive fusion is innate to psychological inflexibility, can lead to destructive behaviors, and may impede an individual from values-based activities [18]. Furthermore, cognitive

Table 20.1 Putting ACT into practice.

Cognitive defusion	- **Purpose:** Get rid of psychological inflexibility by learning to live with negative, automatic thoughts in the moment - **Exercise:** *Milk, Milk, Milk* – ask the patient to pick an uncomfortable word, name all of the negative connotations associated with the word, and then repeat the word for a minute. Reassess for negative connotations
Acceptance	- **Purpose:** Validate a negative thought for what it is in the moment - **Exercise:** Encourage the patient to pay attention to the thoughts, feelings, and sensations that occur when not giving in to a negative thought
Mindfulness	- **Purpose:** Be aware of self and environment without any judgment - **Exercise:** Focus on the present moment by asking about feelings in the moment and redirecting to the present moment
Sense of self	- **Purpose:** Access a sense of self that goes beyond criticisms and one single concept of self - **Exercise:** "Furniture in the house" metaphor – the house is more valuable than its individual contents
Values identification	- **Purpose:** Identify values that align with a sense of self - **Exercise:** Ask the patient what their values might be if nobody were to ever know about their accomplishments
Commitment to values-based goals	- **Purpose:** Commit to action behaviors over the long term that are in alignment with identified values - **Exercise:** Encourage the patient to practice defusion to move forward with values-based behaviors when barriers to goals seem insurmountable

fusion seems to be intrinsically linked to the language employed to express the experience [19]. However, in order to gain psychological flexibility, the patient must learn cognitive defusion, or the process of separating themself from the automatic negative and self-defeating thoughts about his appearance that may be driving their requests for additional interventions. The goal of defusion is not to get rid of these negative thoughts, but to reduce their influence on behaviors and to learn to live with them in the moment [20].

Cognitive defusion changes an overwhelming, ruminative, and restrictive thought into a thought that is nothing more than a single thought among many others. Furthermore, cognitive defusion allows the patient to separate thought from fact and to detach from those thoughts. There are many ways to uncouple the influence of negative thoughts from a more objective reality, though not every method will be effective for every individual. For example:

- A patient may opt to say these thoughts aloud in silly voices to minimize their gravity [12]
- A patient may conceptualize these thoughts as bullies and attack them verbally [12]
- A patient may imagine themself on the banks of a river watching their negative thoughts as debris floating down the river [12]
- A patient can write negative thoughts down on index cards [21]
- A patient can change the phrasing of the thought, i.e. "I am ugly" becomes "I am having the thought that I am ugly." [21]

Another technique, known in the literature as "Milk, Milk, Milk," aims to defuse cognition from meaning through repetition [22]. Described over a hundred years ago [23], a word repeated aloud tends to lose literal meaning as it loses its context. For some, it may be helpful to pick an uncomfortable word (e.g. "wrinkle" or "sagginess"), ask the patient to name any connotations or associations that the

word holds, and then ask the patient to repeat the word for about a minute. Following repetition, ask the patient to name connotations or associations that the word holds. It is likely that the word will no longer hold the same weight as it did only moments before and that cognitive defusion has occurred [21].

These are just a few ways in which people can learn to disengage negative thoughts from the self and move forward toward new values-oriented behaviors. And it is likely that repetition and practice of cognitive defusion techniques will lead to attainment of defusion. It may be helpful to introduce a patient to a cognitive defusion technique and encourage the patient to continue to practice the technique on a daily basis and in between appointments.

Acknowledging, embracing, and accepting disruptive thoughts and feelings *as they occur* is an important precursor to mindfulness. Acceptance is not a resignation from reality, a manipulation or denial of emotion, but rather is a willingness to embrace the uncomfortable [19]. In psychological inflexibility, a negative emotion or thought may trigger harmful, impulsive behaviors to avoid the negative emotion. Acceptance of negative thoughts is an active and thoughtful process, learning to coexist with the negative while simultaneously focusing on other aspects of one's existence. Acceptance does not mean distracting one's self from the negative thought or channeling the negative energy into a constructive or productive task. Acceptance is validating the negative thought for what it is in the moment that it is experienced.

Some brief techniques to practice acceptance include:

- Asking a patient to think about an experience that has been difficult to accept, allowing the patient to imagine being in a tug-of-war with a monster, feeling and focusing on the strain of pulling against something that will not let go of the other end of the rope, and finally imagining letting go of the rope and observing how it feels to let go of the struggle [24].

- Asking a patient to take a few moments to consider their weekend plans and follow up by asking the patient what form these plans take – images, thoughts, or bodily sensations [12].
- Encouraging the patient to pay attention to the feelings, thoughts, and emotions that occur when not giving in to the automatic response to a negative thought [17].

Mindfulness is a popular buzz word and seems to be a modality of treatment for just about everything, from stress reduction [25] to athletic performance enhancement [26]. Given its far-reaching functionality, definitions of mindfulness vary somewhat, from being an outcome to a process to a technique [23]. However, in ACT, mindfulness is "the defused, accepting, open contact with the present moment and the private events it contains as a conscious human being experientially distinct from the content being noticed" [24]. Thus, to be mindful is not only to be constantly present in the moment, but also to be aware of internal and external stimuli at all times without qualitative judgment of the self or the environment, the future, or the past. Engaging in mindfulness allows one to continue to develop and fulfill a robust sense of self.

Mindfulness exercises are abundant and easily found. For purposes of the esthetics clinic, briefer exercises in recognizing mindfulness are likely to be the most useful. For example:

- Try asking, "How are you feeling right now?" This simple question will bring the patient back into the moment, especially if asked following an exchange that disappoints the patient [17].
- When dialogue shifts to the past or the future – i.e. how I want to look/how I will look – ask the patient to be aware of the present moment [17].

A healthy sense of self is an ever-changing myriad of formative experiences, both good and bad, integrated into a whole; it is not only one quality, feeling, or emotion, though to the psychologically inflexible it may seem as such. One cannot be psychologically flexible and be concurrently wedded to a strict view of self, especially if that view is a predominantly negative one. A concept of self should be broad enough to encompass all of an individual's thoughts, emotions, and experiences [19]. Hence, one of the tools to accessing psychological flexibility is accessing a sense of self that goes beyond criticisms of self and does not revolve around one single concept of self. If the patient has been predominantly identifying with what he perceive to be physical flaws in his appearance, it may be useful to remind the patient that he is greater than what meets the eye [17]. Once he can distinguish between the conceptualized version of themself and the context in which these versions of themself occur, he will have become more psychologically flexible [17].

One approach to fostering a healthy sense of self is to utilize "the furniture in the house" metaphor [17]. A house contains all kinds of furniture – ugly, beautiful, and in between – and yet the quality, the character, and the sturdiness of the house as a whole is always considered more valuable than its individual contents. In this example, the house is able to contain everything, including its less attractive contents. Perhaps, the house is defined as a sum of its total parts, but the house also still stands regardless of its contents. For the patient who is motivated to seek out cosmetic augmentation due to a poor sense of self, this exercise may be helpful in distinguishing the total self from its separable parts.

Identifying values that are aligned with a sense of self is the fifth and final practice toward increasing psychological flexibility. Values are "chosen qualities of purposive action that can never be obtained as an object but can be instantiated moment by moment" [20]. It is the patient with a true sense of self who is able to understand that values are the end product of defusion, acceptance, and mindfulness. Asking a patient to identify inherent, life-guiding values will help him, set goals that align with his sense of self beyond the procedural suite and reinforce the richness that can be the human experience. Recognizing and naming core values and setting goals can be particularly motivating for behavioral change, especially when a patient is erroneously fixated on how a cosmetic procedure may be beneficial. Again, there are many ways to elicit these responses from a patient, from having him list concrete goals and barriers to those goals to asking him what their values would be if nobody could ever know of his achievements. It is the expectation of ACT that through identifying life values and goals, one may be able to see his self and his life beyond what a cosmetic procedure may be able to offer.

Some ways in which to help a patient define values are as follows:

- Ask the patient to close his eyes and imagine that he have been told that they only have a year left to live but that he will be physically incapable of living his last year how he might wish. Ask the patient to then describe how he might live his life differently [12].
- Clarify values in all of the patient's life domains. After values have been successfully clarified, ask the patient to list concrete goals, concrete actions, and concrete barriers to reaching those goals [17].

Lastly, ACT compels its participants to commit to action behaviors that are in alignment with identified values. Commitment to value-based goals through behavior change is most feasibly attained over the long term [20]. Commitment to action includes not only behavioral change to achieve goals but also the practices of mindfulness and acceptance when in unchangeable situations where resources, capabilities, or context may be lacking [19]. When barriers to goals seem insurmountable, it is again important for the practitioner to encourage the patient to practice defusion in order to move forward with values-based behaviors [19].

Case Study

Case 20.1   Unrealistic Expectations

A 55-year-old female patient presents to your office for follow-up. She is a very reliable cosmetic patient and sees you for neurotoxin and laser treatments regularly. Recently, she has been repeatedly requesting soft tissue lip augmentation to enhance volume lost with age. The patient is adamant about wanting to look like a young celebrity whose facial proportions are vastly different from her own. She feels like the only way to "regain her life" is to change her appearance. You place an appropriate amount of product to increase the volume of her lips and she leaves the clinic feeling excited and "brimming with opportunity." She returns to the clinic three weeks later, requesting more filler. After several tense appointments, she expresses disappointment with the enhanced volume of her lips, stating that her lips "should be" bigger than they are and that "nothing" has changed for her since her injections.

Clinical Relevance and Implications

Though it is never fun to (wrongly) take the blame for a patient's unrealistic expectations, there are many ways in which a brief, modified version of ACT could be utilized in this scenario to increase this patient's psychological flexibility. It is clear that this patient is exhibiting cognitive fusion between herself and her perception of her physical appearance and that she is not willing to accept the uncomfortableness of aging. Here, it might be reasonable to ask the patient if she is able to uncouple her negative beliefs about her appearance from whom she is fundamentally, asking her to identify values that go beyond her appearance and encouraging mindfulness about negative self-thoughts. It may also be useful to guide this patient through a cognitive defusion technique and an acceptance exercise. Ultimately, applying the principles of ACT to this patient scenario will result in improvements in sense of self for the patient, more realistic anticipation about her next injection, and potentially even enhanced rapport between patient and practitioner.

Finally, many people have heard of cognitive behavioral therapy (CBT) and may have even engaged in CBT treatment. Though they share many overlapping similarities and equivalent outcomes in many settings, ACT is not CBT. The primary difference between ACT and CBT is that ACT strives primarily to change the behavior through increasing psychological flexibility, while CBT aims to change the cognitions driving the behavior [15]. Cognitive restructuring, the hallmark of CBT, may inhibit acceptance, a bedrock of psychological flexibility [27]. For instance, in the above example, a patient seeking lip fillers may reduce the frequency of her contact with the clinic after employing ACT, fully knowing that her distress about the aging process may never go away. On the other hand, a CBT model would encourage this patient to change her negative thoughts about aging to potentially reduce the motivation for additional procedures. Given that aging tends to be an ongoing and negative experience for many, in this example the patient's upsetting beliefs about herself may actually benefit more from an ACT framework that promotes acceptance of negative thoughts and an improvement in sense of self.

Special Populations to Note

In a "selfie" and social-media-driven world, concern for addiction to cosmetic enhancement is a relevant topic of discussion as social media continues to drive cosmetic augmentation. For most who seek it out, cosmetic enhancement offers the opportunity to turn back the clock on aging or feel more attractive [28]. Most people who seek out cosmetic procedures will seek out enhancements that complement their own natural anatomy [3, 29].

However, as cosmetic procedures become easier to access, particularly nonsurgical procedures, so does the risk for dependence. Not unlike the highs offered by substances, gambling, or sex, cosmetic surgery offers the prospect of a better life and possibly even physical perfection [30]. Furthermore, not unlike alcohol or drug dependency, there can be serious consequences for the patient with an unhealthy relationship to cosmetic procedures, including disfigurement and even death [31–33]. So as to avoid any harmful interventions, it is best to obtain a thorough history and physical examination for every patient in the clinic and to refer those with questionable dependency to a higher level of mental healthcare while rejecting any requests for augmentation. For additional information on the cosmetic "addict" and a potential approach to engaging such a patient in mental health treatment see Chapter 22.

Additionally, there is a subset of patients in aesthetic medicine who may meet criteria for body dysmorphic disorder (BDD) and for whom ACT is unlikely to be an adequate form of treatment [34]. Cosmetic consultation is not helpful for these individuals and may actually worsen BDD [35]. Ideally, these individuals should be treated for their underlying psychiatric illness, which involves a combination of intensive therapy as well as medication [36–38]. Given their high risk for suicide, it is best to refer these clients to a psychiatrist as soon as possible [39]. See Chapter 15 for additional information on approaches to the patient with suspected BDD.

Conclusions

For the motivated practitioner, ACT can provide an intuitive and useful modality to incorporate into the aesthetic office. While time constraints may limit the full utilization of ACT, elements of ACT can help when there is disagreement on treatment between practitioner and patient. If there is concern that brief and modified ACT is not helping a patient, it is reasonable to consider recommending or referring to a therapist or a psychiatrist who may be able to offer additional assistance. For those with additional interest in practicing ACT there are many mindfulness workbooks, podcasts, and practice exercises that can be found online or in bookstores. Though the aesthetics clinic is not the psychiatrist's office, it is very possible to modify brief ACT exercises for use with aesthetics patients who may benefit from improved psychological flexibility, mindfulness intervention, and clarification of values and personal goals.

References

1 Garner, D., Kearney-Cooke, A. (1996 March). Body image 1996. Psychology Today.

2 The Aesthetic Society. Aesthetic Plastic Surgery National Databank Statistics 2019 https://www.surgery.org/media/statistics (accessed 27 May 2020).

3 Sommer, B., Zschocke, I., Bergfeld, D. et al. (2003). Satisfaction of patients after treatment with botulinum toxin for dynamic facial lines. *Dermatologic Surgery* 29: 456–460. https://doi.org/10.1046/j.1524-4725.2003.29113.x.

4 Honigman, R.J., Phillips, K.A., and Castle, D.J. (2004). A review of psychosocial outcomes for patients seeking cosmetic surgery. *Plastic and Reconstructive Surgery* 113: 1229–1237. https://doi.org/10.1097/01.PRS.0000110214.88868.CA.

5 Sarwer, D., Gibbons, L., Magee, L. et al. (2005). A prospective, multi-site investigation of patient satisfaction and psychosocial status following cosmetic surgery. *Aesthetic Surgery Journal* 25: 263–269. https://doi.org/10.1016/j.asj.2005.03.009.

6 Buhrman, M., Skoglund, A., Husell, J. et al. (2013). Guided internet-delivered acceptance and commitment therapy for chronic pain patients: a randomized controlled trial. *Behaviour Research and Therapy* 51: 307–315. https://doi.org/10.1016/j.brat.2013.02.010.

7 Lee, E.B., An, W., Levin, M.E., and Twohig, M.P. (2015). An initial meta-analysis of acceptance and commitment therapy for treating substance use disorders. *Drug and Alcohol Dependence* 155: 1–7. https://doi.org/10.1016/j.drugalcdep.2015.08.004.

8 Shayeghian, Z., Hassanabadi, H., Aguilar-Vafaie, M.E. et al. (2016). A randomized controlled trial of acceptance and commitment therapy for type 2 diabetes management: the moderating role of coping styles. *PLoS One* 11 https://doi.org/10.1371/journal.pone.0166599.

9 Juarascio, A., Shaw, J., Forman, E. et al. (2013). Acceptance and commitment therapy as a novel treatment for eating disorders: an initial test of efficacy and mediation. *Behavior Modification* 37: 459–489. https://doi.org/10.1177/0145445513478633.

10 Hayes, S.C., Strosahl, K.D., Bunting, K. et al. (2004). What is acceptance and commitment therapy? In: *A Practical Guide to Acceptance and Commitment Therapy* (eds. S.C. Hayes and K.D. Strosahl), 3–29. Boston, MA: Springer https://doi.org/10.1007/978-0-387-23369-7_1.

11 Hayes, S.C., Strosahl, K.D., and Wilson, K.G. (1996). *Acceptance and Commitment Therapy: An Experiential Approach to Behavior Change.* New York: Guilford Press.

12 Harris, R. (2007). Acceptance and Commitment Therapy (ACT) Introductory Workshop Handout. www.thehappinesstrap.com/acceptance-and-commitment-therapy-worksheets/.

13 Wilson, K.G. and Murrell, A.R. (2004). Values work in acceptance and commitment therapy: setting a course for behavioral treatment. In: *Mindfulness and Acceptance: Expanding the Cognitive Behavioral Tradition* (eds. S. Hayes, V. Follette and M. Linehan), 120–151. New York: Guilford Press.

14 Scott, W. and McCracken, L.M. (2015). Psychological flexibility, acceptance and commitment therapy, and chronic pain. *Current Opinion in Psychology* 2: 91–96. https://doi.org/10.1016/j.copsyc.2014.12.013.

15 McCracken, L.M. and Morley, S. (2014). The psychological flexibility model: a basis for integration and progress in psychological approaches to chronic pain management. *Journal of Pain* 15: 221–234. https://doi.org/10.1016/j.jpain.2013.10.014.

16 Kanter, J.W., Baruch, D.E., and Gaynor, S.T. (2006). Acceptance and commitment therapy and behavioral activation for the treatment of depression: description and comparison. *Behavior Analyst* 29: 161–185.

17 Hayes, S.C., Strosahl, K.D., Bunting, K. et al. (2004). What is acceptance and commitment therapy? In: *A Practical Guide to Acceptance and Commitment Therapy* (eds. S.C. Hayes and K.D. Strosahl), 3–29. Boston, MA: Springer https://doi.org/10.1007/978-0-387-23369-7_1.

18 Ferreira, C., Palmeira, L., and Trindade, I.A. (2014). Turning eating psychopathology risk factors into action. The pervasive effect of body image-related cognitive fusion. *Appetite* 80: 137–142. https://doi.org/10.1016/j.appet.2014.05.019.

19 Pearson, A.N., Heffner, M., and Follette, V.M. (2010). *Acceptance & Commitment Therapy for Body Image Dissatisfaction: A Practitioner's Guide to Using Mindfulness, Acceptance & Values-Based Behavior Change Strategies.* Oakland, CA: New Harbinger Publications.

20 Hayes, S.C., Luoma, J.B., Bond, F.W. et al. (2006). Acceptance and commitment therapy: model, processes and outcomes. *Behaviour Research and Therapy* 44: 1–25. https://doi.org/10.1016/j.brat.2005.06.006.

21 O'Donohue, W.T. and Fisher, J.E. (2009). *General Principles and Empirically Supported Techniques of Cognitive Behavior Therapy.* Hoboken, NJ: Wiley.

22 Masuda, A., Hayes, S.C., Sackett, C.F., and Twohig, M.P. (2004). Cognitive defusion and

self-relevant negative thoughts: examining the impact of a ninety year old technique. *Behaviour Research and Therapy* 42: 477–485. https://doi.org/10.1016/j.brat.2003.10.008.

23 Titchener, E.B. (1916). *A Text-Book of Psychology.* New York: Macmillan.

24 Fletcher, L. and Hayes, S.C. (2005). Relational frame theory, acceptance and commitment therapy, and a functional analytic definition of mindfulness. *Journal of Rational-Emotive & Cognitive-Behavior Therapy* 23: 315–336. https://doi.org/10.1007/s10942-005-0017-7.

25 Grossman, P., Niemann, L., Schmidt, S., and Walach, H. (2004). Mindfulness-based stress reduction and health benefits. *Journal of Psychosomatic Research* 57: 35–43. https://doi.org/10.1016/S0022-3999(03)00573-7.

26 Sappington, R. and Longshore, K. (2015). Systematically reviewing the efficacy of mindfulness-based interventions for enhanced athletic performance. *Journal of Clinical Sport Psychology* 9: 232–262. https://doi.org/10.1123/jcsp.2014-0017.

27 Collard, J.J. (2019). ACT vs CBT: an exercise in idiosyncratic language. *Journal of Cognitive Therapy* 12: 126–145. https://doi.org/10.1007/s41811-019-00043-9.

28 Carter Singh, G., Hankins, M.C., Dulku, A., and Kelly, M.B.H. (2006). Psychosocial aspects of botox in aesthetic surgery. *Aesthetic Plastic Surgery* 30: 71–76. https://doi.org/10.1007/s00266-005-0150-9.

29 Weinkle, S.H., Werschler, W.P., Teller, C.F. et al. (2018). Impact of comprehensive, minimally invasive, multimodal aesthetic treatment on satisfaction with facial appearance: the HARMONY study. *Aesthetic Surgery Journal* 38: 540–556. https://doi.org/10.1093/asj/sjx179.

30 Furnham, A. and Levitas, J. (2012). Factors that motivate people to undergo cosmetic surgery. *Canadian Journal of Plastic Surgery* 20: e47–e50.

31 Rongioletti, F., Atzori, L., Ferreli, C. et al. (2015). Granulomatous reactions after injections of multiple aesthetic micro-implants in temporal combinations: a complication of filler addiction. *Journal of the European Academy of Dermatology and Venereology* 29: 1188–1192. https://doi.org/10.1111/jdv.12788.

32 Lin, C.-H., Chiang, C.-P., Wu, B.-Y., and Gao, H.-W. (2017). Filler migration to the forehead due to multiple filler injections in a patient addicted to cosmetic fillers. *Journal of Cosmetic and Laser Therapy* 19: 124–126. https://doi.org/10.1080/14764172.2016.1248441.

33 Markey, C.N. and Markey, P.M. (2009). Correlates of young women's interest in obtaining cosmetic surgery. *Sex Roles* 61: 158–166. https://doi.org/10.1007/s11199-009-9625-5.

34 American Psychiatric Association (2013). *Diagnostic and Statistical Manual of Mental Disorders: DSM-5,* 5e. Washington, DC: American Psychiatric Association.

35 Phillips, K.A. (2006). The presentation of body dysmorphic disorder in medical settings. *Primary Psychiatry* 13 (7): 51–59.

36 Ribeiro, R.V.E. (2017). Prevalence of body dysmorphic disorder in plastic surgery and dermatology patients: a systematic review with meta-analysis. *Aesthetic Plastic Surgery* 41: 964–970. https://doi.org/10.1007/s00266-017-0869-0.

37 Crerand, C.E., Franklin, M.E., and Sarwer, D.B. (2006). Body dysmorphic disorder and cosmetic surgery. *Plastic and Reconstructive Surgery* 118: 167e–180e. https://doi.org/10.1097/01.prs.0000242500.28431.24.

38 Phillipou, A., Rossell, S.L., Wilding, H.E., and Castle, D.J. (2016). Randomised controlled trials of psychological & pharmacological treatments for body dysmorphic disorder: a systematic review. *Psychiatry Research* 245: 179–185. https://doi.org/10.1016/j.psychres.2016.05.062.

39 Angelakis, I., Gooding, P.A., and Panagioti, M. (2016). Suicidality in body dysmorphic disorder (BDD): a systematic review with meta-analysis. *Clinical Psychology Review* 49: 55–66. https://doi.org/10.1016/j.cpr.2016.08.002.

21

Behavioral Modification for Acne Excoriée and Skin Picking

Karen M. Ong[1], Mary D. Sun[2], and Evan A. Rieder[3]

[1] Department of Internal Medicine, University of Texas Medical Health, Galveston, TX, USA
[2] Icahn School of Medicine at Mount Sinai, New York, NY, USA
[3] The Ronald O. Perelman Department of Dermatology, New York University Grossman School of Medicine, New York, NY, USA

Introduction

Although our perception of ourselves and our physical appearance is intimately intertwined, some behaviors can serve to worsen appearance, causing psychological distress not only because of a perception of decreased aesthetic appearance ("feeling ugly") to others, but also because of feelings of shame and embarrassment that these charges are self-inflicted ("I did it to myself"). Feelings of shame and concern about being judged by a medical practitioner may hinder a patient's ability to seek treatment for the initial cause (such as habitual scratching initially triggered by an itchy skin condition). While a practitioner's first instinct may be to simply instruct a patient with repetitive behaviors to cease those behaviors, such advice not only is generally ineffective but also can lead to a cycle of additional shame and withdrawal of a patient from medical care. Effective and evidence-based treatment is available to treat repetitive motion behaviors with the caveat that success depends on patient motivation and that behavior modification therapy, while simple, is not widely available. This chapter aims to teach the basic principles of behavioral therapy for the aesthetic practitioner; this treatment modality is simple and structured, and requires minimal training to implement. More severe cases may be cause for a referral to a trusted mental health professional.

Case Study

Case 21.1   Acne Picking
CK, a 23-year-old man, presents to you for the treatment of acne and acne scars. He feels tremendously self-conscious regarding the appearance of his face, saying he "feels ugly and embarrassed" about how he looks. He has tried many over-the-counter therapies as well as prescription topical and oral treatments, including oral antibiotics and isotretinoin, without much success. As he is describing his past attempts at acne treatment, you notice that he begins to pick at his face. After asking more questions you learn that he often picks incessantly at facial acne until it bleeds, then disturbs the scabs that form, creating scarring and, in some cases, additional inflammation and infection. Sometimes he is conscious of this behavior, at other times

(Continued)

Case 21.1 (Continued)

(as in the office setting) he picks without awareness. Even when he is having success with physician-guided acne treatment, he still finds the raised texture of the acne distressing and attempts to smooth his face by picking. When you point out to him that he is actively scratching through your examination, he admits that sometimes he unconsciously picks at his skin while "zoning out" in activities like watching his favorite television shows. Despite this, he reports that he functions well socially and is able to work without his acne and scarring causing impairment. It is just "this one issue" that is limiting him.

Clinical Relevance and Implications

Diseases that affect the skin are more than medical diseases as they affect the patient's perception of self. In particular, diseases whose pathology involves a component of scratching and/or skin picking often involve shame or guilt that some component may be self-inflicted. While you may entertain several psychiatric diagnostic possibilities as you evaluate CK, your job as an aesthetic provider is not to provide psychiatric diagnosis and treatment but to recognize problematic behaviors that might affect the provider–patient relationship, the patient's engagement in treatment, and the effectiveness of treatment modalities. While the patient presented to you for the treatment of acne and acne scarring, you recognize that the major limiting factor to the healing of his acne and scarring is his behavior. As importantly, you know that until this behavior is extinguished, any medical or aesthetic acne treatment is likely to be in vain.

From your understanding of the psychology literature, you are familiar with behavioral therapy and related techniques. You know that these modalities, while not widely available, can be profoundly helpful for patients who are struggling with body-focused repetitive behavior disorders. You know that they are easy to enact for patients and easy to learn for interested providers. For motivated patients, behavioral therapy can provide a framework through which to approach daily activities. As importantly, *behavioral therapy does not require that the patient understand the psychology of why they are picking*; it simply gives the patient the tools to recognize, identify, and extinguish these behaviors. Once solidified and learned, the tools that people can gain from behavioral therapy become automatic and can be quickly put into action regardless of the situation and without the need for a prescription from a doctor.

Differential Diagnosis

Skin picking may be automatic or intentional and has been associated with simple skin conditions such as acne or atopic dermatitis. However, the differential diagnosis is broad. Psychiatric disorders that may lead to skin picking include obsessive compulsive disorder (OCD), trichotillomania, body dysmorphic disorder, skin-picking disorder, anxiety/depression, delusional infestation, body-focused repetitive behavior disorders, and other obsessive compulsive and related disorders [1] (see Chapter 15). Nondermatologic medical conditions include itching induced by substances or medications, contact dermatitis and allergies, and toxin-related itching from conditions such as kidney failure or hyperbilirubinemia (gallbladder- or liver-related conditions). The differential diagnosis of skin picking is broad and includes both medical and psychiatric conditions, which should be referred to the appropriate provider for medical, psychiatric, or multidisciplinary care. Such extreme conditions are out of the scope of this chapter, which aims to provide basic guidelines for recognizing and treating acne and skin picking. However, you may wish to consider a targeted screen for high-yield medical or psychiatric conditions

Table 21.1 Screening questions.

Skin picking/excoriation disorder	• How much time do you spend picking at your skin?
	• Have you noticed damage to the skin?
	• Have you tried to decrease or stop skin picking?
	• Have you noticed any feelings of a loss of control, embarrassment, or shame?
	• Has this affected your ability to study, work, or participate in leisure activities?
	• Have you noticed yourself avoiding social situations because of your acne or skin condition?
Body dysmorphic disorder	• Do you pick at your skin because of how it looks?
	• Has this affected your ability to study, work, or participate in leisure activities?
	• Is there any other part of your body that you find to be particularly unattractive?
Obsessive compulsive and related disorders (i.e. trichotillomania)	• Do you experience intrusive or unwanted thoughts, urges, or impulses to wash your hands or pull your hair?
	• Do you feel compelled to perform repetitive behaviors (e.g. hand washing, ordering, checking) or mental acts (e.g. praying, counting, repeating silently) in response to these unwanted urges?
Substance/medication related	• Do you use any stimulants such as methylphenidate (e.g. Ritalin), prescription amphetamines (e.g. Adderall), crystal methamphetamine, or cocaine?
	• Have you started using any new prescription medications?
Medical conditions	• Do you have a history of liver/kidney disease?

(Table 21.1) which occur with high frequency in people who pick at their skin [2].

Estimates of prevalence of skin picking range from about 1.4 to 5% of the population [1–3], with associations found with depression [2], anxiety [2, 3], and OCD [2], as well as affective, eating, substance use, and impulse control disorders [3]. Skin picking most often starts during adolescence and frequently begins with a dermatologic condition such as acne; it usually has a chronic course, with improvement and worsening over time if untreated. It is more common in individuals with OCD or a family history of OCD than in the general population. Skin picking is associated with distress and social and occupational impairment, including daily or weekly interference with work, missing school, or having difficulties studying, with affected individuals spending at least one hour daily on picking, thinking about picking, or resisting urges to pick. Complications of skin picking include tissue damage, scarring, and infection. If the skin picking is primarily secondary to another medical condition, such as scabies, excoriation disorder cannot be diagnosed, but an excoriation disorder can be started by or worsened by another dermatologic condition [4]. In the case of CK, we assume he has simple skin picking associated with acne.

Excoriation disorder is characterized by recurrent skin picking that results in lesions accompanied by repeated attempts to stop or decrease this behavior. Feelings of anxiety, boredom, tension, or other emotions may precede or accompany the behavior, although it is not triggered by obsessions or preoccupations. Notably, skin picking may result in gratification, pleasure, or relief. Individuals with excoriation disorder may or may not have conscious awareness of the behavior, with some focusing on tension before and relief after skin picking, but others seemingly unaware of it [4].

Skin picking can also be caused or exacerbated by itching, a common symptom that is experienced by a quarter of the population during their lifetime and nearly half of all skin disease patients [5, 6]. These symptoms are reported as severe in nearly 30% of dermatology patients and can significantly reduce quality of life [6, 7], worsen academic and professional performance, and create feelings of anxiety and depression. In the "itch–scratch" cycle, scratching provokes inflammation and additional itching, which then can worsen skin problems [8]. Current clinical practices tend to focus on topical and oral therapies for symptom management [9] with little emphasis on itch management, despite evidence that behavioral modification therapies [10], stress-reduction techniques [11, 12] that interrupt the itch–scratch cycle, and patient-education programs can improve skin condition, prevent increased disease severity, and reduce scratching, medication use, and distress [10–13]. Furthermore, such behavioral modification strategies can be enacted in motivated populations with relative ease [9, 14–16].

Behavioral Modification

The Basics and Getting Started

Although your job as an aesthetic practitioner is primarily to assist patients with improving their appearance, it will not be possible to do so as long as a patient is picking at their skin. In the case of patient CK, the additional damage, inflammation, and scarring will interfere with attempts to medically treat his acne or ultimately to improve the scarring with modalities such as laser treatment. Additionally, diseases that involve a component of scratching and/or skin picking often involve shame or guilt that may be self-inflicted. These emotions can result in the patient self-sabotaging treatment and being less adherent in following provider recommendations. Of note, it is not necessary to

have a full-blown diagnosis of excoriation disorder to benefit from behavioral modification. Most of our patients do not meet criteria for this diagnosis, but many, particularly esthetically inclined patients, may obsess over or pick at minor imperfections of their skin. This can be quite damaging when enacted on the face.

Behavioral modification is a treatment that requires patience, persistence, and diligent follow-up on behalf of the patient to complete "homework." However, patients do not need any specific skills other than the ability to follow a treatment plan. While this may not be an appropriate treatment for all patients struggling with skin picking, it can be incredibly helpful for the motivated patient; the patient learns skills to stop skin picking and scratching and gives the skin time to heal. As the patient sees their skin improving, this ideally starts a virtuous cycle where the improvement creates additional motivation to continue the course of therapy. However, persistence is required in overcoming setbacks. For example, a patient who manages to reduce their skin picking by 80% one week might end up undoing that progress with a single episode of picking. Patients should be reminded that changing habits is a gradual process, and as long as they are diligent, patient, and persistent in practicing new habits, their skin will ultimately improve and be better than if they did not attempt to change their behavior. After a patient's behaviors are controlled and their underlying dermatologic conditions (e.g. acne) appropriately treated, aesthetic treatments become appropriate and more likely to lead to lasting improvements.

Stages of Behavioral Modification Therapy

The basic stages of behavioral modification therapy, modified from the original seminal paper by Azrin and Nunn [17], are as follows:

1) Goal setting
2) Awareness training
3) Pattern-trigger detection

4) Development of a competing response
5) Stimulus control

The first stage, *goal setting*, means working with a patient to determine what goals should be set for behavioral modification. For example, a goal for CK might be to reduce scarring on his face from acne by learning to refrain from picking.

During the second stage, *awareness training*, the patient begins to develop greater awareness and management of the emotions surrounding itching/scratching episodes. This awareness is critical to improvement, since scratching triggers sometimes occur outside the patient's conscious awareness (subconsciously). One tool that can help patients accomplish this awareness includes keeping a daily picking or scratching log in a notepad or on a mobile device. Every time the person finds themself manipulating the skin, they should write down the "*where, when, and what:*" their location, the time of day (or night), and the content of their thoughts at the time. Mindfulness exercises such as progressive muscle relaxation, deep abdominal breathing, and guided imagery can help patients manage the feelings of distress and physical discomfort caused by itch (see Chapter 18). These can be sequentially added with prescribed "homework" to practice each technique twice daily to decrease physiological stress responses. Of all the stages, developing awareness is expected to take the longest amount of time to master.

In the third stage, *pattern-trigger detection*, patients learn to identify common patterns or situations that trigger scratching. They learn how to identify different warning signs that indicate the onset of an episode such as thoughts, feelings, physical cues, and bodily sensations. The log of scratching episodes initiated in the second stage will continue to be important and can help to identify triggers.

In the fourth stage, *development of a competing response*, patients learn to substitute scratching with a socially acceptable behavior that makes it impossible to actually scratch.

Examples of behavioral substitutes include creating two fists, sitting on both hands, and squeezing a stress ball. The patient enacts this behavior and holds it in place as the desire to scratch peaks and gradually wanes. Alternatively, patients can teach themselves to practice a mindfulness activity when they feel the sensation of itch. Other substitutes include keeping a log of the negative side effects of scratching and reading or adding to this log when the urge to scratch is felt. Although the negative effects associated with scratching may seem obvious (i.e. scarring, pain, infections), patients often experience gratification or even pleasure from scratching and may not be ready to immediately let go of the behavior.

In the fifth stage, *stimulus control*, the patient learns to identify and modify environmental factors ("stimuli") that may trigger skin picking. Some examples of stimulus control include minimizing exposure to bathrooms, throwing away tweezers, comedone extractors, and magnifying mirrors, and covering large mirrors if, for example, patients find themselves repeatedly picking in front of a bathroom mirror.

Results of learning or completing a course in behavior modification include an increased sense of awareness and control of scratching behaviors, a reduction in scratching behavior, a reduction in anxiety and distress associated with scratching, an improvement in quality of life, an improvement in skin condition, and an improved sense of well-being [10, 13]. These results support the patient's ultimate goal of improving their skin. In the case of CK, significantly reducing his scratching will help control his acne. After scratching reduction is achieved, it would be appropriate to discuss aesthetic interventions such as laser and soft tissue filler treatments to improve residual scarring.

Conclusions

If a patient presents to your practice with some element of skin picking, it may be reasonable to move forward with appropriate medical treatments. However, until patients stop picking at their skin, new scarring is likely to continue. Aesthetic treatments may be considered if scratching behavior occurs primarily in response to symptoms caused by acne (e.g. itch, burning, pain). However, if the patient's skin picking has become independent of the cutaneous concern, which is more frequently the case, it may be appropriate to consider psychiatric care or behavior modification therapy in addition to skin-focused treatments.

While not all providers will be interested in performing behavioral modification for their patients, it is important for all aesthetic providers to have an awareness of the existence of this modality and the framework of treatment. Sometimes a brief intervention can be effective in helping a patient to stop picking and allowing them to move forward with aesthetic procedures. As importantly, it is important for aesthetic providers to know that disruptive behaviors have the propensity to disrupt the treatment relationship, plan, and aesthetic outcome. Before we embark on our patients' aesthetic journey, we must recognize that our patients need a healthy baseline. Without the concomitant medical management of active skin conditions and psychological management of skin manipulation, long-term and durable improvements in skin cannot be achieved. Behavioral therapy can serve as an easy link between active medical conditions and the aesthetic treatments that our patients want to look and feel their best.

References

1 Keuthen, N.J., Koran, L.M., Aboujaoude, E. et al. (2010). The prevalence of pathologic skin picking in US adults. *Comprehensive Psychiatry* 51 (2): 183–186.

2 Hayes, S.L., Storch, E.A., and Berlanga, L. (2009). Skin picking behaviors: an examination of the prevalence and severity in a community sample. *Journal of Anxiety Disorders* 23 (3): 314–319.

3 Odlaug, B.L., Lust, K., Schreiber, L.R.N. et al. (2013). Skin picking disorder in university students: health correlates and gender differences. *General Hospital Psychiatry* 35 (2): 168–173.

4 American Psychiatric Association (2017). Diagnostic and Statistical Manual of Mental Disorders (DSM-V). Springer-Verlag.

5 Matterne, U., Apfelbacher, C., Vogelgsang, L. et al. (2013). Incidence and determinants of chronic pruritus: a population-based cohort study. *Acta Dermato-Venereologica* 93 (5): 532–537.

6 Verhoeven, L., Kraaimaat, F., Duller, P. et al. (2006). Cognitive, behavioral, and physiological reactivity to chronic itching: analogies to chronic pain. *International Journal of Behavioral Medicine* 13 (3): 237–243.

7 Jin, X.Y. and Khan, T.M. (2016). Quality of life among patients suffering from cholestatic liver disease-induced pruritus: a systematic review. *Journal of the Formosan Medical Association* 115 (9): 689–702.

8 Mack, M.R. and Kim, B.S. (2018). The itch–scratch cycle: a neuroimmune perspective. *Trends in Immunology* 39 (12): 980–991.

9 Deckersbach, T., Wilhelm, S., and Keuthen, N. (2003). Self-injurious skin picking: clinical characteristics, assessment methods, and treatment modalities. *Brief Treatment and Crisis Intervention* 3 (2): 249–260.

10 Ehlers, A., Stangier, U., and Gieler, U. (1995). Treatment of atopic dermatitis: a comparison of psychological and dermatological approaches to relapse prevention. *Journal of Consulting and Clinical Psychology* 63 (4): 624–635.

11 Schut, C., Mollanazar, N., Kupfer, J. et al. (2016). Psychological interventions in the treatment of chronic itch. *Acta Dermato-Venereologica* 96 (2): 157–161.

12 Fortune, D.G., Richards, H.L., Kirby, B. et al. (2002). A cognitive-behavioural symptom management programme as an adjunct in psoriasis therapy. *British Journal of Dermatology* 146 (3): 458–465.

13 Evers, A., Duller, P., Jong, E. et al. (2009). Effectiveness of a multidisciplinary itch-coping training programme in adults with atopic dermatitis. *Acta Dermato-Venereologica* 89 (1): 57–63.

14 Cully, J.A. and Teten, A.L. (2008). A Therapist's Guide to Brief Cognitive Behavioral Therapy. Department of Veterans Affairs.

15 van Os-Medendorp, H., Ros, W.J.G., Eland-de Kok, P.C.M. et al. (2007). Effectiveness of the nursing programme "coping with itch": a randomized controlled study in adults with chronic pruritic skin disease. *British Journal of Dermatology* 156 (6): 1235–1244.

16 Watson, D.L., Tharp, R.G., and Krisberg, J. (1972). Case study in self-modification: suppression of inflammatory scratching while awake and asleep. *Journal of Behavior Therapy and Experimental Psychiatry* 3 (3): 213–215.

17 Azrin, N.H. and Nunn, R.G. (1973). Habit-reversal: a method of eliminating nervous habits and tics. *Behaviour Research and Therapy* 11 (4): 619–628.

22

Motivational Interviewing for Identification and Triage of the Cosmetic Addict

Richard G. Fried[1] and Evan A. Rieder[2]

[1] Yardley Dermatology Associates, Yardley, PA, USA
[2] The Ronald O. Perelman Department of Dermatology, New York University Grossman School of Medicine, New York, NY, USA

Introduction

Performing a cosmetic procedure on "the wrong" patient can initiate a cascade of stressful interactions and events that can have ruinous potential. These include patient dissatisfaction, anger, demandingness, and retributions that can damage your quality of life and reputation. Avoiding cosmetic entanglement with these patients should be a priority during the assessment of all cosmetic patients. While personality disorders are discussed in Chapter 13, the "cosmetic addict" can become an ethical–moral conundrum for the clinician, particularly if the escalating desire for procedures becomes an overpowering driver pushing them to procedures that can be physically or emotionally harmful. Cosmetic addiction can sometimes lead to a form of "identity theft" in which multiple cosmetic procedures dramatically change patients' unique defining characteristics (sometimes to a caricature-like proportion), robbing them of the unique aspects of their appearance. Such transformations are in direct contradiction to thoughtfully chosen and well-performed cosmetic procedures that restore a more youthful appearance while maintaining or enhancing the unique characteristics that define the individual.

Case Study

Case 22.1   The Cosmetic Addict

A 51-year-old Caucasian woman with no past medical history presents to your office requesting cosmetic filler to the lips. She is a longstanding patient of yours and has followed you from practice to practice, as you have worked your way through employed positions and ultimately to opening your own boutique aesthetic practice. She is very reliable about her appointments, consistently showing up on time, paying bills in full at the time of service, and never complaining about treatments or costs. She is consistently interested in obtaining cosmetic procedures at her appointments and consistently asks about new procedures and devices that your practice offers.

She comes to the office alone and she is very quiet and demure in her demeanor. Although she asks you about procedures, she

(Continued)

Case 22.1   (Continued)

nearly always defers to your expertise. However, she never leaves the office without doing some type of procedure – a neurotoxin, a laser, a peel, or a soft tissue filler. Though she transiently feels better after having a procedure, she comes back – often sooner than expected, asking for more interventions, often when they are not indicated.

During your years of treating her, you have been able to develop a bond with her and learn about her life. You know that she does not work outside the home, is married to a very successful man who works in finance, and lives in a wealthy suburb just outside a major metropolitan city. Her two children left the house several years ago and attend a prestigious boarding school. Although you do not know the intricacies of her relationships, you have always been curious about the nature of her relationship with her husband.

She says that he will often travel for work or stay in the city on weeknights when working late and return to their suburban house on the weekends. There are times when you find it difficult to extricate yourself from the examination room; she often talks at length about issues that are not related to aesthetics. Although you genuinely like her and enjoy having her as a patient, you begin to wonder if she would be better off seeing a mental health professional, as much of your time is spent in conversation. You suspect that there might be some marital strife, but do not feel comfortable asking about these issues as you feel that they are out of your scope of practice. Even more troubling is your gut sense that there is a chronic sense of emptiness and unfulfillment. Sadly, it seems that the only fulfilled part of her is her skin, which is "fully filled."

Clinical Relevance and Implications

This scenario is likely very familiar to you if you have a cosmetic practice. While most patients seek aesthetic enhancement and rejuvenation therapies in a healthy attempt to delay the aging process and improve their appearance, others may look to cosmetic procedures to ameliorate underlying intrapsychic or psychosocial conflict. Anxiety, depression, unstable social/romantic situations, body dysmorphic disorder, and personality disorders can all lead people to seek a cosmetic practitioner in the hope of feeling better about themselves and their life situation.

Though it has only been described once in the peer-reviewed medical literature, experienced aesthetic practitioners are familiar with the "cosmetic addict" phenotype [1]. These patients are individuals who seek innumerable cosmetic procedures that by self-report never seem to adequately fill an insatiable appetite for "improvement" or reversal of "imperfection" and "aging." Though some

defer to the aesthetic practitioner's expertise, others are perpetually left feeling frustrated and disappointed. They are often described by clinicians and staff as "frequent flyers," with some commenting that "they just can't seem to stop." As their dissatisfaction with imperfect outcomes grows, there may be growing resentment for monetary outlays. An expectation of discounted and free procedures often increases in these patients due to an underlying feeling that they have been misled, shortchanged, or incompetently treated.

The cosmetic addict can usurp time and emotional energy from the clinician. Such patients have difficulty with the concept of "when enough is enough" with respect to cosmetic procedures. Analogous to substance users, cosmetic addicts are driven to achieve the "next high." Despite some ephemeral happiness, they are often left feeling empty and again avidly seek the next "magical" provider or procedure. Unfortunately, they are disappointed not only by the failure of the following procedure to meet their expectations, but also by the failure of the practitioner who performed the procedure. Such patients may seek cosmetic procedures in an attempt to treat an underlying psychiatric disorder or for a primary gain, i.e. in order to satisfy a subconscious psychological need. Such needs are varied, but might include receiving personal attention, touch, and care from a practitioner, particularly when these patients are not having their needs met at home or in the workplace.

Astute clinicians intuitively know that after a certain point, cosmetic procedures are no longer adequate or appropriate to meet the seemingly insatiable expectations and needs of these patients. However, despite the insight and intellectual awareness, clinicians often have difficulty setting limits for these patients. It can be easier to acquiesce to a cosmetic request than to initiate a conversation regarding their need for psychological intervention.

Using Elements of Motivational Interviewing to Identify and Redirect Inappropriate Cosmetic Patients

While traditionally used by mental health professionals for the treatment of substance abuse, motivational interviewing (MI) has been adopted by primary care physicians, predominantly in the treatment of chronic medical conditions that require major lifestyle changes [2]. Though unexplored in the world of aesthetics, MI has been employed in dermatology settings enhancing outcomes in patients living with psoriasis and atopic dermatitis [3]. MI may prove to be a useful technique in certain patients with purported cosmetic addiction. As there are no evidence-based treatments currently in use for patients with the phenotype of cosmetic addiction, MI is a novel modality in that it both allows for the continuation of the practitioner–patient relationship and affords patients substantial autonomy in their care.

What Is Motivational Interviewing?

MI is a patient-centered, goal-directed therapeutic approach that helps patients to gain awareness of distressing and ambivalent thoughts and feelings, and ideally elicit motivations for change [4]. More specifically, MI is a talk therapy consisting of short dialogues between a clinician and a patient in which the clinician explores the patient's insights and perspectives, builds rapport, and gains an understanding of the patient's motivations and expectations. The clinician helps redirect the patient to more useful areas of concern and ultimately the commitment to change. The dialogue focuses on a partnership in which the clinician provides support and gives information when asked to do so, leaving patients with an enhanced sense of control. This approach allows patients to maintain autonomy in their choices and behavior.

Specific Techniques

The technique of MI is based on four steps: (i) *engaging*, (ii) *focusing*, (iii) *evoking*, and (iv) *planning* [4]. Through this process the clinician guides the patient from initial recognition of the need to change, deciding to make a change, and committing to a healthy and realistic plan.

i) *Engaging* establishes the clinician–patient bond by setting an environment of mutual respect and trust, where the patient can feel comfortable and understood. The use of open-ended questions and reflective listening can help foster bonds. Questions such as "How will this cosmetic procedure impact your life?" and "What are your hopes and expectations?" can shed light on patient motivations while simultaneously facilitating engagement.

ii) *Focusing* allows for a singular topic of conversation during cosmetic treatment planning. With guidance from the clinician, focusing helps the patient to identify areas of greatest concern and to embrace specific changes that are appropriate, i.e. avoiding or decreasing the frequency of cosmetic procedures. This particular step of MI has the advantage of allowing the clinician to assess whether a patient is ready to take appropriate action(s) rather than the clinician directing the patient to make a change that they are not ready for.

iii) In *evoking*, clinicians again evaluate the patient's motives and willingness for making a change. By exploring the patient's perspective, the patient is encouraged to talk about how they believe that they or their life will change as a result of their actions.

iv) During *planning* the clinician helps the patient to make a plan by providing information, making suggestions, and taking the patient's own ideas and solutions into account. In an ideal therapeutic relationship, the flow of the conversation is comfortable and the patient feels that they have made an educated and emotionally beneficial appropriate decision.

Why MI?

MI has been utilized in medical dermatology to help people improve their choices and adherence to treatment regimens and ameliorate chronic, intermittently relapsing skin conditions. MI also helps clinicians such as dermatologists and their associates assess whether or not patients are motivated and committed to change their behaviors, and not waste time on those who are not interested in engaging. Although not trained as psychiatrists or psychologists, clinicians can utilize MI techniques to assist their own assessment of patients and help these struggling patients move through the stages of change [5]. Importantly, with a motivated patient, MI routinely achieves effects within one to four 20-minute treatment sessions. The educational background of the clinician does not appear to play a significant role; with training, physicians, counselors, and other staff can effectively deliver this modality [5].

Why MI in the Cosmetic Addict?

Individuals with "cosmetic addiction" present unique challenges to aesthetic providers. Such patients may be very reliable, coming to their appointments and consistently paying their bills. And for much of the time they may be aligned with their treating practitioner with respect to mutually agreed-upon aesthetic goals. However, such patients, even once the aesthetic goals have been achieved, may request more treatments.

The cosmetic practitioner should avoid performance of procedures on these patients when possible. The clinician should express empathy throughout the interaction by actively listening and providing support in a nonjudgmental, collaborative manner. Combative challenges of motivations and diagnostic labeling are usually ineffective in helping patients to seek mental health services and are usually perceived as pejorative and degrading. Instead, the use of reflective listening and open-ended questions can help patients feel understood and allow them to open up and start talking about their concerns and feelings.

While aesthetic interventions may transiently tamper psychological distress, cosmetic procedures are often only temporary fixes that do not resolve a patient's core conflict. In such cases, it is important for an aesthetic practitioner to encourage patients to seek help from a trained therapist, rather than further cosmetic treatment. We encourage the use of the euphemism "skin emotion specialist" to nonjudgmentally designate a behavioral health professional who both uniquely understands the interaction of the skin and the psyche and has the tools to improve the effects of this interaction. To engender motivation and commitment to change from cosmetic seeking to mental health and wellness-focused behaviors, MI may be a promising technique to guide such a patient population effectively.

A Proposed MI Technique

When used correctly, MI can help patients identify unhealthy ideation and expectation, thus avoiding excessive interventions that will likely lead to suboptimal emotional outcomes. To achieve true change, the aesthetic provider must provide a clear strategy and a strong, goal-oriented purpose. Unlike a classic provider–patient relationship in which the clinician makes recommendations for the patient to follow, MI focuses on guiding and a collaborative communication style known by the acronym *OARS*:

- *O*pen questions that encourage further elaboration and consideration
- *A*ffirmations that foster positive feelings in the consultation
- *R*eflections that indicate that the clinician has heard and accurately understood the patient
- *S*ummaries that extend the basic reflections to include a sense of momentum or build interest in changing direction [6].

As this friendly and open dialogue proceeds, several principles are important to keep in mind and employ as the provider–patient relationship progresses:

- *Express empathy*: clinicians must build rapport with their patients to both understand them and assess if they are ready to change their behavior.
- *Develop discrepancy*: in a nonjudgmental way, clinicians should attempt to reconcile how a patient's behavior lines up with their goals. For example, a provider might say: "Tell me more about how your repeated cosmetic filler injections fit with your plans to help with your mood and anxiety."
- *Roll with resistance*: understanding that many people may not be ready to change is part of the process. Direct confrontation is

not an effective method to elicit change. A clinician might say: "So I understand how you enjoy having a cosmetic injection performed as a means to maintain your self-confidence, and it seems as though having three to four procedures performed per month is ok for you. Are there any downsides to all the work you have been having done?"

- *Support self-efficacy*: the clinician should understand that it is ultimately a patient's decision to make a change. Clinicians should help facilitate this by guiding and supporting the patient's belief that a change is possible [6].

Exploration

When encountering a patient suspected of being a "cosmetic addict," the aesthetic practitioner should first explore the patient's motivation for cosmetic procedures. This should occur both through words and through a tandem clinician–patient examination of the patient's physical appearance using a mirror. The physician should try to use open-ended questions so that the patient is encouraged to elaborate on their thoughts. While the cosmetic practitioner encourages the patient to open up and talk, they should be assessing the patient's readiness to change from their overuse of cosmetic procedures. The cosmetic practitioner should listen attentively to assess whether the patient has insight into their excessive use or fixations with skin imperfections and cosmetic interventions.

Table 22.1 Principles of motivational interviewing.

Express empathy
Develop discrepancy
Roll with resistance
Support self-efficacy

Change Talk

Any verbalizations from the patient that signal reasons, desires, and/or motivations to change are considered *change talk* [4]. Change talk is a principle of MI in which the patient offers their own intentions and directions of behavioral change. The patient might talk about anything troubling – their situation at home or at work, or anxiety and insecurities that the clinician can pursue and help the patient to explore further. Change talk is essential because it involves the patient's own words, thoughts, and feelings and gives the patient a sense of autonomy over the content of the conversation.

When an astute provider elicits change talk in a tactful way, the patient believes that these ideas are their own, takes ownership of the content, and may be more likely to develop motivation for change. When the content of change talk relates to a psychosocial conflict, it is much easier to make a transition to introducing the concept of outside intervention with talk therapy. In other situations, the patient might also talk about obsessiveness or fixation on a particular body part that they find to be particularly unattractive. In the event that the treating practitioner is not able to visualize this or sees it as only subtle or minimally noticeable, the clinician should consider the diagnosis of an obsessive compulsive spectrum disorder, such as body dysmorphic disorder (see Chapter 15). The clinician at this point may suggest to the patient that they are concerned that the patient's focus and preoccupations are consuming more of their time than is healthy for them. Again, a suggestion of outside psychotherapeutic intervention can be made, with the concomitant reassurance that the aesthetic practitioner–patient relationship continues.

Reflection

When resistance emerges, rather than being confrontational, MI can help the aesthetic practitioner respond in a way that can take advantage of the situation by redirecting the patient's resistance into self-suggestion for change. Reflection is a very useful technique in which the clinician rephrases what the patient said by adding an experience the patient has had but has not verbalized. For example:

> "So let me see if I understand you correctly. You understand the importance of the media in the setting of beauty goals and trends, yet you also see that some of those expectations of perfection are unrealistic. Despite this intellectual understanding, I am concerned that you believe in your heart of hearts that these mostly unattainable outcomes are possible."

> "It sounds like your home life is pretty stressful and that coming here to talk to me on a regular basis has been somewhat helpful. I'm not an expert in talk therapy, but essentially what we've been doing is a form of supportive talk therapy. I'm wondering if talking with an expert can help you even more than we're accomplishing here. This could help both of us to make the best decisions for your emotional and cosmetic wellness."

Breaking Barriers

Once the change talk is presented, the clinician can then transition to developing a change plan. With gentle clinician support and guidance, the patient can maintain a sense of control in the decision-making process. The clinician can help the patient to identify obstacles and try to overcome them.

> "Are there any barriers getting in the way of you seeing a therapist or exploring that option? How can we help you overcome those obstacles?"

It can be helpful to frame the therapist as a coach, life planner, or skin emotion specialist to destigmatize seeking psychological counsel and assistance.

Committing to Change

Once the plan has been made, commitment to the plan is the last step in the MI encounter and crucial for the behavioral change to occur.

> "Could you commit to talking to a therapist once prior to our next visit to help with optimal and safe decisions on your behalf?"

Setting a goal together at the visit can help the patient commit to the plan and see it through.

Throughout this encounter the relationship between the aesthetic practitioner and the patient is essential in the patient's care. The therapist–patient relationship is framed as adjunctive to the aesthetic practitioner–patient relationship. With a good therapist–patient relationship, the primary and adjunctive relationships will invert over time, with the therapist–patient relationship taking primacy and the aesthetic practitioner–patient relationship becoming secondary. During this period of transition, the clinician should take their time with the patient and schedule regular follow-up visits. Rather than abandoning the patient and excluding them from the aesthetic practice, the clinician can help the patient to transition to a role in which a psychologist, psychiatrist, or other therapist can take the lead.

Conclusions

It is essential to avoid performing cosmetic procedures on the wrong patient. MI techniques have a long history of use in the treatment of addictions and increasingly in general medical and dermatological conditions in which people demonstrate ambivalence about changing unhelpful behaviors. The incorporation of simple MI techniques has the potential to assist the aesthetic practitioner in both identifying and motivating the inappropriate cosmetic patient to seek the most appropriate treatment modalities. With training and interest, a variety of practitioners of different educational backgrounds can efficiently and effectively use the techniques of MI without substantially lengthening the therapeutic encounter.

For more information and training see:

Rollnick S, Miller WR, Butler CC. Motivational Interviewing in Health Care: Helping Patients Change Behavior. New York: Guildford Press; 2008.

Rosengren BD. Building Motivational Interviewing Skills: A Practitioner Workbook. New York: Guildford Press; 2009.

References

1 Shah, P., Rangel, L.K., Geronemus, R.G., and Rieder, E.A. (2020). Cosmetic procedure use as a type of substance-related disorder. *J. Am. Acad. Dermatol.* 84 (1): 86–91.
2 Lundahl, B., Moleni, T., Burke, B. et al. (2013). Motivational interviewing in medical care settings: a systematic review and meta-analysis of randomized controlled trials. *Patient Educ. Couns.* 93: 157–168.
3 Larsen, M., Krogstad, A., Aas, E. et al. (2014). A telephone-based motivational interviewing intervention has positive effects on psoriasis severity and self-management: a randomized controlled trial. *Br. J. Dermatol.* 171 (6): 1458–1469.
4 Miller, W. and Rollnick, S. (2002). Motivational Interviewing, Preparing People to Change Addictive Behavior. New York: Guilford Press.
5 Rubak, S., Sandbaek, A., Lauritzen, T., and Christensen, B. (2005). Motivational interviewing: a systematic review and meta-analysis. *Br. J. Gen. Pract.* 55: 305.
6 Ingersoll, K. (2020). Motivational interviewing for substance use disorders. UpToDate. https://www.uptodate.com/contents/motivational-interviewing-for-substance-use-disorders (accessed 23 February 2020).

23

Beauty Through the Life Continuum

Doris Day

Day Dermatology & Aesthetics, New York, NY, USA
The Ronald O. Perelman Department of Dermatology, New York University Grossman School of Medicine, New York, NY, USA

Introduction

The reason why has been (and probably will always be) hotly debated, but it is widely acknowledged that women, and increasingly some men, will go to extremes to achieve beauty. The journey from good to great to that ever-elusive "perfect" is typically paired with unrealistic expectations. The challenge is that beauty, or the perceived loss of it, is measured in millimeters. Overfilling or filling areas out of proportion to others decreases balance and diminishes overall beauty. While there are well-studied mathematical components to beauty (the systematization of human proportion dates back thousands of years) [1], there is a large degree of subjectivity involved. When prompted, most individuals can think of someone they know and consider to be beautiful, but can only perceive flaws in their own reflection when they look in the mirror.

While essential elements of facial beauty and anatomy and approaches to patients with overt psychiatric disease have been addressed in previous chapters, there are several more subtle, though no less critical, elements of the clinician–patient relationship that are worthy of attention. These include communication, trust, and a few key factors that are essential to

the development of long-term healthy relationships with beauty.

Communication

A critical role of the aesthetic provider starts with the assessment. This can be even more difficult to teach than treatment technique. It begins at first introduction to the patient, and requires analysis of many aspects, including an understanding of anatomy, skin structure and function, and, most importantly, assessment of the subtle yet powerful influence of verbal and nonverbal communication (Table 23.1).

Nonverbal communication is a crucial aspect of aesthetic medicine. It gives the practitioner insight into the patient's self-esteem, confidence, and mood. Staying alert to variances in body language can illuminate unspoken characteristics about your patient and help you discern key clues that will guide your interaction. For example, someone sitting with crossed arms can often be closed off. This patient may have a more complex motivation for seeking treatment, or might disagree or be less likely to comply with the treatment plan. A patient who is overeager, adoring, and your "biggest fan" might be less inclined to communicate their own vision and more likely to follow any

Table 23.1 Nonverbal and verbal communication.

Nonverbal communication:
- Presence or lack of eye contact
- Facial expressions throughout the discussion
- Patient attire/accessories
- Patient posture

Verbal communication:
- What is their area of focus (e.g. eyes, mouth, neck, hair)?
- How do they describe their issues?
- Tone of voice [3]
- Do they have a special event coming up?
- Do they have a written list of issues?
- Did they bring in photos to demonstrate wants/concerns?

suggested treatment option. Later, this can lead to cognitive dissonance, leaving the patient feeling that the choice to get treated was not entirely their own. In more extreme situations, their initial complimentary tone may be a foreshadowing of personality pathology or (at minimum) a later difficult interpersonal interaction between provider and patient. Be sure to note extremes on the spectrum of nonverbal behavior, because this can often indicate that someone could go from satisfied to dissatisfied quickly. All of these cues can tell you how you should approach the patient so that you can offer the best care and manage expectations. Such cues also lead to questions that you may want to ask to better understand the patient and their vision or goals for the treatments. Take care to notice your own body language as well, as this is proven to affect the way the patient perceives you and how much they are willing to share, which ultimately can affect their outcome [2].

Truly listening to and analyzing verbal communication is crucial. Patients often schedule a visit in anticipation of, or after recovering from, a life-defining event. Whether it is a wedding, divorce, birth of a grandchild, or death of a loved one, these patients are seeking to look and feel their best. It is advantageous to always probe the patient to discern their motivation for seeking treatment. Be wary of treating patients with unrealistic expectations, such as a woman interested in rejuvenation treatments to look younger for the upcoming wedding of her child. This might seem completely reasonable. But if after digging deeper she mentions that her ex-husband will be there with a much younger girlfriend or wife, she might be looking for a solution to evoke jealousy or regret, or even win her husband back. This will likely not be the outcome. Tone of voice is another subconscious indicator that can offer a plethora of information. It is even more difficult for the patient to adjust than verbal communication or facial expression [3]. A patient might tell you one thing, but have difficulty controlling drastic inflections in their voice. This could be an indicator of deception or nervousness [4].

Trust

Arguably the most important emotional component of the assessment is the establishment of trust. This starts even before the patient checks in for their visit. They may have already seen you on social media, on TV, or in magazines, or read reviews online. Managing your public image is imperative. What you allow the public to see tells a story about you. This can be challenging, but you can ultimately control much of this content. Be sure that the images and videos you present are authentic and accurately represent you and your brand. If you have a team managing your social media, be sure to review and edit the content. You should know what is being posted and how comments and questions are being answered. I believe social media is the great equalizer. It offers the public access to information that might otherwise be difficult to obtain, and provides professionals with the opportunity to convey and control their image. Posting before and after photos can be helpful, but I think what many followers really want is to get to know you. They are interested in determining whether your image, value system, and approach are consistent with their own. It is okay to be vulnerable, as this is often the element that fosters the best human-to-human connection [2], especially for a physician because doctors are often perceived as authoritative and less approachable. For this reason, I do all of my own posting and writing. It takes time, but the more I do it, the easier it gets and the more I learn about what resonates with my colleagues and patient population. It is also important to be social on social media. Comment on colleagues' and friends' posts and respond quickly to comments on your own pages and platforms. If you are not comfortable posting about yourself, that is also acceptable. It is most important to stay true to yourself and post what feels right for you, because ultimately it is your image that you are creating and fostering.

Establishing trust once the patient comes into the office means listening to them, making sure they feel heard and understood, and guiding them to the treatments that are most appropriate for them. Patients should feel they can be their authentic selves. Studies have evaluated what patients, especially new patients, want from their provider, and much of it is centered around allowing patients to ask questions [5] and being open to hearing their hopes and fears before, during, and after the treatment. This benefits both the patient and practitioner, because the more information you gain as a clinician, the more likely you are to select the right combination of treatments. Trust also means the patient understands that you will protect them from treatments that are inappropriate for them and that you will not take advantage of the relationship for your own gain.

Along this same vein, one of the most important words you can use is "no." I am often surprised at how relieved a patient can be when I tell them they do not need a treatment. Of course, some patients are disappointed when you dissuade them from getting additional treatments because they are

dissatisfied with how they look and are more interested in a quick fix. I do not let these individuals convince me to treat when my aesthetic experience is telling me otherwise. One of the most valuable lessons I have learned in my 20+ years of practice is to follow my own judgment. It is crucial to be confident in your own ability to create an accurate assessment and treatment plan, without adding treatments at the patient's request that you know will not achieve the goal they have in mind. It can be difficult to leave a patient wanting more. However, that is always better than dealing with discontent later when the patient realizes that the treatment did not give them the results they hoped for, because they either needed a different approach or because their expectations were impractical. Sometimes, they may even end up finding another provider who is willing to do the treatment they asked for. In this situation, I am neither offended nor upset, because I can acknowledge that I am not the right doctor for every patient.

Another aspect of establishing trust is to guide patients to seeing themselves in a positive way. You can practice retraining their eye to notice what makes them beautiful. When you hand them a mirror, help them see their attractiveness and their "hero" features, not their flaws. The goal is always to go from beautiful to more beautiful, not from flawed to less flawed. Patients should feel beautiful even before you start to treat. As you assess and review the treatments you have in mind for them, choose your words carefully and keep the conversation positive. Use "we can enhance" or "we can augment" instead of "your problem is that you're sunken in these areas." It helps to have before and after photos, because patients are not wired to see things through the eyes of an artist, and they may only see their flaws rather than how much better they look. There is a case for taking photos as part of establishing trust: a picture speaks a thousand words . . . .

Case Study

Case 23.1   Establishing Trust Through Photography

A 50-year-old woman drove four hours to see me in consultation. Her husband came with her and was not supportive of her receiving aesthetic treatments. He did not want her to spend the money and felt she looked fine as she was. He was also worried something bad could happen or that she would look like she'd had treatments done. She was insistent that I was the doctor for her. She had heard me on my radio show and she followed me on social media. From this she saw that I had a reputation for being "conservative" (I usually correct that and say that I am not conservative, I am appropriate …). We discussed her goals and reviewed treatment options. When it came time for taking photos she asked if we could skip that step. I explained that photos were an important part of the visit and I could not perform any treatment without first taking pictures. My practice uses a detailed consent form that gives the patient options as to how the photos are used. Patients are able to select whether the photos can be shared for education or media, or if they prefer they are seen only by those who have access to their medical record. Some patients are excited to share their photos to encourage others to seek similar treatment. Either way, we respect the patient's choice.

This patient's primary concern was her nasolabial folds. We reviewed her anatomy first, which allowed me to point out her beautiful high cheekbones and strong jawline. I explained that we could best address the issue with her nasolabial folds by adding fillers to areas more lateral in the face as well as to the nasolabial folds themselves. We also needed to balance her chin to restore her proportions. She was initially anxious but followed my advice, understanding that she may need more than one treatment to optimize the outcome. Thankfully, she was open to the idea that going slow was the best approach, especially considering this was her first session. The treatment

went well and she left feeling happy. I was relieved that she followed my guidance and I was satisfied with the results as well.

An hour or so after she left the office, she called in a panic and asked to speak with me right away. She said she looked "terrible" and that her husband was telling her that she had made a big mistake in getting the treatments and that she no longer looked like herself. She said she could see and feel her chin "swelling" as we spoke and she was "horrified." Fortunately, she was still in town and was able to come back in for an evaluation. As soon as she walked in I asked my staff to take another set of photos right away, even before I went in to see her. They created a side-by-side comparison of her photos and I brought them in with me when I saw her again.

When I walked into the room she was slouched in the chair and her eyes were cast downward. She did not look up or make eye contact with me. I smiled, took a close look at her skin to make sure there were no signs of vascular compromise or other adverse effects, and asked if she wanted to see the before and after photos from that day. She did. When she looked at the photos her jaw dropped. She said, "that's my before?" with disbelief in her tone. As she looked at the photos I could see her confidence rise and her attitude shift from defeat to elation. She asked, "Can I keep these photos?" I said yes, of course. Now she became downright chatty. She spoke of how much softer her face and features are and how much younger she looked. She confessed that her husband had been hard on her about doing the treatment and she was self-conscious about it. But after seeing the photos she knew she had done the right thing and was ecstatic with the results. She thanked me repeatedly for the treatment and for the photos, saying she needed to show them to her husband. She left, walking out tall and proud.

Case 23.1   (Continued)

I loved seeing the change in her posture and her attitude. The photos definitely saved me. If I had let her skip the pictures I would never have been able to show her how much improvement there was and she would not have been able to see or appreciate her results. A good outcome would have meant nothing because she would not have been able to see it (Table 23.2).

Table 23.2   Establishing trust.

- Manage your public presence and image
- Be honest and listen
- Take before and after photos
- Say no when no is the right thing to say
- Take time in conversation with the patient to understand their concerns around the treatments [5]
- Start with "hero" features, not flaws

Developing a Long-Term Healthy Relationship with Beauty

Long-Term Relationships

One of the most rewarding aspects of being in the healthcare field, especially focusing on skin and aesthetics, is developing long-term relationships with patients. Sometimes we even get the privilege of watching patients grow, coming in first as children accompanying their parents, then as teens for acne remedies, and later as adults looking for treatments before an important milestone. It is an honor to take this journey with them. We are healers, and it is through our lasting relationships and the associated trust we build that we are able to keep our patients not just looking their best, but also feeling their best and living healthy, fulfilled lives. Longer lasting relationships provide us with the opportunity to truly get to know our patients, along with their goals and values. Patients also benefit from these relationships, because they gain a sense of power in knowing that their care is handled by someone with whom they have a more personal relationship. It is our responsibility to keep their best interest in mind, protecting them against treatments and procedures that are not appropriate for them.

Ethical/Moral Views: How Young Is Too Young and When to Say No

Rejuvenation medicine is still in its infancy. It is as much of an art as it is a science. There has been an explosion of US Food and Drug Administration (FDA)-cleared devices and FDA-approved products to address concerns relating to beauty and aging. Unfortunately, ethics have not kept up with product development and the products are being commoditized. The patient is often treated as a "client" who can dictate what treatment is done and what they will look like afterwards, instead of the physician or trained injector being the one to ascribe the treatment protocol. This has led to distorted and unnatural outcomes, where patients have exaggerated lips, overfilled cheeks, and partial or complete loss of "normal" facial balance or proportion. It has also created a younger market, as products and treatments are advertised on social media where there is a heavier presence of those in their late teens and early 20s. The idea that many of these treatments are reversible makes it tempting for teens, who look up to and often idolize social media influencers and reality stars who use misleading filters to their advantage. Younger patients often think they can "try out" bigger lips or exaggerated proportions because the effects wear off. They are unaware that the treatments may last longer, by many years, than stated in clinical trials and package labels, and that they can change how they see themselves for the rest of their lives. There are also risks to treatments; those risks are especially concerning when the treatment is being done for reasons that are ethically questionable.

There are those who believe that if the "client" asks for a treatment, if the treatment is FDA approved, and the provider is capable, then it is a personal decision that the provider should accommodate. Others believe that the treatments are designed for restoration and realistic augmentation, to address changes due to trauma, manifestation of genetic factors, or predictable changes occurring from natural aging. This field of thought supports rejuvenation and enhancement, without changing natural and authentic features.

The discrepancy may be due to inadequate training of the injector, or an injector who follows the request of the patient rather than properly assessing the patient, informing them of the recommended treatment plan, and refusing to perform a treatment that will distort their natural features. If the patient asks for it and understands the risks, are we entitled to decide whether or not to do the treatment, or should the patient ultimately have the final say? If they want to look more "cat-like" or to have extra-large lips because they have seen others with the same, do we do it just because we can? These questions have not been adequately studied and discussed and further research is needed to define boundaries for treatment. Texts do exist that attempt to outline the ethical considerations we are facing in aesthetic medicine [6], but this has become more challenging and nuanced as the field has progressed. We also face challenges from patients who may subscribe to alternative definitions of beauty that society does not see as within the bounds of "normal." If such patients desire and are happy with outcomes that distort their facial features or involve the use of implants to make them appear less human, should we accommodate their requests or does that violate our code of ethics? Every injector must make such determinations for themselves. However, I believe that as physicians and aesthetic practitioners, we must continue to define new guidelines that help us protect our patients from achieving a specific goal while simultaneously defeating the purpose of the treatment.

Counterfactual Emotions of Beauty

Finally, I want to remark on counterfactual emotions of beauty. I define this concept as the feelings that spur people's minds into creating alternative realities about their appearance to avoid the pain of loss. For most people, looking and feeling younger may actually equate to physically combatting aging. Well-designed studies are needed to assess this theory, but I (and many of my colleagues practicing aesthetic dermatology) have observed this trend over many years. It may be that people who feel they look better begin to make changes in their diet, sleep, and activity levels. It could also be that feeling more beautiful is causing a cascade of hormonal changes, due to the mind–body connection, that initiate a positive change in the physiological process of aging. This is a wide-open area ripe for research that can help transform both the value and quality of aesthetic treatments as well as encourage the need for a discussion of the ethics of treatments and boundaries around the "extremes" of beauty.

Conclusions

The future of aesthetics is bright, but as available treatments become more numerous and as these treatments become more commoditized, understanding the long-term effects on both the individual and society as a whole has never been more important. Training is key. Mastering anatomy and the structure and function of the skin is a minimum. Understanding the nuance of verbal and nonverbal communication as well as developing trust will allow us to develop long-term, healthy, gratifying relationships with our aesthetic patients. Going further, we must better equip providers with education pertaining to the aesthetic nuances of gender, cultural variation, the age continuum, and the technique of delivery that is unique to each product or device. Training must be lifelong and it should also include the psychology of aesthetic treatments. We must master how to help our patients get the most out of any treatment and

how to identify a patient with unrealistic expectations or untreated psychiatric illness in order to avoid contributing to their pathology. When all of these aspects are taken into account, and with ongoing continuing education, we can offer our patients the best outcomes and help them to age beautifully so that every decade is their best.

References

1 Gallucci, H.J. (2020). Commentary on Dürer's "Four Books on Human Proportion". Cambridge: Open Book Publishers.

2 Matsumoto, D.R. and Hwang, H.S. (2013). Body and gestures. In: Nonverbal Communication: Science and Applications (eds. G. Frank and H.S. Hwang). California: SAGE Publications. Chapter 4. Available from: http://sk.sagepub.com/books/nonverbal-communication/n4.xml.

3 Zuckerman, M., DePaulo, B., and Rosenthal, R. (1981). Verbal and nonverbal communication of deception. *Advances in Experimental Social Psychology* 14: 1–59. Available from: https://www.sciencedirect.com/science/article/pii/s006526010860369x.

4 Matsumoto, D.R. and Hwang, H.S. (2013). Deception. In: Nonverbal Communication: Science and Applications (eds. G. Frank and H.S. Hwang). California: SAGE Publications. Chapter 6. Available from: http://sk.sagepub.com/books/nonverbal-communication/n6.xml.

5 Bich, D.N., Westbook, R.A., Njue, S.M., and Giordano, T.P. (2017). Building trust and rapport early in the new doctor–patient relationship: a longitudinal qualitative study. *BMC Medical Education* 17 (1): 32. https://doi.org/10.1186/s12909-017-0868-5.

6 Door Goold, S. and Lipkin, M. Jr. (1999). The doctor–patient relationship: challenges, opportunities, and strategies. *Journal of General Internal Medicine* 14 (1): S26–S33. https://doi.org/10.1046/j.1525-1497.1999.00267.x.

Index

Essential Psychiatry for the Aesthetic Practitioner, First Edition. Edited by Evan A. Rieder and Richard G. Fried.
© 2021 John Wiley & Sons Ltd. Published 2021 by John Wiley & Sons Ltd.